PHARMACOLOGY - RESEARCH, SAFETY TESTING AND REGULATION

AN INTRODUCTION TO P-GLYCOPROTEIN

Pharmacology - Research, Safety Testing and Regulation

Additional books and e-books in this series can be found on Nova's website under the Series tab.

PHARMACOLOGY - RESEARCH, SAFETY TESTING AND REGULATION

AN INTRODUCTION TO P-GLYCOPROTEIN

M. WAHAJUDDIN
RAVINDRA VARMA ALLURI
AND
RAHUL DEV JAYANT
EDITORS

nova
Medicine & Health
New York

NOTICE TO THE READER

Library of Congress Cataloging-in-Publication Data

Names: Wahajuddin, M., editor. | Varma Alluri, Ravindra, editor. | Dev Jayant, Rahul, editor.
Title: An introduction to p-glycoprotein / M. Wahajuddin, PHD, FHEA, FRSB, FRSC, Principal Scientist, CSIR-Central Drug Research Institute, Lucknow (U.P.), India, Ravindra Varma Alluri, PHD, Associate Principal Scientist, Clinical Pharmacology and Safety Sciences, AstraZeneca R&D, Cambridge, UK, Rahul Dev Jayant, PHD, Assistant Professor, Texas Tech University Health Sciences Center, Texas, USA, editors.
Identifiers: LCCN 2021023436 (print) | LCCN 2021023437 (ebook) | ISBN 9781536194883 (hardcover) | ISBN 9781536197280 (adobe pdf)
Subjects: LCSH: Drug resistance in cancer cells. | P-glycoprotein. Classification: LCC RC271.C5 A614 2021 (print) | LCC RC271.C5 (ebook) | DDC 616.99/4061--dc23 LC record available at https://lccn.loc.gov/2021023436
LC ebook record available at https://lccn.loc.gov/2021023437

Published by Nova Science Publishers, Inc. † New York

CONTENTS

PREFACE

P-glycoprotein (P-gp), encoded by the multidrug-resistance (MDR)-1 gene is one of the best studied efflux transporter that is linked to multidrug resistance in cancer chemotherapies. P-gp belongs to ATP-binding cassette (ABC) transporter family of proteins that utilizes energy derived from hydrolysis of ATP to efflux endogenous and exogenous xenobiotics, metabolites and toxins from the intracellular space to the outside, thereby providing a general protective role. P-gp is expressed on the apical plasma membrane of all major drug eliminating organs such as the intestine (enterocytes), liver (bile canaliculi), kidney (proximal tubules), brain (endothelia of blood-brain barrier) and in certain tumour types. In the intestine and BBB, P-gp limits entry of drugs by actively pumping drugs back into the lumen or blood, respectively. In the liver and kidney, P-gp actively efflux's drugs, endogenous substances and metabolites into bile or urine, thereby removing them from the body. Upregulation of P-gp in tumour cells is noted in several cancers and is a hallmark for drug resistance. Additionally, P-gp is also shown to play a role in neurogenesis and maintaining homeostasis in the brain. Alteration of P-gp expression is observed in neurodegenerative diseases, highlighting its importance in maintaining normal brain health.

Due to its central role in defining oral pharmacokinetics, systemic clearance, tissue exposure, organ health and chemoresistance, much of the research has been focused on modulating P-gp. Chemical inhibitors, formulation based and epigenetic approaches are applied to modulate P-gp activity with a goal to improve oral pharmacokinetics, increase tumour and brain penetration, minimize organ toxicity and also potentially treat neurodegenerative diseases.

Although enormous research on P-gp has been published, a book chapter exclusively and comprehensively covering diverse aspects of P-gp, including the recent developments in the field is required. With much enthusiasm from the publisher, we have collaborated to bring together wide-ranging topics on P-gp. This book contains 12 chapters covering the structure, function, regulation, distribution and expression of P-gp, its pharmacological importance in health and disease and role in pharmacokinetics and drug-drug interactions. Also included are computational approaches to identify selective inhibitors, tactics to modulate P-gp function using chemical inhibitors (synthetized or isolated from marine sources), formulations strategies or epigenetics approaches. The last chapter describes various methods to quantify P-gp expression levels and function in *in vitro, in situ* and *in vivo* setting. It is our sincere hope that this material will serve as an important desk reference for students, researchers and clinical scientists in academia, medical research and pharmaceutical industry working in various fields such as pharmacology, pharmacy, toxicology, medicinal chemistry, pharmaceutical sciences, pharmacokinetics and computational biology.

Acknowledgments

We wish to acknowledge the contributions of all the authors who passionately contributed to this book. We also extend our gratitude to the editorial staff and production manager at Nova Publishers. Lastly, but most importantly we thank our families for their continued support during this journey.

In: An Introduction to P-Glycoprotein ISBN: 978-1-53619-488-3
Editors: M. Wahajuddin et al.

Chapter 1

INTRODUCTION: STRUCTURE AND FUNCTION

Anupam Dhasmana[1,2], Sudhir Kotnala[1,2], Murali M. Yallapu[1,2], Subhash C. Chauhan[1,2,*] and Meena Jaggi[1,2,†]

[1]Department of Immunology and Microbiology, School of Medicine, University of Texas Rio Grande Valley, McAllen, TX, US

[2]South Texas Center of Excellence in Cancer Research, School of Medicine, University of Texas Rio Grande Valley, McAllen, TX, US

ABSTRACT

P-glycoprotein (P-gp/MDR1), is an important ATP-driven transmembrane transporter, this protein is translated by the ABCB1 gene. P-gp is capable of effluxing a wide-ranging of structurally distinct and functionally irrelevant compounds like organic cations, carbohydrates,

* Corresponding Author's Email: subhash.chauhan@utrgv.edu.
† Corresponding Author's Email: meena.jaggi@utrgv.edu.

amino acids, and some antibiotics to macromolecules such as polysaccharides and proteins out of the cell. Multidrug resistance (MDR), generally linked with the high-expression of P-gp or ABCB1 gene. There are a large number of single nucleotide polymorphisms (SNPs) that have been noticed in P-gp. These SNPs are responsible for altered oral bioavailability of drugs by limiting intestinal absorption, drug resistance, and a susceptibility to some human diseases. In this chapter, we have flashed the light on the structure and functional features of P-gp, which will be helpful for the better understanding of rational drug design in developing new and effective MDR modulators.

Keywords: P-gp/MDR1/ABCB1, structure, topology, function, pathway enrichment, xenobiotics

INTRODUCTION

P-gp is a glycoprotein based multidrug efflux pump present in the plasma membrane of the cells. It is an ATP-Binding Cassette (ABC) and particularly located at the interface tissues such as intestinal, renal, hepatic, brain barriers, and responsible for efflux of drugs towards the body clearance. P-gp acts as a physiological barrier by extruding toxins and xenobiotics out of cells, thereby, protecting the organs from toxic compounds [1, 2].

The small gene family of p-gp comprises of two classes of isoforms viz. class I (MDR1/ABCB1), which is involved in the transport of drug whereas class II (MDR2/3/ABCB4) transports out phosphatidylcholine into the bile [2, 3]. Moreover, P-gp is known to interact with immunosupressants, anticancer drugs, steroidal hormones and β-adrenoreceptor blockers [2, 4] and hence, it plays a crucial role in absorption, distribution, metabolism, elimination and toxicity (ADMET) properties of drugs of pharmacological importance [5, 6]. Due to its wide range of tissue distribution, p-gp also exudates endogenous metabolites, exogenous substrates, and toxins into the urine, bile, and feces, thereby serving a dual role by protecting the organisms as well as eliminating the cellular wastes [7, 8]. Additonally, p-gp is located in the BBB (blood brain barrier) preventing the infiltration of cytotoxins and restricting the cellular uptake of drugs from the blood into the brain [9, 10].

P-gp is overexpressed in cancer patients; especially those who have undergone chemotherapy. Moeover its over-expression has been associated with HIV, cystic fibrosis, acute myeloid leukemia (AML) and myelodysplastic syndrome (MDS). The function of P-gp is altered during various diseases like epilepsy, Alzheimer's disease (AD), depression, Parkinson. As per the statistics available in the PubMed, it was found that most of the publications related to the P-gp are influenced with Cancer (12506) followed by HIV (662), Epilepsy (463), AD (217) and Cystic Fibrosis (163), were the top studied indications (Figure 1).

Being said about the roles of P-glycoprotein, it is important to closely understand the structure and its distributed functions. Here in this chapter we tried to discuss the primary and secondary structures along with 3D and topological structures of P-glycoprotein. We also discuss the potential modes of action for drug disposition by P-glycoprotein (P-gp). Moreover, various molecular and biological functions as well as the role of P-gp has been reviewed in this chapter.

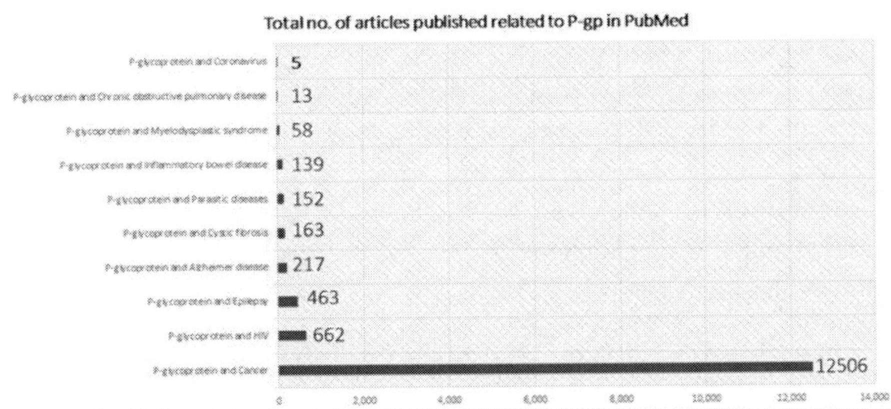

Figure 1. Publication statistics of P-gp in different indications.

STRUCTURE

While identification of only amino acid sequence of protein is not sufficient. In Stanford, the concept of secondary (2°) structure was initially established by Kaj Ulrik Linderstrøm-Lang (1952). Secondary structure of the proteins is also equally important for prediction of back-bone and skeleton of protein structures. The common 2° structural characteristics are α helices, β sheets, extended strand and random coil. The 2° structure of proteins is defined by the pattern of hydrogen bonding which form between the amino hydrogen and carboxyl oxygen atoms in the peptide backbone[11]. P-gp, a 170-kDa consist of 1,280 amino acids encoded by the human MDR1 gene [12]. P-gp (UniProtKB ID: P33527) primary amino acid sequence was procured from the UniPort database and GOR IV (https://npsa-prabi.ibcp.fr/cgi-bin/npsa_automat.pl?page=/NPSA/npsa_gor 4.html) was used for the prediction of secondary structure databases where we have found the α helices 38.86% extended strand 20.17% and random coil 40.43% (Figure 2) were present in P-gp protein. The P-gp is an ATP-binding cassette exporter accountable for drug resistance. P-gp squeeze out xenobiotic molecules from cells through ATP-operated conformational changes. In the Figure 3 here we have demonstrated the inward (Figure 3A) & outward (Figure 3B) facing conformation of P-gp. In these 3D structures both NBD shape a closed dimer blocking two ATP molecules. The drug-binding site was observed redirection toward the extracellular space and condensed to prevent substrate binding in the inward-facing. This remark implies that binding of ATP, negative hydrolysis and stimulates substrate discharge [13].

Topological Features of P-gp

The commonly accepted model for the topologic structure of P-gp/MDR1 is a single polypeptide made up of two homologous halves that occurred from gene duplication. Each half comprises six TMHs (transmembrane helices) and one NBD located on the cytoplasmic side of the membrane, which are connected by a cytoplasmic linker as shown in Figure 4. The TMDs has role to form a pathway via drug or other organic molecules traverse the membrane. Both NH2- and COOH-terminal, and NBDs, are sited inside the cell, and the first extracellular loop is N-glycosylated [14]. All NBD comprises of two fundamental consensus motifs mentioned as Walker A and B motifs of ABC transporters [15]. All motifs are usually observed in a broad range of ATPases enzymes and are precisely implicated in the attaching and hydrolysis of nucleotides molecules. The 'linker region' splits the two highly charged half molecules, which is phosphorylated at numerous locations by protein kinase C [16].

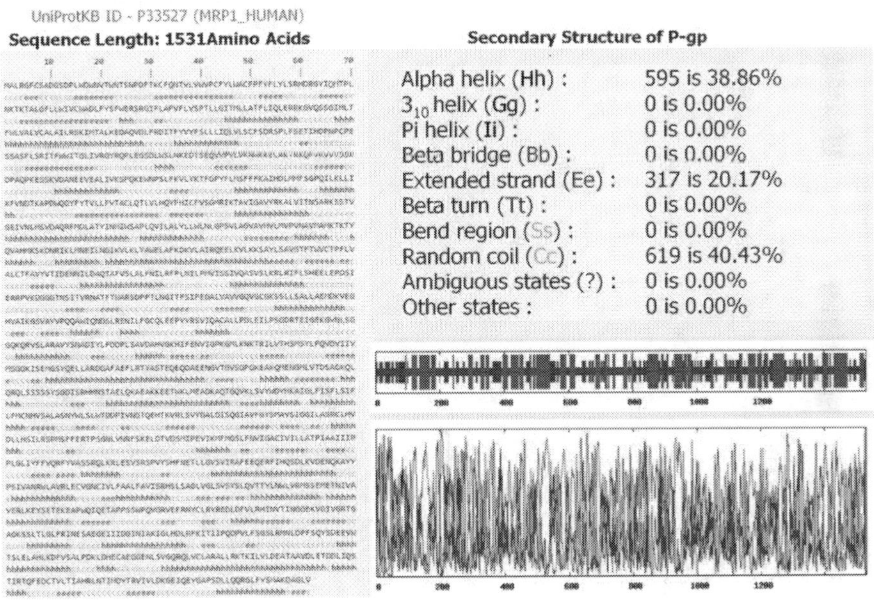

Figure 2. Secondary structure analysis of P-gp.

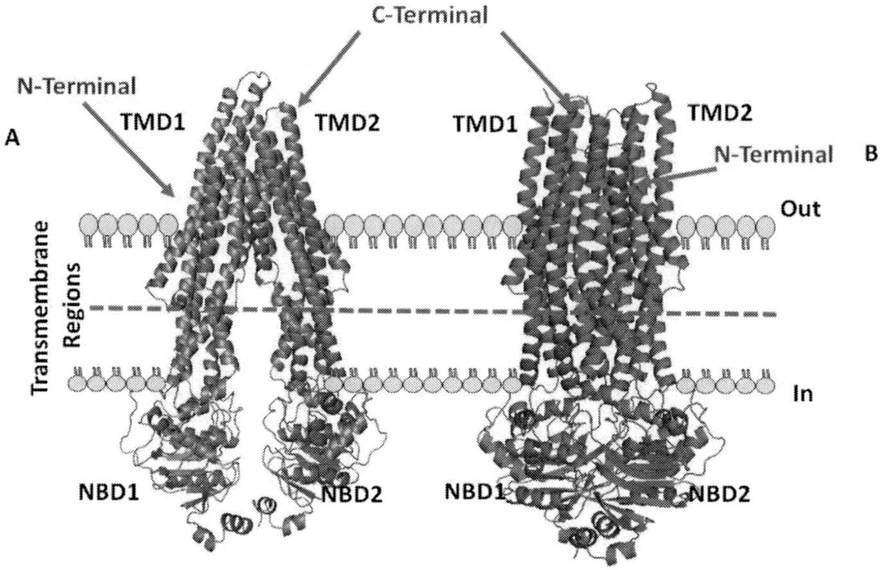

Figure 3. The overall 3D structure of the P-gp in different confirmation style. The N-terminal half (TMD1 and NBD1) is colored in orange and the C-terminal half (TMD2 and NBD2) in green. As illustrated the structures of P-gp representative inward-facing P-gp (A: PDB ID:6QEX) and the outward-facing P-gp (B: PDB ID: 6C0V).

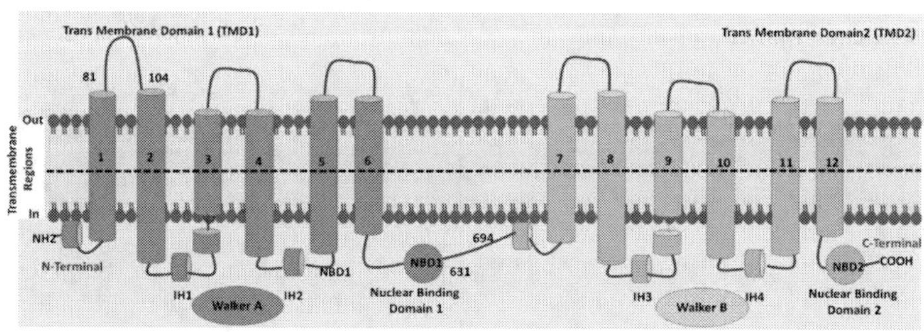

Figure 4. Topology diagram of P-gp. OUT, outer cell membrane & IN, inner cell membrane.

FUNCTIONS OF P-GLYCOPROTEIN

P-glycoprotein (ABCB1) was the first ABC transporter to be cloned and, it is known to be the ABC transporter superfamily's best defined protein attributable in part to its essential feature in the establishment of multidrug resistance (MDR) phenotype to cancer cells that have gained tolerance to chemotherapy drugs [17, 18]. Quite a few secretory cell types such as the kidney, liver, intestine, adrenal gland, and the blood-brain barrier are known to express P-gp/MDR1 in their apical membrane. The function of P-gp/MDR1 comprises of excretion of drugs and their metabolites or simply in other words it is involved in the drug disposition [7, 17]. P-gp has been identified for its dual function in that it defends vulnerable tissues from potentially harmful xenobiotics and, at the same time, induces MDR in tumors and other disorders, thereby preventing successful therapies.

Potential Mechanism of Action for Drug Disposition by P-Glycoprotein (P-gp)

P-gp is involved in the drug disposition/transport of the cytotoxic drugs out of the cells against a concentration gradient, hence minimizing the accumulation of drugs inside the cell and inhibiting drug mediated cell death. The two proposed models for drug disposition via P-gp are pump drug transport model and flippase drug transport model (Figure 5A & 5B respectively). The pump drug transport model involves the formation of hydrophilic passage or a pore which allows the drug efflux to the extracellular environment, preventing the interaction of the substrate from the hydrophobic lipid bilayer [19]. Whereas, in flippase drug transport model the P-gp diverts the drug from the inner leaflet of the lipid bilayer to the outer leaflet followed by its extracellular transport [20, 21].

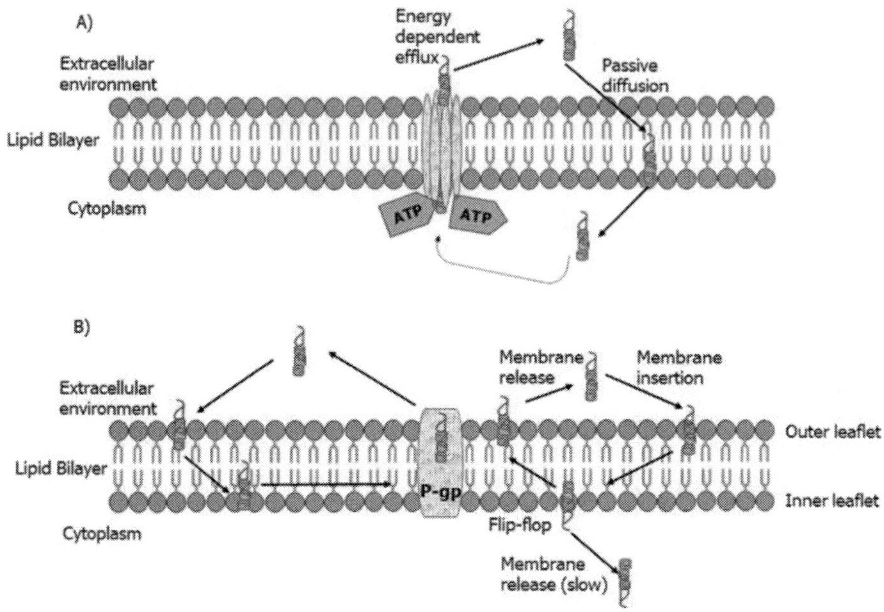

Figure 5. Potential processes for P-gp drug efflux. A) Represents the pump drug transport model of P-gp, which comprises of a single drug pore (blue). The P-gp is involved in the ATP-dependent transport of drugs such as chemotherapeutics (brown), to diffuse out of the cell through the lipid membrane. B) Represents the flippase drug transport model, where the drug first interacts with the lipid bilayer prior to P-gp and then is diffused out to the extracellular environment. Contrary to this, drugs can intercalate in the inner leaflet of lipid bilayer and flips into the outer leaflet and diffuses out to the extracellular environment rapidly. Whereas the release of the drug from the inner leaflet of the lipid bilayer to the cytoplasm is comparatively slow.

Molecular and Biological Functions of P-gp

P-gp is known to have various molecular and biological functions. It is involved in mediating the export of organic anions and drugs from the cytoplasm. Moreover, p-gp is involved in the translocation of glucosylceramide from the cytoplasmic to the luminal membrane leaflet of golgi, thereby playing a physiological role in the biosynthesis of glycosphingolipids [22]. It is also involved in ATP-dependent transport of, leukotriene C4, estradiol-17-beta-o-glucuronide, methotrexate and antiviral drugs [23-27]. P-gp have ABC-type transmembrane transporter activity which means it catalyzes the reaction: ATP + H2O = ADP + phosphate, to precisely propel the active transport of a substance through a membrane (GO:0140359). It also have ATPase-coupled lipid transmembrane transporter activity which enables the transfer of a solute or solutes from one side of a membrane to the other according to the reaction: ATP + H2O + lipid(in) = ADP + phosphate + lipid(out) (GO:0034040). P-gp mediates ATPase-coupled glutathione S-conjugate transmembrane transporter activity and the catalysis of the reaction is: ATP + H2O + glutathione S-conjugate(in) -> ADP + phosphate + glutathione S-conjugate(out) (GO:0015431). P-gp also confers ATPase-coupled vitamin B12 (Cobalamin) transmembrane transporter activity and the catalysis of the reaction is: ATP(4-) + cob(I)alamin + H2O <=> ADP(3-) + hydrogen phosphate + cob(I)alamin + H+ (GO:0015420). P-gp is also known to mediate ATPase-coupled xenobiotic transmembrane transporter activity following the reaction: ATP + H2O + xenobiotic(in) = ADP + phosphate + xenobiotic(out) (GO:0008559). Moreover, P-gp catalyzes the export of sphingosine 1-phosphate from mast cells independently of their degranulation [28].

Role of P-gp in Various Pathologies

Given that P-gp dysregulation is closely related to many biological processes, great anticipation of ways to theoretically and correctly regulate P-gp expression should inspire and promote the analysis of P-gp based chemical regulators for future therapeutic applications. It has been confirmed that up-regulation of P-gp is implicated in multidrug-resistant malignant tumor cells, resulting in significant demand for effective compounds that precisely block P-gp activity [29]. Because most clinical studies include patients with cancer, there is a strong association between production of P-gp and a lower risk of relapse and a higher occurrence of refractory disease, indicating the therapeutic importance of this Pgp-dependent MDR process.

In fact, multiple reports have shown that P-gp expression in some malignancies such as neuroblastoma, childhood sarcoma, and breast cancer can be a prognostic indicator which might be due to the antineoplastic resistance that enhances the cellular apoptotic threshold [30, 31]. However, P-gp is also known to express in some normal cells of intestine, kidney, liver, and brain microvascular endothelia. According to this hypothesis, the production of P-gp in such tissues prevents xenobiotics from being absorbed/eliminated or avoids sensitivity of susceptible tissues to xenobiotics [32]. The dynamic biochemical function of P-gp in the human body puts significant difficulty in the successful usage of P-gp-targeted MDR reversing agents. Awareness of useful structural knowledge in combination with substrate specificity is therefore especially essential for the efficient identification of possible P-gp-related MDR reversal agents with appropriate anti-cancer applications [33]. Work on systemic P-gp inhibitors is now thriving and there have been several attempts to evaluate such P-gp inhibitors [34-36].

Similar to the mechanism of P-gp mediated MDR in cancer progression, it has been seen that in HIV infected cells the upregulated P-gp expression leads to decreased intracellular concentrations of anti-retroviral agents in the plasma, thereby limiting the therapeutic efficacy of antiviral agents [37, 38]. P-gp protein also functions as a transporter in the blood-brain barrier (BBB). However, studies have shown that ATP-dependent drug efflux pump due to P-gp at BBB restricts the brain distribution of protease inhibitors and their subsequent delivery to central nervous system [39]. The overexpression of P-gp has been significantly associated in conferring the MDR to the HIV-infected cells, however, the modulators for P-gp acts as chemosensitizers in HIV therapy [40, 41]. P-gp significantly reduces the absorption rate of several anti-HIV drugs thereby inhibiting their therapeutic use.

The MDR contributed in part due to P-gp has also widely affected the therapeutic efficacy of anti-parasitic drugs. Parasitic diseases like malaria and leishmaniasis has affected the peoples across the world time and again and factors conferring MDR increases the resistance to therapeutic [42]. Increased drug efflux by membrane transporter P-gp, contributes to resistance to anthelmintics [43]. The effective P-gp modulators to combat with protozoan parasites are still unavailable. However, it has been shown that the calcium-channel blocker verapamil (VPL), which is P-gp modulator used as a cancer therapeutic, is found to be effective to some extent in the treatment of parasitic diseases [43].

Cystic fibrosis (CF) is an autosomal recessive disease which involves the mutations in the cystic fibrosis transmembrane conductance regulator (CFTR) gene. CF involves the inflammatory processes and is considered as a multisystem disorder that is not constricted to lungs, but it affects other vital organs too which leads to several co-morbidities [44]. The most common mutations among Caucasians are ΔF508, G542X, G551D, N1303K and W1282X [45-47]. P-gp shares structural and functional homologies with CFTR and can be used as a therapeutic option for the treatment of cystic fibrosis to acts as a pharmacological chaperone. Study have shown that, the P-gp modulator quinazoline derivative CFcor- 325 can be used as a therapeutic agent for CF treatment. Therefore, controlled over-expression of P-gp can induce the release of cellular ATP, and might be therapeutically beneficial for the treatment of CF.

Alzheimer disease (AD) is characterized by the accumulation of amyloid-β (Aβ) in the extracellular spaces of the brain. The removal of Aβ from CNS through efflux transport across BBB has been implicated to be beneficial for the treatment of AD. The P-glycoprotein, which is an efflux pump that is highly expressed at the endothelial cells of the BBB, has been shown to transport amyloid-β across BBB. In a study it has been shown that, the decreased P-gp function may be involved in the pathogenesis of Alzheimer's disease [48].

The role of P-gp has also been associated with acute myeloid leukemia (AML) [49] and myelodysplastic syndrome (MDS) [50], which is in part due to over-expression of P-gp leading to MDR. Moreover, inflammatory disorders such as inflammatory bowel disease (IBD), Crohn's disease, and ulcerative colitis might be due to the aberrant expression of P-gp [51].

Lazarowski et al., have found that P-gp is consistently expressed in the cardiomyocytes of chronically ischemic porcine myocardium. Therefore, the modulation of P-gp activity might be useful for the therapy of ischemic cardiomyocytes [52].

Coronaviruses are a wide group of viruses which can cause animal and human disease. Coronavirus disease 2019 (COVID-19) is a respiratory illness that was identified in Wuhan, China, and is now being spread throughout the world. In the COVID-19 pandemic, co-administration of antimalarial chloroquine or anti-rheumatic hydroxychloroquine with antibacterial azithromycin is reportedly recommended as a remedy [53]. Moreover, due to its antibacterial property, azithromycin is presently proposed as a potential therapeutic option during the COVID-19 pandemic and a substrate of P-gp which is localized in endosomes and lysosomes with a polarized substrate transport from the cell cytosol into the vesicle interior. Scherrmann J. M. in a recent study have hypothesized that P-gp could have a potential role as an enhancer for the synergistic effect of azithromycin on hydroxychloroquine [54]. P-gp is expressed in lysosome/endosome membranes as well as on plasma cellular membranes of the lung epithelial cells. Moreover, the transport of the P-gp substrates is targeted from the cell cytoplasm to the extracellular environment at the lipid bilayer membrane level and to the lysosomes. Therefore, the intracellular transport of substrate via P-gp might result in up-regulated endolysosomal accumulation of P-gp substrates. A proposed scheme by Scherrmann J. M. [54] for the potential role of the synergistic effect of P-gp with azithromycin and hydroxychloroquine for SARS-CoV-2 drugs has been described in Figure 6.

P-gp possibly is involved in the alteration of SARS-CoV-2 replication implicated by synergizing the lysosomotropic effect of azithromycin and hydroxychloroquine and involving endolysosomal pathway. The proposed schematic represents the diffusion of unionized drugs across lysosomal membranes. A vacuolar proton-type adenosine triphosphatase membrane (v-ATPase), pumping protons into the interior of the vesicle, helps to preserve the ideal pH medium for lysosomal enzymes. The drug species becomes protonated due to lysosomal acidic environment, thereby hindering their backward backward diffusion into the cytosol. The efficient uptake of azithromycin as a substrate of P-gp leads to the amplification of this trapping impact under these acidic conditions and the neutralization of the acidic pH. These synergistic effects induces a cascade of anti-inflammatory and antiviral activities. AZM = Azithromycin; HCQ = Hydroxychloroquine;

ATP = Adenosine Tri-phosphate, v-ATPase = Vacuolar proton-type adenosine triphosphatase.

Interactome Analysis of P-Gp and Associated Metabolic Pathways Using Protein Interaction Analysis and Pathway Enrichment Analysis

In this study we have used the STRING DB [55] server to identify the closest protein interactors of P-gp/ABCB1. As per the interactome analysis total 7 nodes with 15 edges were found in P-gp/ABCB1 (Figure 7). TP53, EP300, ABCB4, MAPK8, TAF1 and RPA1 were found the close interactor proteins of P-gp1/ABCB1 and all these proteins were well connected with each other. In continuation of network study, the pathway enrichment of interactome was done and 31 associated pathways have been identified (Table 1).

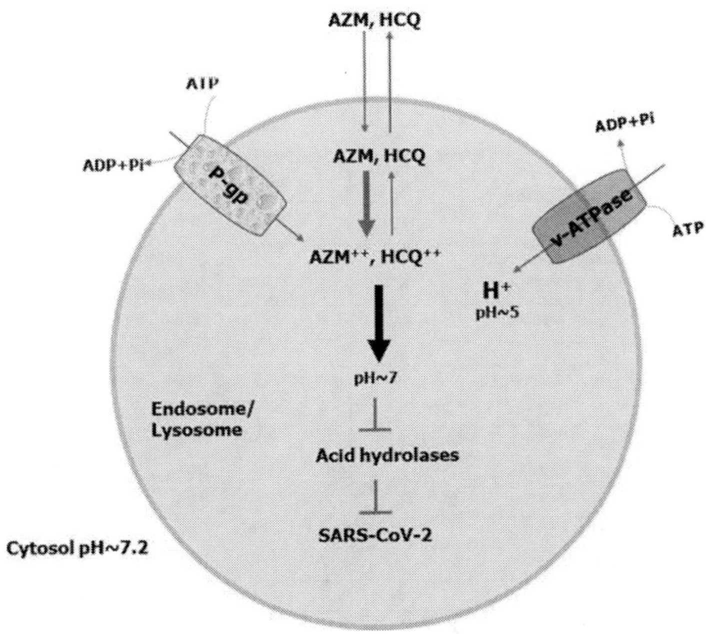

Figure 6. A proposed schematic model for the potential role of P-gp in COVID-19.

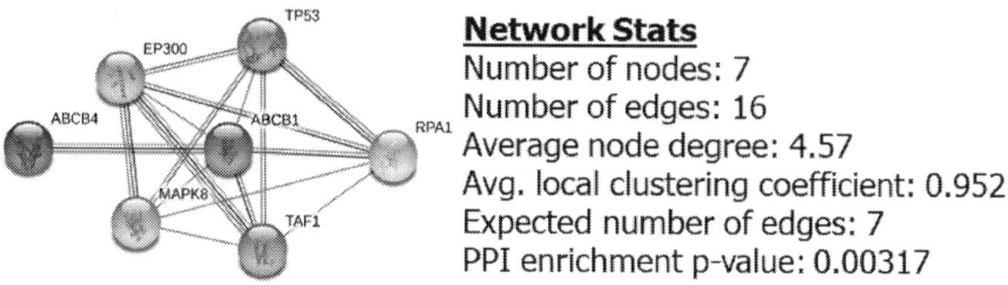

Figure 7. Interactome analysis of P-gp/ABCB1.

Table 1. Pathway enrichment analysis of P-gp and associated proteins

KEGG Pathway ID	Pathway	Observed Gene Count	Background gene count	False discovery rate	Proteins in network
hsa04310	Wnt signaling pathway	3	143	0.0014	EP300, MAPK8, TP53
hsa05161	Hepatitis B	3	142	0.0014	EP300, MAPK8, TP53
hsa05166	HTLV-I infection	3	250	0.0014	EP300, MAPK8, TP53
hsa05167	Kaposi's sarcoma-associated herpesvirus infection	3	183	0.0014	EP300, MAPK8, TP53
hsa05168	Herpes simplex infection	3	181	0.0014	EP300, MAPK8, TP53
hsa05169	Epstein-Barr virus infection	3	194	0.0014	EP300, MAPK8, TP53
hsa05206	MicroRNAs in cancer	3	149	0.0014	ABCB1, EP300, TP53
hsa02010	ABC transporters	2	44	0.0015	ABCB1, ABCB4
hsa04137	Mitophagy - animal	2	63	0.0026	MAPK8, TP53
hsa04976	Bile secretion	2	71	0.003	ABCB1, ABCB4
hsa05212	Pancreatic cancer	2	74	0.003	MAPK8, TP53
hsa05210	Colorectal cancer	2	85	0.0035	MAPK8, TP53
hsa01522	Endocrine resistance	2	95	0.0041	MAPK8, TP53
hsa05215	Prostate cancer	2	97	0.0041	EP300, TP53
hsa05200	Pathways in cancer	3	515	0.0042	EP300, MAPK8, TP53
hsa04071	Sphingolipid signaling pathway	2	116	0.0048	MAPK8, TP53
hsa04110	Cell cycle	2	123	0.0048	EP300, TP53

KEGG Pathway ID	Pathway	Observed Gene Count	Background gene count	False discovery rate	Proteins in network
hsa04722	Neurotrophin signaling pathway	2	116	0.0048	MAPK8, TP53
hsa04919	Thyroid hormone signaling pathway	2	115	0.0048	EP300, TP53
hsa04068	FoxO signaling pathway	2	130	0.0049	EP300, MAPK8
hsa04210	Apoptosis	2	135	0.0049	MAPK8, TP53
hsa05160	Hepatitis C	2	131	0.0049	MAPK8, TP53
hsa05418	Fluid shear stress and atherosclerosis	2	133	0.0049	MAPK8, TP53
hsa05226	Gastric cancer	2	147	0.0052	ABCB1, TP53
hsa05164	Influenza A	2	168	0.0064	EP300, MAPK8
hsa05152	Tuberculosis	2	172	0.0065	EP300, MAPK8
hsa05203	Viral carcinogenesis	2	183	0.007	EP300, TP53
hsa04024	cAMP signaling pathway	2	195	0.0075	EP300, MAPK8
hsa05016	Huntington's disease	2	193	0.0075	EP300, TP53
hsa04010	MAPK signaling pathway	2	293	0.0158	MAPK8, TP53
hsa05165	Human papillomavirus infection	2	317	0.0178	EP300, TP53

CONCLUSION AND FUTURE PERSPECTIVES

It is now commonly accepted that ABC multidrug efflux pumps play a key function in shielding tissues from exogenous and endogenous toxins. However, cellular mechanism by which it translocates the various number of molecules out of the cell are still unexplainable. Moreover, P-gp plays important role on the absorption, distribution, and elimination of drugs; however, we do have a lot to know regarding the dynamic connection networks between drugs and such drug transporters. A thorough understanding of structure and function of P-gp will be helpful in elucidating the catalytic reactions and drug transport mechanism of multidrug efflux pumps. The information obtained can thus be used in manipulating the therapeutic potential of P-gp transporters that can be made readily available as a novel diagnostic and therapeutic target for drug therapy.

REFERENCES

[1] Srivalli, K. M. R., Lakshmi, P. K., Overview of P-glycoprotein inhibitors: a rational outlook. *Brazilian Journal of Pharmaceutical Sciences* 2012, 48, 353-367.

[2] Sharom, F. J., The P-glycoprotein multidrug transporter. *Essays Biochem* 2011, 50 (1), 161-78.

[3] Ruetz, S., Gros, P., Phosphatidylcholine translocase: a physiological role for the mdr2 gene. *Cell* 1994, 77 (7), 1071-81.

[4] Varma, M. V., Ashokraj, Y., Dey, C. S., Panchagnula, R., P-glycoprotein inhibitors and their screening: a perspective from bioavailability enhancement. *Pharmacol Res* 2003, 48 (4), 347-59.

[5] Lin, J. H., Drug-drug interaction mediated by inhibition and induction of P-glycoprotein. *Adv Drug Deliv Rev* 2003, *55* (1), 53-81.

[6] Leslie, E. M., Deeley, R. G., Cole, S. P., Multidrug resistance proteins: role of P-glycoprotein, MRP1, MRP2, and BCRP (ABCG2) in tissue defense. *Toxicol Appl Pharmacol* 2005, 204 (3), 216-37.

[7] Thiebaut, F., Tsuruo, T., Hamada, H., Gottesman, M. M., Pastan, I., Willingham, M. C., Cellular localization of the multidrug-resistance gene product P-glycoprotein in normal human tissues. *Proc Natl Acad Sci U S A* 1987, 84 (21), 7735-8.

[8] Schinkel, A. H., Mayer, U., Wagenaar, E., Mol, C. A., van Deemter, L., Smit, J. J., van der Valk, M. A., Voordouw, A. C., Spits, H., van Tellingen, O., Zijlmans, J. M., Fibbe, W. E., Borst, P., Normal viability and altered pharmacokinetics in mice lacking mdr1-type (drug-transporting) P-glycoproteins. *Proc Natl Acad Sci U S A* 1997, 94 (8), 4028-33.

[9] Ma, J. D., Tsunoda, S. M., Bertino, J. S., Jr., Trivedi, M., Beale, K. K., Nafziger, A. N., Evaluation of *in vivo* P-glycoprotein phenotyping probes: a need for validation. *Clin Pharmacokinet* 2010, 49 (4), 223-37.

[10] Cordon-Cardo, C., O'Brien, J. P., Casals, D., Rittman-Grauer, L., Biedler, J. L., Melamed, M. R., Bertino, J. R., Multidrug-resistance

gene (P-glycoprotein) is expressed by endothelial cells at blood-brain barrier sites. *Proc Natl Acad Sci U S A* 1989, 86 (2), 695-8.

[11] Schellman, J. A., Schellman, C. G., Kaj Ulrik Linderstrøm-Lang (1896-1959). *Protein Sci* 1997, 6 (5), 1092-100.

[12] Bodor, M., Kelly, E. J., Ho, R. J., Characterization of the human MDR1 gene. *Aaps j* 2005, 7 (1), E1-5.

[13] Kim, Y., Chen, J., Molecular structure of human P-glycoprotein in the ATP-bound, outward-facing conformation. *Science* 2018, 359 (6378), 915-919.

[14] Zhou, S. F., Structure, function and regulation of P-glycoprotein and its clinical relevance in drug disposition. *Xenobiotica* 2008, 38 (7-8), 802-32.

[15] Walker, J. E., Saraste, M., Runswick, M. J., Gay, N. J., Distantly related sequences in the alpha- and beta-subunits of ATP synthase, myosin, kinases and other ATP-requiring enzymes and a common nucleotide binding fold. *Embo j* 1982, 1 (8), 945-51.

[16] Higgins, C. F., Callaghan, R., Linton, K. J., Rosenberg, M. F., Ford, R. C., Structure of the multidrug resistance P-glycoprotein. *Semin Cancer Biol* 1997, 8 (3), 135-42.

[17] Dean, M., Hamon, Y., Chimini, G., The human ATP-binding cassette (ABC) transporter superfamily. *J Lipid Res* 2001, 42 (7), 1007-17.

[18] Romsicki, Y., Sharom, F. J., The ATPase and ATP-binding functions of P-glycoprotein. Modulation by interaction with defined phospholipids. *European Journal of Biochemistry* 1998, 256 (1), 170-178.

[19] Gottesman, M. M., Pastan, I., Biochemistry of multidrug resistance mediated by the multidrug transporter. *Annu Rev Biochem* 1993, 62, 385-427.

[20] Johnstone, R. W., Ruefli, A. A., Smyth, M. J., Multiple physiological functions for multidrug transporter P-glycoprotein? *Trends Biochem Sci* 2000, 25 (1), 1-6.

[21] Higgins, C. F., Gottesman, M. M., Is the multidrug transporter a flippase? *Trends Biochem Sci* 1992, 17 (1), 18-21.

[22] Sharom, F., Complex Interplay between the P-Glycoprotein Multidrug Efflux Pump and the Membrane: Its Role in Modulating Protein Function. *Frontiers in Oncology* 2014, 4 (41).

[23] Conseil, G., Deeley, R. G., Cole, S. P. C., *Functional importance of three basic residues clustered at the cytosolic interface of transmembrane helix 15 in the multidrug and organic anion transporter MRP1 (ABCC1).* 2006, Vol. 281, pp. 43-50.

[24] Leier, I., Jedlitschky, G., Buchholz, U., Cole, S. P. C., Deeley, R. G., Keppler, D., *The MRP gene encodes an ATP-dependent export pump for leukotriene C4 and structurally related conjugates.* 1994, Vol. 269, pp. 27807-27810.

[25] Robbiani, D. F., Finch, R. A., Jäger, D., Muller, W. A., Sartorelli, A. C., Randolph, G. J., *The leukotriene C4 transporter MRP1 regulates CCL19 (MIP-3β, ELC)-dependent mobilization of dendritic cells to lymph nodes.* 2000, Vol. 103, pp. 757-768.

[26] Sjölinder, M., Tornhamre, S., Claesson, H. E., Hydman, J., Lindgren, J. Å., *Characterization of a leukotriene C4 export mechanism in human platelets: Possible involvement of multidrug resistance-associated protein 1.* 1999, Vol. 40, pp. 439-446.

[27] Stride, B. D., Grant, C. E., Loe, D. W., Hipfner, D. R., Cole, S. P. C., Deeley, R. G., *Pharmacological characterization of the murine and human orthologs of multidrug-resistance protein in transfected human embryonic kidney cells.* 1997, Vol. 52, pp. 344-353.

[28] Mitra, P., Oskeritzian, C. A., Payne, S. G., Beaven, M. A., Milstien, S., Spiegel, S., *Role of ABCC1 in export of sphingosine-1-phosphate from mast cells.* 2006, Vol. 103, pp. 16394-16399.

[29] McDevitt, C. A., Callaghan, R., *How can we best use structural information on P-glycoprotein to design inhibitors?* 2007, Vol. 113, pp. 429-441.

[30] Lee, B. D., Li, Z., French, K. J., Zhuang, Y., Xia, Z., Smith, C. D., *Synthesis and Evaluation of Dihydropyrroloquinolines That Selectively Antagonize P-Glycoprotein.* 2004, Vol. 47, pp. 1413-1422.

[31] O'Connor, R., *The pharmacology of cancer resistance.* 2007, Vol. 27, pp. 1267-1272.

[32] Thomas, H., Coley, H. M., Overcoming multidrug resistance in cancer: an update on the clinical strategy of inhibiting p-glycoprotein. *Cancer Control* 2003, 10 (2), 159-65.

[33] Shen, X., Chen, G., Zhu, G., Fong, W. F., *(±)-3'-O, 4'-O-dicynnamoyl-cis-khellactone, a derivative of (±)-praeruptorin A, reverses P-glycoprotein mediated multidrug resistance in cancer cells.* 2006, Vol. 14, pp. 7138-7145.

[34] Kars, M. D., Işeri, O. D., Gunduz, U., Molnar, J., *Reversal of multidrug resistance by synthetic and natural compounds in drug-resistant MCF-7 cell lines.* 2008, Vol. 54, pp. 194-200.

[35] Li, Y., Yuan, H., Yang, K., Xu, W., Tang, W., Li, X., *The Structure and Functions of P-Glycoprotein.* 2010, Vol. 17, pp. 786-800.

[36] Ren, Y., Wang, Y., Zhang, Y., Wei, D., *Overcoming multidrug resistance in human carcinoma cells by an antisense oligodeoxynucleotide-doxorubicin conjugate in vitro and in vivo.* 2008, Vol. 5, pp. 579-587.

[37] Merenstein, D., Yang, Y., Schneider, M. F., Goparaju, L., Weber, K., Sharma, A., Levine, A. M., Sharp, G. B., Gandhi, M., Liu, C., *Association of complementary and alternative medicine use with highly active antiretroviral therapy initiation.* 2008, Vol. 14, pp. 18-22.

[38] Petriz, J., Gottesman, M., Aran, J., *An MDR-EGFP Gene Fusion Allows for Direct Cellular Localization, Function and Stability Assessment of P-Glycoprotein.* 2005, Vol. 1, pp. 43-56.

[39] Shaik, N., Giri, N., Pan, G., Elmquist, W. F., *P-glycoprotein-mediated active efflux of the anti-HIV1 nucleoside abacavir limits cellular accumulation and brain distribution.* 2007, Vol. 35, pp. 2076-2085.

[40] Cianfriglia, M., Dupuis, M. L., Molinari, A., Verdoliva, A., Costi, R., Galluzzo, C. M., Andreotti, M., Cara, A., Di Santo, R., Palmisano, L., *HIV-1 integrase inhibitors are substrates for the multidrug transporter MDR1-P-glycoprotein.* 2007, Vol. 4.

[41] Pal, D., Mitra, A. K. In *MDR- and CYP3A4-mediated drug-drug interactions*, 2006/09//, *J Neuroimmune Pharmacol*: pp. 323-339.

[42] Schwab, A. E., Churcher, T. S., Schwab, A. J., Basáñez, M. G., Prichard, R. K., *An analysis of the population genetics of potential multi-drug resistance in Wuchereria bancrofti due to combination chemotherapy.* 2007, Vol. 134, pp. 1025-1040.

[43] Luscher, A., de Koning, H., Maser, P., *Chemotherapeutic Strategies Against Trypanosoma brucei: Drug Targets vs. Drug Targeting.* 2007, Vol. 13, pp. 555-567.

[44] Collaco, J. M., Cutting, G. R., *Update on gene modifiers in cystic fibrosis.* 2008, Vol. 14, pp. 559-566.

[45] Ostedgaard, L. S., Baldursson, O., Vermeer, D. W., Welsh, M. J., Robertson, A. D., A functional R domain from cystic fibrosis transmembrane conductance regulator is predominantly unstructured in solution. *Proceedings of the National Academy of Sciences of the United States of America* 2000, 97, 5657-5662.

[46] Riordan, J. R., Rommens, J. M., Kerem, B. S., Alon, N. O. A., Rozmahel, R., Grzelczak, Z., Zielenski, J., Lok, S. I., Plavsic, N., Chou, J. L., Drumm, M. L., Iannuzzi, M. C., Collins, F. S., Tsui, L. C., Identification of the cystic fibrosis gene: Cloning and characterization of complementary DNA. *Science* 1989, 245, 1066-1073.

[47] Zhang, Z., Liu, F., Chen, J., Conformational Changes of CFTR upon Phosphorylation and ATP Binding. *Cell* 2017, 170, 483-491.e8.

[48] Cirrito, J. R., Deane, R., Fagan, A. M., Spinner, M. L., Parsadanian, M., Finn, M. B., Jiang, H., Prior, J. L., Sagare, A., Bales, K. R., Paul, S. M., Zlokovic, B. V., Piwnica-Worrns, D., Holtzman, D. M., *P-glycoprotein deficiency at the blood-brain barrier increases amyloid-β deposition in an Alzheimer disease mouse model.* 2005, Vol. 115, pp. 3285-3290.

[49] Benderra, Z., Faussat, A. M., Sayada, L., Perrot, J. Y., Tang, R., Chaoui, D., Morjani, H., Marzac, C., Marie, J. P., Legrand, O., *MRP3, BCRP, and P-glycoprotein activities are prognostic factors in adult acute myeloid leukemia.* 2005, Vol. 11, pp. 7764-7772.

[50] Ross, D. D., *Modulation of drug resistance transporters as a strategy for treating myelodysplastic syndrome.* 2004, Vol. 17, pp. 641-651.

[51] Buyse, M., Radeva, G., Bado, A., Farinotti, R., *Intestinal inflammation induces adaptation of P-glycoprotein expression and activity.* 2005, Vol. 69, pp. 1745-1754.

[52] Lazarowski, A. J., García Rivello, H. J., Vera Janavel, G. L., Cuniberti, L. A., Cabeza Meckert, P. M., Yannarelli, G. G., Mele, A., Crottogini, A. J., Laguens, R. P., Cardiomyocytes of chronically ischemic pig hearts express the MDR-1 gene-encoded P-glycoprotein. *J Histochem Cytochem* 2005, 53 (7), 845-50.

[53] Gautret, P., Lagier, J. C., Parola, P., Hoang, V. T., Meddeb, L., Mailhe, M., Doudier, B., Courjon, J., Giordanengo, V., Vieira, V. E., Tissot Dupont, H., Honoré, S., Colson, P., Chabrière, E., La Scola, B., Rolain, J. M., Brouqui, P., Raoult, D., Hydroxychloroquine and azithromycin as a treatment of COVID-19: results of an open-label non-randomized clinical trial. *Int J Antimicrob Agents* 2020, 56 (1), 105949.

[54] Scherrmann, J. M., Intracellular ABCB1 as a Possible Mechanism to Explain the Synergistic Effect of Hydroxychloroquine-Azithromycin Combination in COVID-19 Therapy. *Aaps j* 2020, 22 (4), 86.

[55] Szklarczyk, D., Gable, A. L., Lyon, D., Junge, A., Wyder, S., Huerta-Cepas, J., Simonovic, M., Doncheva, N. T., Morris, J. H., Bork, P., Jensen, L. J., Mering, C. V., STRING v11: protein-protein association networks with increased coverage, supporting functional discovery in genome-wide experimental datasets. *Nucleic Acids Res* 2019, 47 (D1), D607-d613.

In: An Introduction to P-Glycoprotein ISBN: 978-1-53619-488-3
Editors: M. Wahajuddin et al.

Chapter 2

RELATIVE DISTRIBUTION OF P-GLYCOPROTEIN (P-GP) AND ITS PHARMACOLOGICAL RELEVANCE

Nishant S. Kulkarni, Snehal K. Shukla and Vivek Gupta*
Department of Pharmaceutical Sciences,
College of Pharmacy and Health Sciences,
St. John's University, Queens, NY, US

ABSTRACT

Permeability glycoprotein (P-gp)/Multidrug resistance-1 (MDR-1) is a member of the ATP-Binding cassette transporter family and is first of its kind to be cloned and studied for its involvement in multiple disorders. P-gp has been heavily investigated for its role as an efflux transporter along with its involvement in development of cellular resistance for certain molecules. Physiologically, P-gp receptors are present throughout the body with a heavy presence on the intestinal epithelium, liver, kidneys, blood-brain barrier, etc. Being an efflux transporter with presence in the above-mentioned areas, P-gp acts as a first-line defense system against

* Corresponding Author's Email: guptav@stjohns.edu.

xenobiotics and native molecules. Due to this innate feature of P-gp receptors, studies have been conducted in determining its role in development of resistance in conditions like epilepsy, rheumatoid arthritis, ovarian cancer etc. where P-gp is believed to be ejecting potent therapeutic P-gp substrates out of the cells, leading to low therapeutic outcomes. Keeping P-gp's relevance in mind, this chapter summarizes key physiological locations with heavy P-gp presence and its role as cellular gatekeepers in those areas. Moreover, the chapter also summarizes the role of P-gp in altering oral bioavailability for molecules, and its relevance in conditions like cancer, CNS conditions and autoimmune disorders.

Keywords: P-glycoprotein, transporters, pharmacology, distribution, ATP-Binding cassette

Introduction

Permeability glycoprotein/Multidrug Resistance-1 (P-gp/MDR1) is an essential protein belonging to the ATP-binding cassette transporter (ABC-transporters) family [1] and was the first human ABC transporter to be cloned and characterized thoroughly in various disorders [2–4]. P-gp, encoded by the MDR-1 gene, is responsible for transport of native and non-native cellular components and small molecules across the cell membrane at the expense of energy derived from ATP hydrolysis [5]. P-gp is considered to be the first-line cellular defense which can be attributed to its role in energy dependent transport of structurally diverse molecules across cell membranes, especially against toxins and therapeutic agents by limiting their intracellular accumulation via efflux enhancement [1].

P-gp (a 170 kDa membrane protein) is present in diverse locations throughout the body with major sites being the blood-brain barrier (BBB), gastrointestinal tract (GIT), liver, kidneys, placental barrier etc. [5]. Transporters in GIT, liver and kidneys are responsible for drug disposition and interactions whereas transporters present in more intricate areas such as the BBB or placental barrier are responsible for protection of sensitive regions from toxins [2]. Apart from these locations, P-gp is also endogenous to hematopoietic cells such as $CD34^+$ stem cells, cytotoxic $CD8^+$ T cells and

CD56+ natural killer cells, signifying its role in immunomodulation [2]. P-gp is also present on mitochondrial membrane and nuclear membrane in MDR positive cells; and is responsible for flushing out exogenous substrates from the mitochondria and nucleus, respectively, into the cytosol [2].

A vital role of P-gp is to maintain cellular homeostasis via regulating transport across the cell membrane [6]. Based on the physiological locations, various pharmacological applications have been described for P-gp. One of the most essential pharmacological applications comes in the cerebral region where P-gp is present on the endothelial cells of luminal vessels which make up the BBB [7]. Hydrophobic molecules, ideally, should be able to traverse the BBB easily but the presence of P-gp results in efflux of these hydrophobic molecules back in the blood at a tremendous rate, thus severely limiting BBB permeation [8].

Another major implication of P-gp is its overexpression in various types of tumors, causing a substantial increase in drug molecule efflux from the cancer cells [9]. This high efflux rate can affect the treatment strategy drastically due to premature clearance of chemotherapeutics from cells leading to a loss in therapeutic potency. Due to overexpression in tumors, P-gp has also been heavily linked to the acquisition of multidrug resistance in many disorders, thus completely rendering the therapy ineffective, or may even cause development of cross-resistance to unrelated molecules [10]. P-gp also plays a major role in immunomodulation due to its expression on immune cells such as T cells and B cells, where it has been reported to be involved in efflux of inflammatory molecules such as steroids, prostaglandins and cytokines [11]. Dysfunction of P-gp transporters on such immune cells may lead to enhanced efflux of inflammatory molecules leading to various autoimmune conditions such as inflammatory bowel disease or rheumatoid arthritis [12].

With such widespread physiological locations and a high pharmacological relevance, P-gp has often been studied for its applicability as a therapeutic/diagnostic target. Therapeutically, inhibition of P-gp action is ought to be the most accepted strategy, but there are multiple complications such as inhibitor toxicity and enzyme-mediated inhibitor degradation, which have led to the failure of multiple clinical trials involving these P-gp inhibitors [13]. First generation inhibitors of P-gp (verapamil and cyclosporin-A) were not developed to specifically inhibit P-gp and were also interactive with other types of efflux transporters, which led to major unpredictability in pharmacokinetic profiles of these molecules [2, 14]. The second-generation inhibitors (dexverapamil) were less toxic and more potent inhibitors but there were issues relating to enzyme-mediated degradation, which rendered them ineffective [14]. Subsequent generations (tarquidar and elacridar) were developed to be more potent and less toxic which led to clinical investigations. Tarquidar was successful in phase-1, and thus, in phase-3 was combined with commonly used chemotherapeutics (carboplatin, paclitaxel and vinorelbine) to assess the overall effect of P-gp inhibition in chemotherapy. Although tarquidar had promising phase-1 results, phase-3 trial had to be prematurely stopped due to toxicity concerns [14]. Development of newer generation P-gp inhibitors is in progress with at least one molecule (tetrandine) under phase-1 trial. (www.clinicaltrials.gov, NCT03002805). From a diagnostic point of view, P-gp has been explored to study tumor relapse in leukemia patients. It was revealed that P-gp expression is more prominent in relapse conditions than initial diagnosis of leukemia [15].

Earlier chapters highlighted various structural and physiological characteristics of P-gp receptors in detail. The current chapter will focus on delivering in-depth up-to-date advancements in ABCB1 transporter systems, discussing novel discoveries regarding physiological distribution along with an extensive pharmacological applicability of P-gp receptors in various diseased conditions and genetic disorders.

Physiological Distribution of P-glycoprotein in Normal and Diseased Conditions

P-gp is widely distributed in intestinal epithelium, pancreatic ductules, bile ductules, liver, renal proximal tubules, and the blood brain barrier (BBB) [16]. The major role of P-gp can be classified as; a) limiting the entry of xenobiotics after oral administration owing to localization in luminal membrane of intestinal epithelia; b) promoting their elimination/excretion into bile and urine after absorption of xenobiotics in systemic circulation; and c) minimizing the penetration of xenobiotics into sensitive tissues such as brain, placenta, lymphocytes etc. [17]

Intrinsic functionalities of P-gp can be influenced by several factors which impact the therapeutic response of drugs. In this section, alteration in role of P-gp will be discussed in relation to the following topics a) modulation of P-gp due to polymorphism; b) drug-drug interaction/inhibition; and c) variation of P-gp function due to diseased conditions.

Intestinal Epithelium

The presence of P-gp in the intestinal epithelial cells is known to affect the rate and extent of drug absorption and metabolism which impacts bioavailability [18]. This transmembrane protein can effectively pump out wide variety of xenobiotics back in the intestinal lumen after permeation, therefore restricting the systemic absorption of oral drugs. Primarily P-gp is found to be expressed on the apical surface of superficial columnar epithelial cells in the human intestine [19, 20]. Regional difference has been observed in P-gp expression wherein higher expression was reported in ileum and colon while lower expression for stomach, upper parts of small intestine (duodenum, and jejunum) [21, 22]. Several transport studies using P-gp substrates have reported significantly higher efflux rate of the substrate in the ileal region substantiating higher expression of P-gp in ileum [23–25]. In addition to regional differences, high inter and intra-individual variability has also been observed in the basal expression of P-gp in gastrointestinal tract [26].

P-gp expression and activity can be modulated by numerous endogenous and exogenous factors which may differentially trigger metabolic signaling and xenobiotic transport across the intestinal mucosa [27]. The oral bioavailability of P-gp substrates are impacted by the intestinal P-gp absorption and altered by co-administration of drugs, polymorphism and disease state [20]. For instance, tacrolimus, a P-gp substrate, when co-administered with ketoconazole, demonstrated increased in systemic absorption and intestinal permeability due to P-gp inhibition [28]. P-gp efflux is also known to influence the first pass effects of drugs and was believed to be correlated to the enteral cytochrome P-450 (CYP3A) activity [29, 30]. Cyclosporine, a P-gp substrate and a substrate of CYP3A, was reported to have modulated oral bioavailability upon co-administration with other drugs. Bioavailability of cyclosporine is known to significantly increase upon co-administration with ketoconazole (CYP3A inhibitor) and grapefruit juice (containing CYP3A inhibitors) [29, 30]. However, Lown et al., based on clinical pharmacokinetic data, confirmed that P-gp activity is more important in modulating cyclosporine absorption from the intestine than its interaction with CYP3A in liver [31].

It has been reported that P-gp undergoes diverse physiological polymorphic changes leading to genetic differences in individuals, influencing P-gp functionalities [32]. C3435T polymorphism occurring at position 3435 in the exon 26 of MDR-1 (gene encoding P-gp) is one of the most common polymorphisms in the ABCB1 gene known to affect the intestinal expression of P-gp and its activity [33]. The polymorphism of P-gp thereby influences the therapeutic response and toxicity of P-gp substrates [32, 34]. Based on the study performed by Foote et al., C3435T polymorphism was reported to be an independent predictor of cyclosporine pharmacokinetics in post-transplant treatment. Moreover, the patients with C3435T polymorphism demonstrated ~15% decrease in the AUC of cyclosporine, indicating that polymorphism must also be considered as an important tool for deciding dose [35]. In another study by Li et al., a positive association was found between polymorphism of P-gp and tacrolimus levels per dose in renal transplant patients, wherein, P-gp polymorphism resulted in an increase in tacrolimus levels per dose upon genetic change in subjects [36].

Diseased conditions are known to impact expression levels and activity of P-gp in the intestinal epithelium. Iiaza et al., reported reduced expression of P-gp in experimental mouse model of dextran sodium sulfate (DSS)-induced colitis [37]. Downregulation of P-gp expression has also been associated with conditions such as ulcerative colitis [38], inflammatory bowel disease [27]. Several studies have reported reduced expression of P-gp in the inflamed tissues of ulcerative colitis patients as compared to the unaffected mucosa [38–40]. Low level of P-gp expression in diseased conditions alters the xenobiotic transport and exposure of tissues [41]. Interestingly, in Crohn's disease, the expression of P-gp levels doubled in patients as compared to healthy subjects, thereby reducing the absorption and therapeutic efficacy of tacrolimus which led to higher than average required dose in the diseased patients [42]. Preclinical studies performed on obese rat experimental model induced by high fat diet resulted into 1.2-fold increase in nelfinavir bioavailability, possibly due to downregulation of intestinal P-gp [43]. The relationship between P-gp expression and required oral doses of immunosuppressants in organ transplant patients has been widely explored. Liver failure induced after hepatic transplantation including chronic rejection/or cholangitis resulted into increased P-gp levels altering the bioavailability of immunosuppressants [44]. Based on the clinical study performed by Lamhieu et al., persistent diarrhea has been associated with decreased intestinal P-gp activity resulting into increased oral bioavailability of tacrolimus in transplant patients [45]. Intestinal variability of P-gp is also found to be influenced by the circadian rhythms of genetic regulatory pathways, controlled by the MDR1 gene expression [46]. The expression of several circadian genes were found to be altered in ulcerative colitis, inflammatory bowel disease and Crohn's disease which are suggestive of playing an important role in the pathophysiology of the disease [47]. Changes in the circadian expression of P-gp are suggestive of influence on absorption, transport, excretion, and pharmacokinetics of the substrates [48].

Liver

Among these, efflux transporters such as P-gp, MRPs and BRCP belong to the ABC superfamily, widely studied for their inevitable role in hepatic metabolism and absorption with ABCB1/P-gp impacting the drug transport. P-gp receptors utilize ATP to efflux their substrate against concentration gradient [49] and are distributed widely in apical surface of cells present in canalicular membrane of hepatocytes and on the apical region of small biliary ductules [19]. Owing to such localization, P-gp is known to be responsible for hepatobiliary excretion of drugs and therefore plays an important role in bioavailability by preventing intracellular drug accumulation [50, 51]. Upon systemic absorption of drugs from the intestine, drugs readily enter hepatocytes, wherein P-gp, along with other efflux transporters, excrete them into the bile. This biliary excretion is one of the most important xenobiotic excretion routes transporting xenobiotics to the bile or back to the systemic circulation, thus determining the fate of hepatic clearance [49]. Besides, P-gp is also responsible for maintaining homeostasis and transport of various lipids such as cholesterol [52], phospholipids [53] and sphingolipids [17] along with variety of steroids [54]. *In-vivo* studies on P-gp knockdown mouse models have demonstrated about 2-fold reduction in biliary excretion of irinotecan (P-gp substrate) and its metabolites [55]. Other *in-vivo* studies performed using P-gp inhibitors such as verapamil and cyclosporine resulted into improved bioavailability of irinotecan and its metabolites [56, 57]. These results suggest that P-gp induced biliary excretion influences the absorption, metabolism, and pharmacokinetics of the substrates.

Hepatic P-gp expression has also been reported to influence the drug pharmacokinetics due to drug-drug interactions. Lowes et al., performed impact of pregnenolone 16α-carbonitrile on biliary excretion of digoxin in rat model, wherein the excretion of digoxin was increased 2-fold due to increased P-gp expression altering the drug disposition [58]. A significant increase in the ratio of biliary excretion to hepatic uptake of [3H]-vincristine was observed upon concomitant administration of phenothiazine (P-gp inducer) in rats [59]. Similarly, biliary elimination of vinblastine was increased due to increase in P-gp levels upon administration of 2-acetylaminofluorene in cholestasis rat model [60]. In clinical studies, co-administration of rifampicin (P-gp inducer) increased biliary excretion of digoxin resulting into reduced bioavailability [61]. Booth et al., reported that elacridar (GF120918), a P-gp inhibitor, significantly decreased biliary clearance of doxorubicin and its metabolite doxorubinicol [62].

Polymorphism of P-gp is known to impact the hepatic function and hepatobiliary secretion of various endogenous and exogenous compounds [63]. The 3435 polymorphisms of P-gp (C > T allele) is known to be associated with lower hepatic ABCB1 mRNA levels thus downregulating the P-gp expression and activity [64]. Studies performed on patients to evaluate the response and toxicity of irinotecan with respect to p-gp polymorphism indicated that patients homozygous for the 3435T allele showed decreased function of P-gp mediated biliary secretion of irinotecan [65].

Liver plays an important role in clearance of endogenous and xenobiotic molecules, therefore any change in the uptake and efflux transporter activity and expression impacts drug accumulation, metabolism, and excretion [66]. P-gp is responsible for maintaining lipid balance in the body and its impaired functioning contributes into diseased conditions such as hepatic steatosis and obesity. Experimental studies performed on mdr1ab$^{-/-}$ mice model confirmed that P-gp deficiency leads to changes in the lipid availability and metabolic pathways favoring development of obesity [67]. Cholestasis has been shown to increase the MDR-1 gene expression and thereby alter the P-gp levels [60]. *In-vivo* studies on a rodent model of cholestasis demonstrated reduced bioavailability of digoxin, suggestive of P-gp mediated hepatic clearance [68]. Liver dysfunction results into adaptive changes in the signaling mechanisms involved in handling of bile salts and bile acids, transport, metabolism, and excretion of drug. *In-vivo* studies performed on carbon tetrachloride induced acute hepatic failure in rats demonstrated suppressed intestinal P-gp functionality evaluated by the absorption and exsorption of P-gp substrates (digoxin and rhodamine) [69]. On the contrary, P-gp activity was found to be significantly higher for digoxin and rhodamine in studies performed on everted intestine [69]. These results signify the difference in the P-gp function in acute liver failure in *in-vitro* and *in-vivo* conditions. P-gp expression along with other efflux transporters has been extensively reduced in hepatocellular carcinoma as compared to normal hepatocytes [70]. Due to this, P-gp expression was found to be inversely correlated with therapeutic response of the administered anticancer agents [71].

Kidneys

Kidneys are the major elimination organs in human body, responsible for excretion of xenobiotics, maintenance of physiological conditions and secretion of hormones [72]. In human kidneys, P-gp efflux transporters are mainly expressed on the apical surfaces (brush borders) of proximal tubules and sparsely on the thick limb of Henle's loop, glomerular mesangium and the collecting duct [19, 73]. The localization of P-gp in kidneys is consistent with its function of excretory transport of xenobiotics in urine [74]. The physiological function of P-gp in kidneys is associated with removal of xenobiotics, toxic metabolites, several drugs and other endogenous components such as cytokines (interleukins 2) [75]. Inducibility of renal P-gp has been very well explored as a protective mechanism against nephrotoxicity as induced by several compounds. Hauser et al., reported that incubation of tubular and endothelial cells with cyclosporine caused increase in P-gp expression [76]. This study hints at a protective mechanism of P-gp against conditions such as cyclosporine induced renal toxicity. Similarly, *in-vivo* studies have shown that chronic exposure of cadmium caused increase in P-gp expression in proximal tubular cells. This upregulation of P-gp provided anti-apoptotic protection to tubular cells against cadmium-mediated stress [77].

Drug-drug interactions result into induction and/or inhibition of renal P-gp expression and activity which influences the fate of xenobiotics. In a clinical study performed by Rengelshausen et al., coadministration of clarithromycin with digoxin resulted in increased oral bioavailability and reduced non-glomerular renal clearance of digoxin, possibly due to inhibition of renal and intestinal P-gp [78]. *In-vitro* studies performed on isolated perfused rat kidney indicated that tubular secretion of digoxin was reduced upon coadministration of verapamil and quinidine due to inhibition of P-gp activity [79]. Wakasugi et al., also reported increase in serum concentration of digoxin after administration of clarithromycin, which inhibits P-gp mediated tubular excretion [80]. Kyrklund et al., described increase in plasma concentrations of pravastatin upon concomitant administration of gemfibrozil which is attributed to alter transport protein activity [81].

Polymorphism of MDR-1 gene is known to impact the P-gp expression as well as impact the exposure of xenobiotics to the organs resulting into altered absorption, excretion, and toxicity [82]. Siegsmund et al., demonstrated that patients with 3435TT genotype possessed significantly reduced P-gp levels as compared to 3435CC genotypes. This reduced P-gp expression could potentially increase the exposure of toxic substances to the organs and therefore induce severe toxicity and/or organ damage [83]. In a clinical study performed by Yates et al., MDR-1 C3435T genotype determined the oral clearance of cyclosporin wherein patients with at least one 3435T allele had significantly higher clearance than the homozygous wildtype patients [84]. Takeshi et al., reported decreased risk of steroid-induced osteonecrosis after kidney transplantation in patients with 3435TT genotype due to increased P-gp expression [85].

Renal dysfunction and various diseased conditions affect the activity and regulation of renal P-gp. *In-vivo* studies performed in glycerol-induced acute renal failure (ARF) rat model demonstrated significant suppression of renal P-gp function than normal healthy rats [86]. Shibata et al., reported decreased oral bioavailability of cyclosporine in gentamycin induced ARF rat model which may be attributed to altered P-gp expression [87]. Okabe et al., evaluated the impact of renal failure on bioavailability of tacrolimus in cisplatin-induced renal failure model rats. The results demonstrated significantly improved intestinal absorption of tacrolimus due to suppressed P-gp activity in rats [88]. Clinical studies performed by Stangier et al., investigated the effect of renal impairment on pharmacokinetics of dabigatran etexilate. AUC of dabigatran was 6.3-fold higher in severe renal impairment patients as compared to healthy subjects, which may be attributed to downregulation of renal P-gp expression in disease condition [89].

Blood-Brain Barrier (BBB)

Blood-Brain Barrier (BBB) is considered the primary barrier for entry of xenobiotics in the central nervous system. It comprises of a physical or biochemical barrier formed by endothelial cells lining the brain capillaries; and functions to maintain homeostasis of central nervous system, regulate transport of compounds including nutrients, metabolic wastes and protect against toxins [90]. The diffusion across the BBB depends on the physicochemical properties of drug molecules and their interaction with the transporters present at the barrier interface [91]. P-gp, an ATP-dependent efflux transporter is majorly localized on the luminal membrane of the endothelial cells present on the brain microcapillaries [90, 92]. Additionally, P-gp is also found to be localized in various cellular components of brain such as astrocytes, microglia, and neurons [93]. Localization of P-gp in brain components and BBB signifies a very important role of protecting central nervous system against unwanted and harmful agents.

In-vitro studies performed on pentylenetetrazol induced epileptic rat models indicated significantly increased expression and activity of P-gp at BBB resulting into reduced distribution of phenobarbital in rat brains. However, administration of cyclosporine, a P-gp inhibitor, resulted in significant increase in brain distribution and anti-epileptic activity of phenobarbital in animals [94]. Kemper et al., demonstrated ~5-fold increase in brain uptake of paclitaxel after pre-treatment with GF120918 (elacridar), a P-gp inhibitor. This increase in paclitaxel uptake was also followed by reduced clearance, attributed to inhibition of P-gp activity in brain [95]. Montesinos et al., studied the impact of coadministration of tariquidar and elacridar (both P-gp inhibitors) on pharmacokinetics and brain distribution of loperamide (P-gp substrate) in rats. A significant increase was observed in the plasma and tissue distribution of loperamide with use of P-gp inhibitor which may be due to suppression of P-gp activity at BBB interface [96]. These results suggest that therapeutic doses of P-gp modulators can help to improve the activity of P-gp substrates.

Single nucleotide polymorphism of MDR-1 gene has been most extensively studied to evaluate the response of several P-gp substrate treatment. In a study performed by Jelen et al., C3435T polymorphisms in the *MDR-1* gene were shown to be strongly associated with a predisposition to depression development, severity of depressive symptoms and effectiveness of therapy with using different groups of antidepressant agents [97]. Patients with CC genotype displayed higher severity of depression symptoms along with reduced treatment response to antidepressant drugs as compared to CT or TT genotype [97]. Kerb et al., reported that patients with TT genotype of C3435 polymorphism showed higher phenytoin plasma levels than CC genotype patients. This fact can be attributed to the suppressed P-gp activity in C3435TT polymorphism patients [98]. Occurrence of Parkinson's disease is known to be impacted by P-gp polymorphism, wherein frequency of 3435T/T genotype was highest in early-onset Parkinson's patients as compared to late-onset or control groups resulting into inhibition of P-gp expression and function [99].

Diseased conditions are known to alter the P-gp expression further influencing the brain uptake of drugs and their therapeutic activity. Increase in P-gp expression has been reported in epileptic patients. Wen et al., investigated the role of chronic exposure of anti-epileptic drugs on P-gp expression. P-gp levels were found to be significantly higher in the cortex, medulla, and capillary endothelial vessels of the rat brains which resulted into decreased brain to plasma ratio of the administered drugs and eventually leading to development of multidrug resistance [100]. P-gp expression is also known to be upregulated in neurodegenerative disorders such as amyotrophic lateral sclerosis (ALS) conferring acquired pharmaco-resistance impacting the therapeutic efficacy of treatment [101, 102].

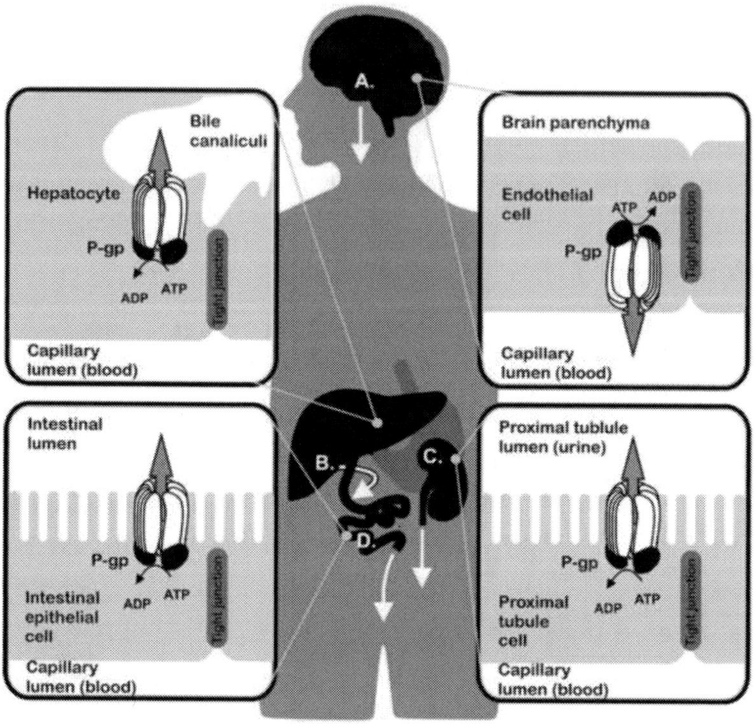

Figure 1. Overview of physiological location of P-gp receptors in liver, brain intestine and kidneys. Reproduced with permission from MDPI, Basel, Switzerland under Creative Commons Attribution License [106].

Concomitant administration of minocycline (P-gp inhibitor) with riluzole for ALS treatment in mice resulted into increased uptake of riluzole in central nervous system as compared to riluzole treatment alone [103]. Ischemic stroke results into hypomethylation of ABCB1 promoter resulting into increased expression and activity of P-gp in patients. This increased P-gp function causes reduced uptake of clopidogrel and therefore its diminished therapeutic response in ischemic stroke patients [104]. Brain tumors have shown variation in expression of drug transporters at the blood-tumor barrier along with the BBB interface. An animal study performed on MDR1a/b$^{(-/-)}$ knockout mice model, showed significant increase in the brain penetration of topotecan in knockout mice as compared to the wildtype subjects emphasizing the influence of P-gp on the effect of drug transport in tumor [105]. Figure 1 summarizes the physiological location and relevance of P-gp receptors in liver, brain, intestine and kidneys [106].

Pharmacokinetics and Pharmacological Relevance

P-gp receptors are known to play a crucial role in pharmacokinetic fate of drugs by influencing their absorption, distribution, metabolism and elimination processes due to its diverse locations throughout the intestinal tract [107]. Thus, it is vital to understand that inhibition of P-gp activity can markedly affect the pharmacokinetic fate of the drug via improving absorption of not only orally administered drugs, but even parentally administered drugs via enhanced intestinal reuptake, and reduced biliary excretion and renal clearance [108]. This inhibition of P-gp can be via saturation of P-gp receptors, which is a major pathway for most of the developed P-gp inhibitors, in addition to inhibiting the ATP hydrolysis and starving the receptors of essential energy required for efflux [107, 108]. One such studied P-gp inhibitor is Verapamil (VP). Verapamil has been reported to improve the plasma concentration and volume of distribution of many drug molecules including doxorubicin which is a known substrate of P-gp [109]. VP competitively binds to P-gp receptors preferentially over substrate drugs, thus improving their intestinal absorption and thereby has a positive influence on their pharmacokinetic profile. Moreover, VP also extends the elimination half-life of doxorubicin, thus leading to an enhanced therapeutic effect [109]. VP is also well-known to improve the premature clearance issues of paclitaxel following oral administration [110]. However, it is important to note that the concentrations of VP required to achieve these stellar effects are cardiotoxic [111]. Thus, safer novel options such as dexverapamil have been developed with negligible cardiotoxic effects, while retaining the P-gp inhibition potency [111].

Efflux Mechanisms and Effect of P-gp in Oral Bioavailability

Efflux Mechanisms

P-gp, an ABCB1 type transporter, is responsible for the transport of a variety of structurally diverse molecules [2]. While the basic mechanism of transport across cell membrane is not yet fully understood, "ATP Switch Theory" is the best explanation till date regarding the molecular transport system. This theory explains that the efflux of ABC substrates takes place in three major steps, as shown in Figure 2 [2]. Briefly, the transport is initiated by binding of the substrate to the transmembrane domain (TMD) of the transporter, initially in an inward facing orientation, with high affinity. The second step is a well-choreographed relay of orientational changes in the TMD. ATP binds to the nucleotide binding domain (NBD) and acts like a glue resulting in formation of a sandwich-like structure with two nucleotide binding sites (NBS) at the interface of NBD. Following this, influx through the TMD is closed, and ATP hydrolysis further leads to generation of chemical potential difference between the substrate and the transporter resulting in an affinity reversal. The high affinity substrate now has very low affinity for the transporter domain. Simultaneously, ATP hydrolysis also results in a net negative charge on the domain which leads to the extracellular part of the domain to open up, thus transporting the substrate outside the cell [112].

An alternative mechanism, termed as the "Hydrophobic Vacuum Cleaner" flushes out hydrophobic molecules which have partitioned into the lower part (towards the intracellular site) of the cell membrane via a concentration gradient effect [113]. Prior to reaching the cytosol, foreign hydrophobic molecules are recognized by the P-gp transporter and flushed out in the aqueous hydrophilic extracellular area, thus protecting the cells from toxins. It has been reported that hydrophobic molecules partitioned in the cell membrane could bind to P-gp binding domains via traversing through "gates" between transmembrane alpha helices 5/8 and 2/11 [113].

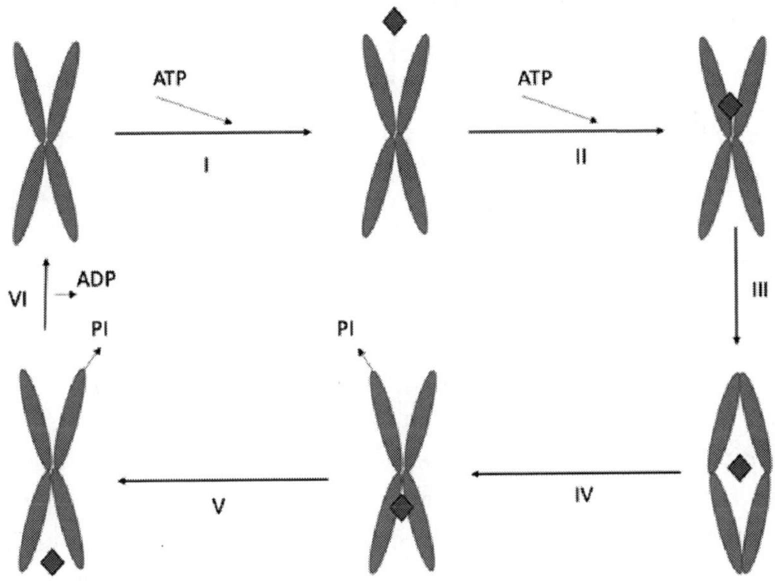

Figure 2. Efflux Mechanism for P-gp transporter.

Effect on Oral Bioavailability

The extent of absorption of orally administered drugs into systemic circulation depends on their ability to permeate through the intestinal epithelium. As discussed, P-gp is present in abundance on the intestinal epithelium with an intrinsic ability to flush out a wide variety of P-gp substrates, prior to their entry in the blood stream. This premature flushing of P-gp substrates from intestinal epithelium leads to a drastic reduction in absorption of these molecules resulting in low systemic bioavailability, and high dose requirement for achieving therapeutic concentrations in the blood stream [2]. A classic example of this phenomenon is the difference in oral bioavailability of paclitaxel in wild-type and ABCB1 knockdown mice models [114]. It was observed that bioavailability of paclitaxel in wild type was 11% and that in the knockdown model was 35%, a drastic enhancement. Furthermore, fecal samples revealed that around 87% of the oral dose of paclitaxel was excreted and less than 3% of dose was excreted from feces in the knockdown models [114]. Having established this, Bardelmeijer et al., tested the effect on bioavailability of paclitaxel when supplemented with elacridar, a potent P-gp inhibitor [115]. It was reported that oral bioavailability of paclitaxel was enhanced from 8.5% to 40% after elacridar supplementation, which is a result of diminished efflux of paclitaxel from the intestinal epithelium [115].

It is important to highlight that P-gp receptors are vulnerable to saturation, which can be explained by the Michaelis-Menten (MM) equation. The theory suggests that P-gp receptors can be saturated if the P-gp substrate's intestinal concentration is above their MM constants. For example, indinavir (oral dose of 800mg) has an MM constant of 140μM and it has been reported that the intestinal concentrations indinavir achieved with such high oral dose exceeds its MM constant [2]. Thus P-gp receptors are saturated and the effect of efflux through the intestinal epithelium is negligible, resulting in no significant impact on oral bioavailability. Although, for extremely low-dose orally administered drugs like digoxin, efflux via intestinal P-gp is very prominent. Oral dose of digoxin is around 0.5-1mg and its MM constant is 58μM. Digoxin can never achieve the MM constant concentration in the intestinal epithelium at therapeutic doses, and thus is easily flushed out of the intestine hampering its systemic absorption and thus reduced bioavailability [2, 116]. Thus, it is essential to consider the MM constant values for drugs being orally administered and correlate that constant with the dose via pharmacokinetic predictions of achievable intestinal concentrations at that dose. It should also be considered that only administering a high oral dose cannot help achieving high intestinal concentrations that exceed the drugs' MM constant. The aqueous solubility of the drug also plays a vital role, as poorly water-soluble drugs consistently fail to achieve high intestinal concentrations in spite of a high orally administered dose. For example, cyclosporine has an oral dose between 200-700 m,g but its intestinal absorption is greatly limited by P-gp efflux due to poor aqueous solubility, cyclosporine cannot achieve high intestinal concentrations to saturate the P-gp receptors and hence is a substrate for P-gp efflux [2].

Cerebral Disorders

As mentioned in an earlier section, P-gp receptors are predominantly present in the endothelial cells that make up the tight junction of the blood-brain barrier (BBB). At BBB, P-gp is responsible to protect the intricate areas of the brain from potential lipophilic toxins and foreign material from entering the brain. It does so via flushing the potential toxins out of the brain prior to their cerebral entry, thus extremely limiting the number of molecules able to traverse the BBB [8]. This excellent ability of P-gp, though, hinders with certain essential therapeutics from entering the brain as well in certain cerebral dysfunctionalities. Thus, multiple studies have been reported to utilize certain P-gp inhibitors that competitively inhibit the function of P-gp, in turn aiding in accumulation of P-gp substrates in the cerebral area, where they can exert therapeutic activity [117, 118]. Certain studies in P-gp knockdown mice have showed up to a 100-fold increase in P-gp substrate accumulation across the BBB, further cementing the need for P-gp's functional inhibition for substrate's therapeutic needs [119]. For instance, an oral injection of ivermectin was administered in MDR1 positive and knockdown mice models. After 24 hours, It was revealed that the penetration of ivermectin in brain in MDR1 positive mice was about 1.5 nanograms and those in MDR1 knockdown mice was 135 nanograms respectively, indicating the importance of P-gp receptors in maintaining cerebral homeostasis [120].

It is important to understand that some physiological dysfunctionalities may alter the expression levels of P-gp in the BBB. For example, occurrence of diabetes or liver failure has been shown to cause a significant decrease in P-gp expression at the BBB [121]. In such conditions, cerebral region becomes more vulnerable to toxins that, ideally, are effluxed by P-gp. Moreover, some CNS disorders also cause an alteration in P-gp expression. For instance, Alzheimer's disease causes a marked decrease in P-gp expression levels in CNS, which in turn makes the brain more susceptible for therapeutics' entry to exert their pharmacological action [122]. But in epileptic conditions, P-gp expression is increased, which results in a limited/negligible entry for therapeutics across the BBB, due to higher P-gp saturation levels [123].

Alzheimer's Disease

Alzheimer's disease (AD) is a chronic disorder associated with degeneration of neural abilities affecting quality of life, memory, personality disorders and behavioral issues. AD is characterized by senile plaques around brain cells due to amyloid-B protein deposition (AB), which is considered to be the main cause for AD occurrence [124]. In a healthy brain, P-gp is responsible for the transport and efflux of AB to maintain homeostasis. But in AD, as mentioned earlier, there have been reports that P-gp levels are significantly lowered, leading to lesser AB transport out of the brain leading to its higher accumulation. This signifies that for successful management of AD, P-gp levels need to be restored to regain homeostasis [124]. Studies have shown that use of molecules such as oleocanthal (a natural phenolic compound in extra-virgin olive oil) promotes P-gp induction along with induction of low density lipoprotein receptor related protein 1 (LRP1) which helps in clearance of AB in rat brains [124]. Although, it is interesting to note that the mechanism of decreased P-gp expression in AD is not yet completely understood. Some reports suggest that there is a negative feedback by extensive AB deposition which inhibits P-gp expression level and this is associated to the Wnt/B-catenin pathway or RAGE-Nf-kB pathway [4]. In a recent study by Zhang et al., AD was induced in mice and it was observed that inflammatory factors were significantly upregulated along with upregulation of P-gp levels [4]. Keeping these inflammatory pathways in mind, the team deployed ibuprofen for restoring levels of tumor necrosis factor-alpha (TNF-a), interleukin-1b (IL-1b) and Nf-kB. Their AD mice model had elevated levels of TNF-a, IL-1b and Nf-kB with suppressed levels of P-gp. Treatment with ibuprofen successfully lowered levels of the two inflammatory markers along with Nf-kB and this in turn increased the levels of P-gp. Thus, it was established that there is a correlation between inflammatory pathways and P-gp expression;

and suppression of inflammatory markers can help in improving AD prognosis via P-gp regulation [4].

Epilepsy

Epilepsy is a chronic disorder associated with uncontrolled occurrence of seizures in patients [125]. These seizures may sometime be periodic or can be chaotic, depending on the progression of the disease. Epilepsy is often managed in patients by long-term usage of anti-epileptic drugs (AEDs). While effective, patients do not respond to AEDs after a brief treatment period in about 30% cases; and these patients started experiencing uncontrolled seizures [125]. Upon investigation, it was revealed that there is an overexpression of drug transporters in the region of the brain which was subject to development of experimentally induced seizures. Among these transporters, P-gp transporters are widely studied and with multiple AEDs being substrates of P-gp, the failure in achieving therapeutic outcomes can be implied to the overexpression of P-gp receptors. This P-gp overexpression may be due to seizures themselves, genetic factors, or certain AEDs like carbamazepine may increase the expression levels [123]. It has been reported that expression levels of P-gp vary among patients, and genetic build-up of these patients have been cited as the major reason for these variances. P-gp overexpression in pharmaco-resistant epileptic patients was first reported by Tishler et al., [126], which has since been corroborated by multiple studies involving evaluation of P-gp levels in epileptic rat models using techniques such as real-time reverse transcription polymerase chain reaction (RT-PCR) and western blotting [127, 128]. Recent study by Yuan et al., demonstrated the presence of P-gp in rat amygdala kindling model, which better mimics epileptic seizures in humans as compared to cell induced epileptic models [129]. Furthermore, the team investigated the effect of P-gp inhibitor verapamil (VP) when given alongside carbamazepine (CBZ) and phenytoin (PT). Initial assessment of neural tissues from rat models proved the overexpression of P-gp at the BBB and this was followed by measurement of drug concentrations in the cortical fluids with or without VP. When supplemented with VP, the levels of AEDs in the cortical fluids were comparable to non-epileptic rat models, but the levels of AEDs in neural tissues of the epileptic rat models were lower. This study confirms the fact that P-gp levels are in fact partly responsible for development of resistance to AEDs in epilepsy [129].

Although significant strides have been taken in studying the role of ABCB1 transporters in dysfunctions of the central nervous system, extensive research is still on-going to establish the mechanism of MDR via P-gp expression. Clinical studies are currently in progress to better understand the physiological behavior and functions of P-gp involving polymorphism of the receptor which may further complicate its involvement in acquisition of MDR in CNS disorders.

Tumors

Cancer is a disease which is prevalent throughout the world, victimizing millions of people annually. Extensive research in the field of cancer has led to stellar discoveries which explain the prognosis of tumors, and yet, there seems to be one perplexing issue that persists till date. Development of resistance by cancer cells towards a particular therapy still remains at the crux of all issues to be resolved by scientists all over the world. One of the major implications of development of resistance is that the therapy is no longer effective and cancer cells continuously divide and proliferate in spite of therapeutic interventions. Development of resistance can occur due to various reasons like genetic mutations or efflux by transporters. Efflux by transporters like ABC transporters has been reported to play a major role in acquisition of drug resistance and this can be attributed to the diverse substrates of ABC transporters which are used in chemotherapy [2]. Among the ABC family, P-gp transporters, coded by the MDR-1 gene, are vital. P-gp has multiple commonly used chemotherapeutic substrates such as vincristine, doxorubicin, docetaxel, paclitaxel, etc. [2]. All these substrates are known to induce the expression levels of MDR-1 gene on cancer cells. Induction of MDR-1 in turn results in increase of P-gp receptors, which may lead to enhanced efflux of chemotherapeutic substrates via this transporter. Thus, chronic exposure of any of the chemotherapeutic substrates of P-gp may lead to ineffective therapy. At the same time, studies have shown that post cessation of chronic drug chemotherapies, levels of P-gp at the site of exposure (kidney, liver, small intestine, etc.) drop down to normal [130, 131]. It is very interesting to understand the transcription factors, epigenetic factors, and post-transcriptional factors involved in this induction in expression levels on exposure to chemotherapeutics [130]. Transcription factors such as Y-box binding protein-1 (YB-1), nuclear factor kappa-B (Nf-kB), specificity protein-1 (SP-1), early growth response protein-1 (EGR-1), Wilms tumor-1 (WT-1) and heat shock factor (HSF) are actively involved in regulating MDR-1 gene that codes P-gp [132–135]. For instance, YB-1 is activated after treatment with paclitaxel [136]. Paclitaxel is involved in relaying protein kinase-c mediated signals, which in turn translocate YB-1 from cytosol to the nucleus where it has access to a T-box binding site present upstream of the MDR-1 gene [136]. Second possible mechanism for alteration of P-gp levels are epigenetic factors. Events such as DNA methylation and histone acetylation are heavily involved in epigenetic regulation which in turn is responsible for regulation of gene expression levels in cells. Clinical studies have revealed that there is an inverse relationship between DNA methylation and MDR-1 gene expression levels [137, 138]. Inversely, studies have shown that histone acetylation and P-gp induction are concurrent [139]. In a study by Baker et al., daunorubicin treated CEM-Bcl2 cells enhanced histone acetylation which in turn resulted in upregulation of P-gp expression levels in these cells [139]. Multiple studies have reported similar conclusions with diverse chemotherapeutic drugs such as valproic acid, apicidin, etc. [140, 141]. In addition, certain post-transcriptional factors such as membrane trafficking, or membrane localization are involved in regulation of P-gp expression levels at the cell membrane, where P-gp exerts its major functional activity [142]. Although extremely relevant, lack of evidence between the correlation of post-transcriptional factors and chemotherapeutics in regulation P-gp levels necessitates further studies in the area.

Ovarian Cancer

Ovarian Cancer (OC) is one of the most threatening malignancies occurring in women and is often associated with a low survival rate of <5 years [143]. As other cancerous conditions, OC is also plagued with the issue of MDR on chronic exposure of chemotherapeutics. The three major components that contribute towards this resistance development are class III beta-tubulin (TUBB3), excision repair cross-commentary gene (ERCC1) and P-gp [144]. As many chemotherapeutic agents are known P-gp substrates, P-gp efflux is believed to be the most important factor in MDR acquisition. Jia et al., recently demonstrated striking difference between the expression levels of P-gp receptors in ovarian cancer patient tissues versus healthy tissues. Briefly, the study was conducted in 166 patients at each stage of ovarian cancer, i.e., from stages I-IV and the tissues were compared to 55 healthy tissues. P-gp levels were measured by RT-PCR technique and it was concluded that the levels of P-gp were higher as the stages of OC progressed. Stage IV had the highest levels of P-gp as compared to Stage I, with all stages showing significantly higher P-gp levels as compared to normal healthy tissues [144]. This study encourages the use of P-gp receptors in ovarian tissue to be used as diagnostic markers to assess the progression of OC in patients. Once it was established that P-gp played a vital role in OC and it is widely present in all OC stages, researchers started to utilize strategies to overcome P-gp induced MDR in OC. The go-to strategy to overcome P-gp mediated resistance is use of P-gp inhibitors which preferentially block the receptors and inhibit the efflux of potent chemotherapeutics. Moreover, researchers are now finding novel techniques to efficiently deliver payload of inhibitors and active ingredients to the site of action. One of the novel techniques utilized widely is nanotechnology [145]. Nanocarriers as drug delivery systems have proven their worth time and again to deliver drugs at the site of action, while helping in higher intracellular accumulation of drugs in cancer cells. Taking inspiration from breakthroughs in nanocarrier-based delivery systems, Zheng et al., fabricated a polyethylene glycol-polylactic acid based nanoparticulate system loaded with doxorubicin (dox) and verapamil (VP). As mentioned earlier, VP is a P-gp inhibitor and has been used extensively in tandem with other potent molecules to suppress the efflux mechanism of P-gp and in turn enhance the efficacy of the potent molecule. It is well known that overexposure of Dox in cancer cause development of resistance via the P-gp efflux (since Dox is a substrate of P-gp). Thus, Zheng and team supplemented Dox with VP with an aim to reverse the Dox resistance. The team developed Dox resistant ovarian cancer cell lines SKOV3-D and A2780-D and tested their nanoformulation *in-vitro*. It was revealed that there was a significant enhancement in intracellular uptake and efficacy of Dox in these cells when supplemented with VP as compared to Dox alone, which displayed negligible effects. These studies were backed by *in-vivo* testing in xenograft mice models with the above-mentioned cells. It was observed that combination of Dox with VP resulted in higher % survival of mice as compared to Dox alone; and there was a significant decrease in the rate of tumor progression with Dox and VP [145]. This signifies that supplementing a P-gp inhibitor with a chemotherapeutic agent can result in enhanced efficacy and reversal of P-gp mediated resistance in ovarian cancer.

Autoimmune Disorders

Autoimmune disorders are associated with major complications and dysfunctionalities of the immune system, wherein rogue physiological immune cells target certain healthy cells leading to complications pertaining majorly to joints, liver, brain, heart, etc. Disorders such as rheumatoid arthritis (RA), systemic lupus erythematosus (SLE) and psoriatic arthritis (PA) are chronic inflammatory autoimmune disorders and till date have been managed using corticosteroids, although not all patients respond to the therapy positively [146]. Moreover, majority of patients over time report development of resistance to corticosteroids. This development of resistance is majorly due to the presence of P-gp receptors on Th17 inflammatory lymphocytes and these receptors, as mentioned earlier, have the ability to efflux corticosteroids and diverse immunosuppressants from immune cells, leading to inefficient therapy [147]. It has been reported that combining P-gp inhibitors can help reverse this efflux of immunosuppressants which may be helpful in achieving desired therapeutic efficacy to manage these inflammatory conditions.

Systemic Lupus Erythematosus (SLE)

SLE is a chronic inflammatory disorder occurring due to high production levels of autoantibodies and self-reactive cells (148). It is one of the most common autoimmune disorder and it hugely affects the quality of life in patients and also make them vulnerable to other conditions due to a weakened immune system, making them 2-3 times more prone to mortality than normal population [147]. It has been reported that in patients with highly active SLE, the expression levels of P-gp on peripheral blood lymphocytes (PBL) have been markedly elevated [149]. To correlate the expression levels of P-gp and SLE, an in-depth clinical study was carried out by Zhang et al., where the team studied 30 healthy subjects and 60 subjects with SLE who received glucocorticoid (GC) treatment for >6 months [150]. As per SLE disease activity index, patients were classified as cases of active SLE and severely active SLE. P-gp expression levels were measured in all patients and it was revealed that the expression levels in SLE patients was significantly higher than the expression levels in healthy subjects. Moreover, as the severity of disease increased, P-gp levels on PBLs were found to be higher as patients with severely active SLE had significantly higher P-gp levels as compared to active SLE patients [150]. This signifies that P-gp levels on PBLs is correlated to disease severity and progression in patients with SLE. Such high levels of P-gp can alter the effectiveness of the GC therapy, studied separately by Kansal et al., The team studied patients that were given GC therapy for 3 months and classified them as resistant to therapy and sensitive to therapy [151]. On continuing the therapy, it was found that P-gp levels on PBLs in GC resistant patients were fairly constant with no significant change. But the levels of P-gp in GC sensitive patients went down, indicating an effective therapy [151]. This further strengthens the role of P-gp in development of resistance to therapy in autoimmune disorders such as SLE. Furthermore, it also portrays the ability of P-gp to successfully detect the therapy progress and thus, can be used as an indicator for a successful/failed GC therapy. Another recent study by Perez-Guerrero et al., included 93 female patients with SLE who were on GC therapy for 6 months or more. The team measured the levels of P-gp in serum as compared to lymphocytes in the previous studies. Similar significant results were obtained for P-gp serum levels i.e., the expression level of P-gp was higher in patients with active SLE versus patients with inactive SLE [152]. Although it was earlier proven by Ragab and Soliman [153] that suppression of P-gp function can be possible by supplementing GC therapy with P-gp substrates like cyclophosphamide (CP). It was observed that P-gp function on CD5 lymphocytes was lowered when CP was supplemented with steroidal therapy as compared to patients who were only on steroidal therapy [153]. Several similar studies have reported that as P-gp levels go down, the effectiveness of therapy improves and thus there are constant efforts in the field of SLE to manage the expression levels and functional activity of P-gp by combining multiple P-gp substrates and steroidal therapy [146]. Moreover, use of P-gp as an indicator for SLE therapy can help establish the course of therapy for patients in the future.

Rheumatoid Arthritis

Rheumatoid Arthritis (RA) is a chronic inflammatory autoimmune disorder which causes inflammation of diarthrodial joints. This progressive disease deteriorates patient's quality of life significantly by eventual joint dysfunction and inflammation. Treatment for RA is often initiated with disease modifying anti-rheumatic drugs (DMARDs) which include drugs like methotrexate (MTX) [154]. MTX is usually prescribed in early detected cases to delay the progression of RA, but MTX was soon reported to be ineffective over long term due to a conspired development of resistance. MTX being an ABCB1 substrate, the usual suspect for resistance development was P-gp. The first detection of P-gp receptors on PBLs in RA patients treated with prednisolone was back in 1996 by Maillefert [155].

Further revelations in the field led to the discovery that P-gp is associated with RA via presence on circulating mononuclear cells and TH1 cells as well [156, 157]. Since then, multiple studies have demonstrated the correlation of failure of MTX therapy and overexpression of P-gp receptors on PBL [158]. The involvement of P-gp in MTX resistance was further confirmed when P-gp inhibitors were supplemented with MTX which led to a better therapeutic outcome in patients [159, 160]. One such study done by Qin et al., demonstrated that MTX, when supplemented with hydroperoxycyclophosphamide (HC) caused a higher anti-P-gp effect via measuring P-gp expression on receptors on fibroblasts like synoviocytes as compared to MTX alone therapy. Further, the group proposed that the anti-P-gp effect was mediated by the JAK2/STAT3 pathway, which is a cellular pathway mediating essential functions such as growth and metabolism [154]. Another study by Perez-Guerrero et al., demonstrated that serum P-gp levels in RA patients are altered based on the therapeutic approach taken for the treatment. Briefly, the study was conducted in 151 patients, classified as patients who were responsive and non-responsive to DMARDs. It was revealed that RA positive patients had significantly higher P-gp levels in the serum as compared to healthy volunteers. Moreover, patients who were responsive to DMARDs therapy had significantly lower levels of P-gp expression in the serum as compared to patients who were non-responsive, indicating the role of P-gp in diminishing the DMARD therapy [161]. Thus, it can be concluded that high levels of serum P-gp can be deleterious to DMARD therapy and serum P-gp can be a potent indicator for selection of therapy in RA patients.

The involvement of P-gp in multiple autoimmune disorders like SLE and RA is noteworthy; and constant research in this field has led to novel revelations that have helped progress the therapy. Supplementing SLE and RA therapies with P-gp inhibitors have proven to be efficient therapies, although more conclusive studies in the field can help gather more evidence to understand the role of P-gp and the mechanisms involved for development of resistance.

Role of P-gp in Development of Multidrug Resistance (MDR)

The development of multidrug resistance remains a major challenge for designing treatment regimens of various diseases. Resistance against drug treatment can be developed by several mechanisms including alteration of drug targets, modified expression of drug transporters, varied detoxification mechanisms and altered cellular proliferation [162]. These mechanisms may result into several changes such as reduced intracellular accumulation, increased efflux, imbalanced cellular functions which determines the development of drug resistance [163]. Resistance develops when the ability to uptake drugs in cells is significantly diminished while the efflux capacity has significantly increased so that the drug is unable to reach the desired therapeutic concentration to show its effectiveness. The best mechanism of development of MDR is explained by overexpression of ABC transporters [164]. Dano et al., discovered the first incidence of ABC transporter mediated MDR in Ehrlich ascites tumor cells against daunorubicin and several other chemotherapeutic agents including vinca alkaloids and anthracyclines [165]. Few years later, the protein responsible for development of multi-drug resistance was identified and named as P-gp (permeability-associated glycoprotein) [166]. Numerous studies have reported the role of P-gp in development of multi-drug resistance in diseased condition and can be used as a potential drug target [167].

Hyperactivation or increased expression of P-gp is associated with reduced intracellular drug accumulation, diminished bioavailability and development of drug resistance [168]. Upregulation of P-gp expression causing MDR in tumor environment is governed by genomic instability and epigenetic interactions [169]. Epigenetic modification of ABCB1 (gene encoding P-gp) promoter region resulting due to demethylation of DNA or acetylation of histone has been reported to increase the P-gp expression resulting into MDR in several leukemias [170–172]. Polymorphism of ABCB1 is also known to impact the development of MDR in various cells. Siddiqui et al., identified the linkage between the ABCB1 C3435T polymorphism and resistance to anti-epileptic drugs. The study reported that patients with CC genotype expressed higher levels of P-gp than TT genotype resulting into reduced systemic concentration of drugs and requiring higher dose for desired therapeutic effect eventually leading to development of drug resistance [173]. Zawadzka et al., reported that lung cancer patients possessed higher TT allele of C3435T polymorphism which is also responsible for higher expression of ABCB1 mRNA resulting into induction of MDR [174]. Teng et al., [175] demonstrated that Zhankuic acids (A, B and C) extracted from *Taiwanofungus camphoratus* reversed MDR by influencing P-gp efflux pumps activity. As shown in Figure 3. Zhankuic acids A, B and C (ZA-A, ZA-B and ZA-C) influenced the P-gp activity through competitive and non-competitive binding. ZA-A and ZA-C demonstrated competitive binding to P-gp efflux receptors in the presence of chemotherapeutic P-gp substrates therefore reducing the efflux of the P-gp substrates and providing improved chemotherapeutic potency. On the other hand, ZA-B illustrated non-competitive binding via binding to the allosteric site of the P-gp receptor and modulating the efflux activity of the P-gp substrate (Figure 3). These results signify that P-gp receptors can be inhibited in several ways to reverse the MDR and improve the activity of the P-gp substrates.

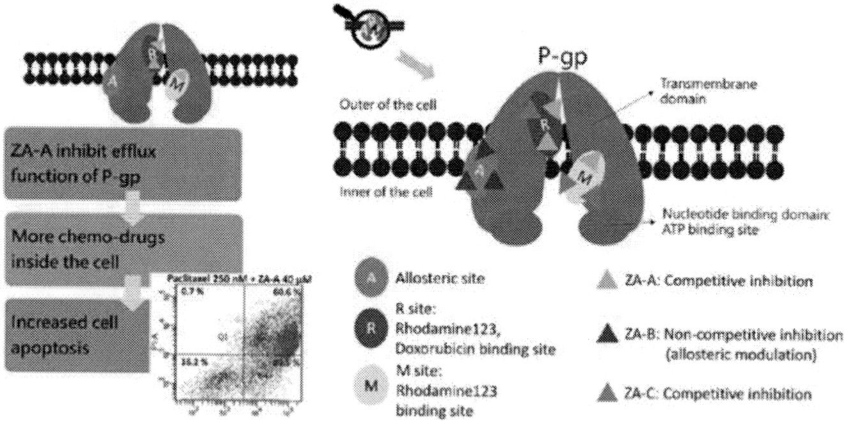

Figure 3. Influence of triterpenoids on P-gp activity via competitive and non-competitive inhibition. Reproduced with permission from MDPI, Basel, Switzerland under Creative Commons Attribution License [175].

Table 1. Role of P-gp in promoting efflux in different diseases and intended outcomes

Disease Conditions	P-gp Relevance	Reference
Cerebral Disorders		
Alzheimer's Disease (AD)	Decreased P-gp levels in AD brain leads to decreased clearance of amyloid deposition in brain, leading to development of AD	[181]
Epilepsy	P-gp overexpression in brain leads to rapid efflux of anti-epileptic drugs (P-gp substrates). This leads to ineffective therapy	[123]
Parkinson's Disease Progression	Patients with Parkinson's disease have been reported to have lower levels of P-gp receptors in the brain, leading to decreased efflux of toxic P-gp substrates leading to disease progression	[182]
Tumors		
Ovarian Cancer	P-gp levels are increased exponentially as severity of ovarian cancer goes up. Stage IV has been reported to have th highest expression levels of P-gp. P-gp substrate chemotherapeutics are cleared from cells leading to ineffective therapy	[144]
Breast Cancer	No correlation of P-gp expression levels and metastases, recurrence or survival was reported in breast cancer leading to the conclusion that increase in P-gp levels are not related to ineffectiveness in therapy	[183]
Autoimmune Disorders		
Systemic Lupus Erythematosus (SLE)	Marked elevation of P-gp levels on peripheral blood lymphocytes in patients with highly active SLE, indicating P-gp's utility as marker for tracking disease severity	[150]
Rheumatoid Arthritis (RA)	P-gp is associated with RA via presence on circulating mononuclear cells and TH1 cells.	[156, 157]

In conclusion, although P-gp expression is known to play a vital role in development of MDR, it is still a major challenge for development of effect therapies for several diseases. Combinatorial treatment regimen with P-gp modulators at therapeutic dose can help to improve the sensitivity of drugs and cause reversal of P-gp induced MDR.

While alteration of P-gp expression and activity has been recognized to play pivotal role in development of MDR, several P-gp modulators have been explored to overcome the induced resistance. In a study performed by Dong et al., confirmed the overexpression of P-gp in sorafenib resistant hepatocellular carcinoma cells as compared to the normal (non-resistant) cells [176]. MDR hepatocellular carcinoma cell line Bel7402/5-FU displayed increased P-gp levels resulting in reduced intracellular concentration of epirubicin and rhodamine-123. However, treatment with baicalein resulted into reversal of MDR and increased accumulation of substrates in the Bel7402/5-FU cells [177]. Kong et al., demonstrated an increase in P-gp and breast cancer resistant protein efflux transporters in MDR mediated hepatocellular carcinoma HepG2 cells resulting into significantly reduced uptake of imatinib [178].

Warmann et al., reported increase in anti-tumor response of doxorubicin in MDR hepatoblastoma cells and hepatocellular carcinoma cells upon incubation with valspodar (P-gp modulator) which may have suppressed the activity of P-gp [179]. Yuan et al., described that P-gp mediated MDR in colon cancer can be effectively reversed by cinobugafin (P-gp modulator) which resulted into increased intracellular accumulation and anticancer activity of doxorubicin [180].

Conclusion

The role of P-gp in maintaining physiological homeostasis, protecting against xenobiotics, and influencing the effectiveness of therapeutics in diseased conditions has been well investigated and summarized in Table 1. Exploratory studies revolving around P-gp transporter system have been heavily focused on its role in diseased conditions and this can be attributed to the fact that many therapeutics deployed for diverse disorders are P-gp substrates. Strategies such as concomitant administration of P-gp substrates along with P-gp inhibitors, development of novel drug delivery systems etc.

have been developed to evade efflux via P-gp in an attempt to improve therapeutic outcomes in diseased conditions. Furthermore, studies have revealed that factors such as polymorphism and epigenetic factors of P-gp receptors contribute towards inter-patient variances in therapeutic response. Thus, understanding genomic framework will unveil the association between patient's response to therapeutic activity of drug at genetic level and cellular alteration in physiological or diseased conditions. This information could help predict the propensity of therapeutic effect in patients and personalized dosing can be prescribed for futuristic therapies.

Declaration of Competing Interests

The authors declare no conflict of interest.

Acknowledgments

This study was supported by start-up funds provided to Dr Vivek Gupta by College of Pharmacy and Health Sciences (CPHS), St. John's University. Nishant S. Kulkarni, and Snehal K. Shukla were supported by research assistantships provided by an NIH Research Enhancement Award (R15), 1R15HL138606-01A1 to Dr. Vivek Gupta.

References

[1] Mora Lagares L, Minovski N, Novič M. Multiclass Classifier for P-Glycoprotein Substrates, Inhibitors, and Non-Active Compounds. *Molecules*. 2019 May 25;24(10):2006.

[2] Liu X, Pan G, editors. Drug Transporters in Drug Disposition, Effects and Toxicity [Internet]. Singapore: Springer Singapore; 2019 [cited

2020 Oct 26]. (Advances in Experimental Medicine and Biology; vol. 1141). Available from: http://link.springer.com/10.1007/978-981-13-7647-4.

[3] del Moral RG, Olmo A, Aguilar M, O'Valle F. P glycoprotein: a new mechanism to control drug-induced nephrotoxicity. Exp Nephrol. 1998 Apr;6(2):89–97.

[4] Zhang C, Qin H, Zheng R, Wang Y, Yan T, Huan F, et al., A new approach for Alzheimer's disease treatment through P-gp regulation via ibuprofen. *Pathol Res Pract.* 2018 Nov;214(11):1765–71.

[5] Chen C, Lee MH, Weng CF, Leong M. Theoretical Prediction of the Complex P-Glycoprotein Substrate Efflux Based on the Novel Hierarchical Support Vector Regression Scheme. *Molecules.* 2018 Jul 22;23(7):1820.

[6] Cole SPC. Multidrug resistance protein 1 (MRP1, ABCC1), a "multitasking" ATP-binding cassette (ABC) transporter. *J Biol Chem.* 2014 Nov 7;289(45):30880–8.

[7] Xu HB, Yu J, Xu LZ, Fu J. Regulation of P-glycoprotein efflux activity by Z-guggulsterone of Commiphora mukul at the blood-brain barrier. *Journal of the Neurological Sciences*. 2016 Apr;363:147–52.

[8] De Klerk OL, Bosker FJ, Luurtsema G, Nolte IM, Dierckx R, Den Boer JA, et al., The role of p-glycoprotein in psychiatric disorders: a reliable guard of the brain? *Cent Nerv Syst Agents Med Chem*. 2011 Sep 1;11(3):197–209.

[9] Aynacıoğlu AŞ, Bilir A, Kadomatsu K. Dual inhibition of P-glycoprotein and midkine may increase therapeutic effects of anticancer drugs. *Medical Hypotheses.* 2017 Sep;107:26–8.

[10] Saneja A, Khare V, Alam N, Dubey RD, Gupta PN. Advances in P-glycoprotein-based approaches for delivering anticancer drugs: pharmacokinetic perspective and clinical relevance. *Expert Opinion on Drug Delivery.* 2014 Jan;11(1):121–38.

[11] Frank MH, Denton MD, Alexander SI, Khoury SJ, Sayegh MH, Briscoe DM. Specific MDR1 P-glycoprotein blockade inhibits human alloimmune T cell activation in vitro. *J Immunol.* 2001 Feb 15;166(4):2451–9.

[12] Tsujimura S, Adachi T, Saito K, Kawabe A, Tanaka Y. Relevance of P-glycoprotein on CXCR4 + B cells to organ manifestation in highly active rheumatoid arthritis. *Modern Rheumatology.* 2018 Mar 4;28(2):276–86.

[13] Breier A, Gibalova L, Seres M, Barancik M, Sulova Z. New Insight into P-Glycoprotein as a Drug Target. *Anti-Cancer Agents in Medicinal Chemistry*. 2012 Dec 1;13(1):159–70.

[14] Syed SB, Arya H, Fu IH, Yeh TK, Periyasamy L, Hsieh HP, et al., Targeting P-glycoprotein: Investigation of piperine analogs for overcoming drug resistance in cancer. *Scientific Reports* [Internet]. 2017 Dec [cited 2020 Nov 6];7(1). Available from: http://www.nature.com/articles/s41598-017-08062-2.

[15] Dhooge C, De Moerloose B. Clinical Significance of P-Glycoprotein (P-gp) Expression in Childhood Acute Lymphoblastic Leukemia. In: Kaspers GJL, Pieters R, Veerman AJP, editors. Drug Resistance in Leukemia and Lymphoma III [Internet]. Boston, MA: Springer US; 1999 [cited 2020 Nov 6]. p. 11–9. (Advances in Experimental Medicine and Biology; vol. 457). Available from: http://link.springer.com/10.1007/978-1-4615-4811-9_2.

[16] Amin MdL. P-glycoprotein Inhibition for Optimal Drug Delivery. *Drug Target Insights.* 2013 Aug 19;7:27–34.

[17] Mizutani T, Masuda M, Nakai E, Furumiya K, Togawa H, Nakamura Y, et al., Genuine functions of P-glycoprotein (ABCB1). *Curr Drug Metab.* 2008 Feb;9(2):167–74.

[18] Kruijtzer CMF, Beijnen JH, Rosing H, ten Bokkel Huinink WW, Schot M, Jewell RC, et al., Increased oral bioavailability of topotecan in combination with the breast cancer resistance protein and P-glycoprotein inhibitor GF120918. *J Clin Oncol.* 2002 Jul 1;20(13):2943–50.

[19] Thiebaut F, Tsuruo T, Hamada H, Gottesman MM, Pastan I, Willingham MC. Cellular localization of the multidrug-resistance gene product P-glycoprotein in normal human tissues. *Proc Natl Acad Sci U S A.* 1987 Nov;84(21):7735–8.

[20] Murakami T, Takano M. Intestinal efflux transporters and drug absorption. *Expert Opinion on Drug Metabolism & Toxicology*. 2008 Jul;4(7):923–39.

[21] von Richter O, Burk O, Fromm MF, Thon KP, Eichelbaum M, Kivistö KT. Cytochrome P450 3A4 and P-glycoprotein expression in human small intestinal enterocytes and hepatocytes: a comparative analysis in paired tissue specimens. *Clin Pharmacol Ther*. 2004 Mar;75(3):172–83.

[22] Mouly S, Paine MF. P-glycoprotein increases from proximal to distal regions of human small intestine. *Pharm Res*. 2003 Oct;20(10):1595–9.

[23] Makhey VD, Guo A, Norris DA, Hu P, Yan J, Sinko PJ. Characterization of the regional intestinal kinetics of drug efflux in rat and human intestine and in Caco-2 cells. *Pharm Res*. 1998 Aug;15(8):1160–7.

[24] Yumoto R, Murakami T, Nakamoto Y, Hasegawa R, Nagai J, Takano M. Transport of rhodamine 123, a P-glycoprotein substrate, across rat intestine and Caco-2 cell monolayers in the presence of cytochrome P-450 3A-related compounds. *J Pharmacol Exp Ther*. 1999 Apr;289(1):149–55.

[25] Stephens RH, O'Neill CA, Warhurst A, Carlson GL, Rowland M, Warhurst G. Kinetic profiling of P-glycoprotein-mediated drug efflux in rat and human intestinal epithelia. *J Pharmacol Exp Ther*. 2001 Feb;296(2):584–91.

[26] MacLean C, Moenning U, Reichel A, Fricker G. Closing the gaps: a full scan of the intestinal expression of p-glycoprotein, breast cancer resistance protein, and multidrug resistance-associated protein 2 in male and female rats. *Drug Metab Dispos*. 2008 Jul;36(7):1249–54.

[27] Cario E. P-glycoprotein multidrug transporter in inflammatory bowel diseases: More questions than answers. *World J Gastroenterol*. 2017 Mar 7;23(9):1513–20.

[28] Tamura S, Tokunaga Y, Ibuki R, Amidon GL, Sezaki H, Yamashita S. The site-specific transport and metabolism of tacrolimus in rat small intestine. *J Pharmacol Exp Ther*. 2003 Jul;306(1):310–6.

[29] Wu CY, Benet LZ, Hebert MF, Gupta SK, Rowland M, Gomez DY, et al., Differentiation of absorption and first-pass gut and hepatic metabolism in humans: studies with cyclosporine. *Clin Pharmacol Ther.* 1995 Nov;58(5):492–7.

[30] Ducharme MP, Warbasse LH, Edwards DJ. Disposition of intravenous and oral cyclosporine after administration with grapefruit juice. *Clinical Pharmacology & Therapeutics.* 1995;57(5):485–91.

[31] Lown KS, Mayo RR, Leichtman AB, Hsiao HL, Turgeon DK, Schmiedlin-Ren P, et al., Role of intestinal P-glycoprotein (mdr1) in interpatient variation in the oral bioavailability of cyclosporine. *Clin Pharmacol Ther.* 1997 Sep;62(3):248–60.

[32] Zakeri-Milani P, Valizadeh H. Intestinal transporters: enhanced absorption through P-glycoprotein-related drug interactions. *Expert Opinion on Drug Metabolism & Toxicology.* 2014 Jun;10(6):859–71.

[33] Hoffmeyer S, Burk O, Richter O von, Arnold HP, Brockmöller J, Johne A, et al., Functional polymorphisms of the human multidrug-resistance gene: Multiple sequence variations and correlation of one allele with P-glycoprotein expression and activity *in vivo*. *PNAS.* 2000 Mar 28;97(7):3473–8.

[34] Karlsson L, Green H, Zackrisson AL, Bengtsson F, Jakobsen Falk I, Carlsson B, et al., ABCB1 gene polymorphisms are associated with fatal intoxications involving venlafaxine but not citalopram. *Int J Legal Med.* 2013 May;127(3):579–86.

[35] Foote CJ, Greer W, Kiberd BA, Fraser A, Lawen J, Nashan B, et al., MDR1 C3435T Polymorphisms Correlate With Cyclosporine Levels in De Novo Renal Recipients. *Transplantation Proceedings.* 2006 Nov 1;38(9):2847–9.

[36] Li D, Gui R, Li J, Huang Z, Nie X. Tacrolimus Dosing in Chinese Renal Transplant Patients Is Related to MDR1 Gene C3435T Polymorphisms. *Transplantation Proceedings.* 2006 Nov;38(9):2850–2.

[37] Iizasa H, Genda N, Kitano T, Tomita M, Nishihara K, Hayashi M, et al., Altered expression and function of P-glycoprotein in dextran

sodium sulfate-induced colitis in mice. *J Pharm Sci*. 2003 Mar;92(3):569–76.

[38] Gutmann H, Hruz P, Zimmermann C, Straumann A, Terracciano L, Hammann F, et al., Breast cancer resistance protein and P-glycoprotein expression in patients with newly diagnosed and therapy-refractory ulcerative colitis compared with healthy controls. *Digestion*. 2008;78(2–3):154–62.

[39] Erdmann P, Bruckmueller H, Martin P, Busch D, Haenisch S, Müller J, et al., Dysregulation of Mucosal Membrane Transporters and Drug-Metabolizing Enzymes in Ulcerative Colitis. *J Pharm Sci*. 2019;108(2):1035–46.

[40] Ufer M, Häsler R, Jacobs G, Haenisch S, Lächelt S, Faltraco F, et al., Decreased sigmoidal ABCB1 (P-glycoprotein) expression in ulcerative colitis is associated with disease activity. *Pharmacogenomics*. 2009 Dec;10(12):1941–53.

[41] Englund G, Rasmusson A, Rorsman F, Artursson P, Kindmark A, Rönnblom A. Efflux transporters in ulcerative colitis: decreased expression of BCRP (ABCG2) and Pgp (ABCB1). *Inflammatory bowel diseases*. 2007 Apr 1;13:291–7.

[42] Sartor RB. Review article: the potential mechanisms of action of rifaximin in the management of inflammatory bowel diseases. *Aliment Pharmacol Ther*. 2016 Jan;43 Suppl 1:27–36.

[43] Sugioka N, Haraya K, Fukushima K, Ito Y, Takada K. Effects of obesity induced by high-fat diet on the pharmacokinetics of nelfinavir, a HIV protease inhibitor, in laboratory rats. *Biopharm Drug Dispos*. 2009 Dec;30(9):532–41.

[44] Masuda S, Goto M, Kiuchi T, Uemoto S, Kodawara T, Saito H, et al., Enhanced expression of enterocyte P-glycoprotein depresses cyclosporine bioavailability in a recipient of living donor liver transplantation. *Liver Transpl*. 2003 Oct;9(10):1108–13.

[45] Lemahieu W, Maes B, Verbeke K, Rutgeerts P, Geboes K, Vanrenterghem Y. Cytochrome P450 3A4 and P-glycoprotein Activity and Assimilation of Tacrolimus in Transplant Patients with

Persistent Diarrhea. *American Journal of Transplantation.* 2005;5(6):1383–91.

[46] Murakami Y, Higashi Y, Matsunaga N, Koyanagi S, Ohdo S. Circadian clock-controlled intestinal expression of the multidrug-resistance gene mdr1a in mice. *Gastroenterology.* 2008 Nov;135(5):1636-1644.e3.

[47] Palmieri O, Mazzoccoli G, Bossa F, Maglietta R, Palumbo O, Ancona N, et al., Systematic analysis of circadian genes using genome-wide cDNA microarrays in the inflammatory bowel disease transcriptome. *Chronobiol Int.* 2015;32(7):903–16.

[48] Iwasaki M, Koyanagi S, Suzuki N, Katamune C, Matsunaga N, Watanabe N, et al., Circadian modulation in the intestinal absorption of P-glycoprotein substrates in monkeys. *Mol Pharmacol.* 2015 Jul;88(1):29–37.

[49] Shugarts S, Benet LZ. The Role of Transporters in the Pharmacokinetics of Orally Administered Drugs. *Pharm Res.* 2009 Sep;26(9):2039–54.

[50] Neumanova Z, Cerveny L, Ceckova M, Staud F. Interactions of tenofovir and tenofovir disoproxil fumarate with drug efflux transporters ABCB1, ABCG2, and ABCC2; role in transport across the placenta. *AIDS.* 2014 Jan 2;28(1):9–17.

[51] Srivalli KMR, Lakshmi PK. Overview of P-glycoprotein inhibitors: a rational outlook. *Braz J Pharm Sci*. 2012 Sep;48(3):353–67.

[52] Garrigues A, Escargueil AE, Orlowski S. The multidrug transporter, P-glycoprotein, actively mediates cholesterol redistribution in the cell membrane. *PNAS.* 2002 Aug 6;99(16):10347–52.

[53] Frijters CMG, Tuijn CJ, Ottenhoff R, Zegers BN, Groen AK. The role of different P-glycoproteins in hepatobiliary secretion of fluorescently labeled short-chain phospholipids. :8.

[54] Kim WY, Benet LZ. P-glycoprotein (P-gp/MDR1)-mediated efflux of sex-steroid hormones and modulation of P-gp expression in vitro. *Pharm Res.* 2004 Jul;21(7):1284–93.

[55] Iyer L, Ramírez J, Shepard DR, Bingham CM, Hossfeld D-K, Ratain MJ, et al., Biliary transport of irinotecan and metabolites in normal

and P-glycoprotein-deficient mice. *Cancer Chemother Pharmacol.* 2002 Apr;49(4):336–41.

[56] Gupta E, Safa AR, Wang X, Ratain MJ. Pharmacokinetic modulation of irinotecan and metabolites by cyclosporin A. *Cancer Res.* 1996 Mar 15;56(6):1309–14.

[57] Arimori K, Kuroki N, Hidaka M, Iwakiri T, Yamsaki K, Okumura M, et al., Effect of P-glycoprotein modulator, cyclosporin A, on the gastrointestinal excretion of irinotecan and its metabolite SN-38 in rats. *Pharm Res.* 2003 Jun;20(6):910–7.

[58] Lowes S, Haslam IS, Fihn BM, Hilgendorf C, Karlsson JE, Simmons NL, et al., The Effects of Pregnenolone 16α-Carbonitrile Dosing on Digoxin Pharmacokinetics and Intestinal Absorption in the Rat. *Pharmaceutics.* 2010 Mar;2(1):61–77.

[59] Watanabe T, Suzuki H, Sawada Y, Naito M, Tsuruo T, Inaba M, et al., Induction of hepatic P-glycoprotein enhances biliary excretion of vincristine in rats. *Journal of Hepatology*. 1995 Oct 1;23(4):440–8.

[60] Schrenk D, Gant TW, Preisegger KH, Silverman JA, Marino PA, Thorgeirsson SS. Induction of multidrug resistance gene expression during cholestasis in rats and nonhuman primates. *Hepatology.* 1993 May;17(5):854–60.

[61] Drescher S, Glaeser H, Mürdter T, Hitzl M, Eichelbaum M, Fromm MF. P-glycoprotein-mediated intestinal and biliary digoxin transport in humans. *Clin Pharmacol Ther*. 2003 Mar;73(3):223–31.

[62] Booth CL, Brouwer KR, Brouwer KL. Effect of multidrug resistance modulators on the hepatobiliary disposition of doxorubicin in the isolated perfused rat liver. *Cancer Res.* 1998 Aug 15;58(16):3641–8.

[63] Wang D, Johnson AD, Papp AC, Kroetz DL, Sadée W. Multidrug resistance polypeptide 1 (MDR1, ABCB1) variant 3435C>T affects mRNA stability. *Pharmacogenetics and Genomics.* 2005 Oct;15(10):693–704.

[64] Kroetz DL. Role for Drug Transporters Beyond Tumor Resistance: *Hepatic Functional Imaging and Genotyping of Multidrug Resistance Transporters for the Prediction of Irinotecan Toxicity.* JCO. 2006 Sep 10;24(26):4225–7.

[65] Michael M, Thompson M, Hicks R, Mitchell P, Ellis A, Milner A, et al., Relationship of Hepatic Functional Imaging to Irinotecan Pharmacokinetics and Genetic Parameters of Drug Elimination. Journal of clinical oncology : *official journal of the American Society of Clinical Oncology*. 2006 Sep 1;24:4228–35.

[66] Malik MY, Jaiswal S, Sharma A, Shukla M, Lal J. Role of enterohepatic recirculation in drug disposition: cooperation and complications. *Drug Metabolism Reviews*. 2016 Apr 2;48(2):281–327.

[67] Foucaud-Vignault M, Soayfane Z, Ménez C, Bertrand-Michel J, Martin PGP, Guillou H, et al., P-glycoprotein Dysfunction Contributes to Hepatic Steatosis and Obesity in Mice. *PLoS One* [Internet]. 2011 Sep 16 [cited 2020 Nov 4];6(9). Available from: https://www.ncbi.nlm.nih.gov/pmc/articles/PMC3174940/.

[68] Thakkar N, Slizgi JR, Brouwer KLR. Effect of Liver Disease on Hepatic Transporter Expression and Function. *J Pharm Sci.* 2017 Sep;106(9):2282–94.

[69] Yumoto R, Murakami T, Takano M. Differential Effect of Acute Hepatic Failure on *in Vivo* and *in Vitro* P-Glycoprotein Functions in the Intestine. *Pharm Res*. 2003 May 1;20(5):765–71.

[70] Zollner G, Wagner M, Fickert P, Silbert D, Fuchsbichler A, Zatloukal K, et al., Hepatobiliary transporter expression in human hepatocellular carcinoma. *Liver Int.* 2005 Apr;25(2):367–79.

[71] Chou YY, Cheng AL, Hsu HC. Expression of P-glycoprotein and p53 in advanced hepatocellular carcinoma treated by single agent chemotherapy: clinical correlation. *J Gastroenterol Hepatol.* 1997 Aug;12(8):569–75.

[72] Atilano-Roque A, Roda G, Fogueri U, Kiser JJ, Joy MS. Effect of Disease Pathologies on Transporter Expression and Function. *The Journal of Clinical Pharmacology*. 2016;56(S7):S205–21.

[73] Tramonti G, Xie P, Wallner EI, Danesh FR, Kanwar YS. Expression and functional characteristics of tubular transporters: P-glycoprotein, PEPT1, and PEPT2 in renal mass reduction and diabetes. *American*

Journal of Physiology-Renal Physiology. 2006 Nov 1;291(5):F972–80.

[74] Schinkel AH, Jonker JW. Mammalian drug efflux transporters of the ATP binding cassette (ABC) family: an overview. *Advanced Drug Delivery Reviews*. 2003 Jan 21;55(1):3–29.

[75] Koziolek MJ, Riess R, Geiger H, Thévenod F, Hauser IA. Expression of multidrug resistance P-glycoprotein in kidney allografts from cyclosporine A-treated patients. *Kidney International.* 2001 Jul 1;60(1):156–66.

[76] Hauser IA, Koziolek M, Hopfer U, Thévenod F. Therapeutic concentrations of cyclosporine A, but not FK506, increase P-glycoprotein expression in endothelial and renal tubule cells. *Kidney International.* 1998 Oct 1;54(4):1139–49.

[77] Thévenod F, Friedmann JM, Katsen AD, Hauser IA. Up-regulation of multidrug resistance P-glycoprotein via nuclear factor-kappaB activation protects kidney proximal tubule cells from cadmium- and reactive oxygen species-induced apoptosis. *J Biol Chem.* 2000 Jan 21;275(3):1887–96.

[78] Rengelshausen J, Göggelmann C, Burhenne J, Riedel KD, Ludwig J, Weiss J, et al., Contribution of increased oral bioavailability and reduced nonglomerular renal clearance of digoxin to the digoxin–clarithromycin interaction. *Br J Clin Pharmacol.* 2003 Jul;56(1):32–8.

[79] Hori R, Okamura N, Aiba T, Tanigawara Y. Role of P-glycoprotein in renal tubular secretion of digoxin in the isolated perfused rat kidney. *J Pharmacol Exp Ther.* 1993 Sep;266(3):1620–5.

[80] Wakasugi H, Yano I, Ito T, Hashida T, Futami T, Nohara R, et al., Effect of clarithromycin on renal excretion of digoxin: Interaction with P-glycoprotein. *Clinical Pharmacology & Therapeutics.* 1998;64(1):123–8.

[81] Kyrklund C, Backman JT, Neuvonen M, Neuvonen PJ. Gemfibrozil increases plasma pravastatin concentrations and reduces pravastatin renal clearance. *Clin Pharmacol Ther.* 2003 Jun;73(6):538–44.

[82] Marzolini C, Paus E, Buclin T, Kim RB. Polymorphisms in Human MDR1 (P-glycoprotein): Recent Advances and Clinical Relevance. *Clinical Pharmacology & Therapeutics.* 2004;75(1):13–33.

[83] Siegsmund M, Brinkmann U, Schǻffeler E, Weirich G, Schwab M, Eichelbaum M, et al., Association of the P-glycoprotein transporter MDR1(C3435T) polymorphism with the susceptibility to renal epithelial tumors. *J Am Soc Nephrol.* 2002 Jul;13(7):1847–54.

[84] Yates CR, Zhang W, Song P, Li S, Gaber AO, Kotb M, et al., The effect of CYP3A5 and MDR1 polymorphic expression on cyclosporine oral disposition in renal transplant patients. *J Clin Pharmacol.* 2003 Jun;43(6):555–64.

[85] Asano T, Takahashi KA, Fujioka M, Inoue S, Okamoto M, Sugioka N, et al., ABCB1 C3435T and G2677T/A polymorphism decreased the risk for steroid-induced osteonecrosis of the femoral head after kidney transplantation. *Pharmacogenetics and Genomics.* 2003 Nov;13(11):675–82.

[86] Murakami T, Yumoto R, Nagai J, Takano M. Factors affecting the expression and function of P-glycoprotein in rats: drug treatments and diseased states. *Pharmazie.* 2002 Feb;57(2):102–7.

[87] Shibata N, Inoue Y, Fukumoto K, Nishimura A, Fukushima K, Yoshikawa Y, et al., Evaluation of factors to decrease bioavailability of cyclosporin A in rats with gentamicin-induced acute renal failure. *Biol Pharm Bull.* 2004 Mar;27(3):384–91.

[88] Okabe H, Yano I, Hashimoto Y, Saito H, Inui K. Evaluation of increased bioavailability of tacrolimus in rats with experimental renal dysfunction. *J Pharm Pharmacol.* 2002 Jan;54(1):65–70.

[89] Stangier J, Rathgen K, Stähle H, Mazur D. Influence of renal impairment on the pharmacokinetics and pharmacodynamics of oral dabigatran etexilate: an open-label, parallel-group, single-centre study. *Clin Pharmacokinet.* 2010 Apr;49(4):259–68.

[90] de Boer A g., van der Sandt I c. j., Gaillard P j. The Role of Drug Transporters at the Blood-Brain Barrier. *Annu Rev Pharmacol Toxicol.* 2003 Apr 1;43(1):629–56.

[91] Tsuji A, Tamai I. Blood-brain barrier function of P-glycoprotein. *Advanced Drug Delivery Reviews.* 1997 May 12;25(2):287–98.

[92] Bendayan R, Lee G, Bendayan M. Functional expression and localization of P-glycoprotein at the blood brain barrier. *Microsc Res Tech.* 2002 Jun 1;57(5):365–80.

[93] Sanchez-Covarrubias L, Slosky LM, Thompson BJ, Davis TP, Ronaldson PT. Transporters at CNS Barrier Sites: Obstacles or Opportunities for Drug Delivery? *Curr Pharm Des.* 2014;20 (10):1422–49.

[94] Liu X, Yang Z, Yang J, Yang H. Increased P-glycoprotein expression and decreased phenobarbital distribution in the brain of pentylenetetrazole-kindled rats. *Neuropharmacology.* 2007 Oct;53(5):657–63.

[95] Kemper EM, van Zandbergen AE, Cleypool C, Mos HA, Boogerd W, Beijnen JH, et al., Increased penetration of paclitaxel into the brain by inhibition of P-Glycoprotein. *Clin Cancer Res.* 2003 Jul;9(7):2849–55.

[96] Montesinos RN, Moulari B, Gromand J, Beduneau A, Lamprecht A, Pellequer Y. Coadministration of P-glycoprotein modulators on loperamide pharmacokinetics and brain distribution. *Drug Metab Dispos.* 2014 Apr;42(4):700–6.

[97] Jeleń AM, Sałagacka A, Żebrowska MK, Mirowski M, Talarowska M, Gałecki P, et al., The Influence of C3435T Polymorphism of the ABCB1 Gene on Genetic Susceptibility to Depression and Treatment Response in Polish Population - Preliminary Report. *Int J Med Sci.* 2015 Nov 20;12(12):974–9.

[98] Kerb R, Aynacioglu AS, Brockmöller J, Schlagenhaufer R, Bauer S, Szekeres T, et al., The predictive value of MDR1, CYP2C9, and CYP2C19 polymorphisms for phenytoin plasma levels. *Pharmacogenomics J.* 2001;1(3):204–10.

[99] Furuno T, Landi MT, Ceroni M, Caporaso N, Bernucci I, Nappi G, et al., Expression polymorphism of the blood-brain barrier component P-glycoprotein (MDR1) in relation to Parkinson's disease. *Pharmacogenetics.* 2002 Oct;12(7):529–34.

[100] Wen T, Liu YC, Yang HW, Liu HY, Liu XD, Wang GJ, et al., Effect of 21-day exposure of phenobarbital, carbamazepine and phenytoin on P-glycoprotein expression and activity in the rat brain. *Journal of the Neurological Sciences.* 2008 Jul 15;270(1):99–106.

[101] Milane A, Fernandez C, Dupuis L, Buyse M, Loeffler JP, Farinotti R, et al., P-glycoprotein expression and function are increased in an animal model of amyotrophic lateral sclerosis. *Neurosci Lett.* 2010 Mar 26;472(3):166–70.

[102] Miller DS. Regulation of P-glycoprotein and other ABC drug transporters at the blood-brain barrier. *Trends Pharmacol Sci.* 2010 Jun;31(6):246–54.

[103] Jablonski MR, Jacob DA, Campos C, Miller DS, Maragakis NJ, Pasinelli P, et al., Selective increase of two ABC drug efflux transporters at the blood-spinal cord barrier suggests induced pharmacoresistance in ALS. *Neurobiol Dis.* 2012 Aug;47(2):194–200.

[104] Yang J, Zhou JS, Zhao YX, Yang ZH, Zhao HD, Zhang YD, et al., ABCB1 hypomethylation is associated with decreased antiplatelet effects of clopidogrel in Chinese ischemic stroke patients. *Pharmazie.* 2015 Feb;70(2):97–102.

[105] Vries NA de, Zhao J, Kroon E, Buckle T, Beijnen JH, Tellingen O van. P-Glycoprotein and Breast Cancer Resistance Protein: Two Dominant Transporters Working Together in Limiting the Brain Penetration of Topotecan. *Clin Cancer Res.* 2007 Nov 1;13 (21):6440–9.

[106] Hano M, Tomášová L, Šereš M, Pavlíková L, Breier A, Sulová Z. Interplay between P-Glycoprotein Expression and Resistance to Endoplasmic Reticulum Stressors. *Molecules.* 2018 Feb 6;23(2):337.

[107] Mollazadeh S, Sahebkar A, Hadizadeh F, Behravan J, Arabzadeh S. Structural and functional aspects of P-glycoprotein and its inhibitors. *Life Sciences.* 2018 Dec;214:118–23.

[108] Lin JH, Yamazaki M. Role of P-glycoprotein in pharmacokinetics: clinical implications. *Clin Pharmacokinet.* 2003;42(1):59–98.

[109] Kerr DJ, Graham J, Cummings J, Morrison JG, Thompson GG, Brodie MJ, et al., The effect of verapamil on the pharmacokinetics of adriamycin. *Cancer Chemother Pharmacol.* 1986;18(3):239–42.

[110] Berg SL, Tolcher A, O'Shaughnessy JA, Denicoff AM, Noone M, Ognibene FP, et al., Effect of R-verapamil on the pharmacokinetics of paclitaxel in women with breast cancer. *J Clin Oncol.* 1995 Aug;13(8):2039–42.

[111] Varma M. P-glycoprotein inhibitors and their screening: a perspective from bioavailability enhancement. *Pharmacological Research*. 2003 Oct;48(4):347–59.

[112] Higgins CF, Linton KJ. The ATP switch model for ABC transporters. *Nature Structural & Molecular Biology*. 2004 Oct;11(10):918–26.

[113] Silva R, Vilas-Boas V, Carmo H, Dinis-Oliveira RJ, Carvalho F, de Lourdes Bastos M, et al., Modulation of P-glycoprotein efflux pump: induction and activation as a therapeutic strategy. *Pharmacology & Therapeutics.* 2015 May;149:1–123.

[114] Sparreboom A, van Asperen J, Mayer U, Schinkel AH, Smit JW, Meijer DKF, et al., Limited oral bioavailability and active epithelial excretion of paclitaxel (Taxol) caused by P-glycoprotein in the intestine. *Proceedings of the National Academy of Sciences.* 1997 Mar 4;94(5):2031–5.

[115] Bardelmeijer HA, Beijnen JH, Brouwer KR, Rosing H, Nooijen WJ, Schellens JH, et al., Increased oral bioavailability of paclitaxel by GF120918 in mice through selective modulation of P-glycoprotein. *Clin Cancer Res.* 2000 Nov;6(11):4416–21.

[116] Gerloff T, Schaefer M, Johne A, Oselin K, Meisel C, Cascorbi I, et al., MDR1 genotypes do not influence the absorption of a single oral dose of 1 mg digoxin in healthy white males: Effect of MDR1 genotypes on digoxin single dose kinetics. *British Journal of Clinical Pharmacology.* 2002 Dec;54(6):610–6.

[117] Pacchioni AM, Gabriele A, Donovan JL, Lindsay DeVane C, See RE. P-glycoprotein inhibition potentiates the behavioural and neurochemical actions of risperidone in rats. *The International Journal of Neuropsychopharmacology.* 2010 Sep;13(08):1067–77.

[118] Davis TP, Sanchez-Covarubias L, Tome ME. P-glycoprotein Trafficking as a Therapeutic Target to Optimize CNS Drug Delivery. In: Advances in Pharmacology [Internet]. Elsevier; 2014 [cited 2020 Nov 6]. p. 25–44. Available from: https://linkinghub.elsevier.com/retrieve/pii/S1054358914000106.

[119] Schinkel AH, Jonker JW. Mammalian drug efflux transporters of the ATP binding cassette (ABC) family: an overview. *Adv Drug Deliv Rev.* 2003 Jan 21;55(1):3–29.

[120] Schinkel AH, Smit JJM, van Tellingen O, Beijnen JH, Wagenaar E, van Deemter L, et al., Disruption of the mouse mdr1a P-glycoprotein gene leads to a deficiency in the blood-brain barrier and to increased sensitivity to drugs. *Cell.* 1994 May;77(4):491–502.

[121] Liu L, Liu XD. Alterations in function and expression of ABC transporters at blood-brain barrier under diabetes and the clinical significances. *Frontiers in Pharmacology* [Internet]. 2014 Dec 10 [cited 2020 Nov 6];5. Available from: http://journal.frontiersin.org/article/10.3389/fphar.2014.00273/abstract.

[122] Chai AB, Leung GKF, Callaghan R, Gelissen IC. P-glycoprotein: a role in the export of amyloid-β in Alzheimer's disease? *FEBS J.* 2020;287(4):612–25.

[123] Stępień KM, Tomaszewski M, Tomaszewska J, Czuczwar SJ. The multidrug transporter P-glycoprotein in pharmacoresistance to antiepileptic drugs. *Pharmacol Rep.* 2012;64(5):1011–9.

[124] Abuznait AH, Qosa H, Busnena BA, El Sayed KA, Kaddoumi A. Olive-Oil-Derived Oleocanthal Enhances β-Amyloid Clearance as a Potential Neuroprotective Mechanism against Alzheimer's Disease: In Vitro and in Vivo Studies. *ACS Chemical Neuroscience*. 2013 Jun 19;4(6):973–82.

[125] Mesraoua B, Deleu D, Kullmann DM, Shetty AK, Boon P, Perucca E, et al., Novel therapies for epilepsy in the pipeline. *Epilepsy Behav.* 2019;97:282–90.

[126] Tishler DM, Weinberg KI, Hinton DR, Barbaro N, Annett GM, Raffel C. MDR1 Gene Expression in Brain of Patients with Medically Intractable Epilepsy. *Epilepsia.* 1995 Jan;36(1):1–6.

[127] Seegers U, Potschka H, Löscher W. Transient increase of P-glycoprotein expression in endothelium and parenchyma of limbic brain regions in the kainate model of temporal lobe epilepsy. *Epilepsy Res*. 2002 Oct;51(3):257–68.

[128] Morimoto K, Sato H, Sato K, Sato S, Yamada N. BW1003C87, phenytoin and carbamazepine elevate seizure threshold in the rat amygdala-kindling model of epilepsy. *Eur J Pharmacol*. 1997 Nov 19;339(1):11–5.

[129] Yuan W, Ma A, Wang C, Chen Y. P-glycoprotein alters blood–brain barrier penetration of antiepileptic drugs in rats with medically intractable epilepsy. *Drug Design, Development and Therapy*. 2013 Dec;1447.

[130] Kobori T, Harada S, Nakamoto K, Tokuyama S. Time-Dependent Changes in the Activation of RhoA/ROCK and ERM/p-ERM in the Increased Expression of Intestinal P-Glycoprotein by Repeated Oral Treatment with Etoposide. *Journal of Pharmaceutical Sciences*. 2013 May;102(5):1670–82.

[131] Demeule M, Jodoin J, Beaulieu É, Brossard M, Béliveau R. Dexamethasone modulation of multidrug transporters in normal tissues. *FEBS Letters*. 1999 Jan 15;442(2–3):208–14.

[132] Geick A, Eichelbaum M, Burk O. Nuclear Receptor Response Elements Mediate Induction of Intestinal *MDR1* by Rifampin. *Journal of Biological Chemistry*. 2001 May 4;276(18):14581–7.

[133] Oda Y, Sakamoto A, Shinohara N, Ohga T, Uchiumi T, Kohno K, et al., Nuclear expression of YB-1 protein correlates with P-glycoprotein expression in human osteosarcoma. *Clin Cancer Res*. 1998 Sep;4(9):2273–7.

[134] Scotto KW, Johnson RA. Transcription of the multidrug resistance gene MDR1: a therapeutic target. Mol Interv. 2001 Jun;1(2):117–25.

[135] Zhou G, Kuo MT. NF-kappaB-mediated induction of mdr1b expression by insulin in rat hepatoma cells. *J Biol Chem. 1*997 Jun 13;272(24):15174–83.

[136] Fujita T, Ito K, Izumi H, Kimura M, Sano M, Nakagomi H, et al., Increased nuclear localization of transcription factor Y-box binding

protein 1 accompanied by up-regulation of P-glycoprotein in breast cancer pretreated with paclitaxel. *Clin Cancer Res*. 2005 Dec 15;11(24 Pt 1):8837–44.

[137] Gryder BE, Sodji QH, Oyelere AK. Targeted cancer therapy: giving histone deacetylase inhibitors all they need to succeed. *Future Med Chem*. 2012 Mar;4(4):505–24.

[138] Shiota K. DNA methylation profiles of CpG islands for cellular differentiation and development in mammals. *Cytogenet Genome Res*. 2004;105(2–4):325–34.

[139] Baker EK, Johnstone RW, Zalcberg JR, El-Osta A. Epigenetic changes to the MDR1 locus in response to chemotherapeutic drugs. *Oncogene*. 2005 Dec;24(54):8061–75.

[140] Eyal S, Lamb JG, Smith-Yockman M, Yagen B, Fibach E, Altschuler Y, et al., The antiepileptic and anticancer agent, valproic acid, induces P-glycoprotein in human tumour cell lines and in rat liver. *Br J Pharmacol*. 2006 Oct;149(3):250–60.

[141] Kim SN, Kim NH, Lee W, Seo DW, Kim YK. Histone deacetylase inhibitor induction of P-glycoprotein transcription requires both histone deacetylase 1 dissociation and recruitment of CAAT/enhancer binding protein beta and pCAF to the promoter region. *Mol Cancer Res*. 2009 May;7(5):735–44.

[142] Kobori T, Harada S, Nakamoto K, Tokuyama S. Mechanisms of P-Glycoprotein Alteration During Anticancer Treatment: Role in the Pharmacokinetic and Pharmacological Effects of Various Substrate Drugs. *Journal of Pharmacological Sciences*. 2014;125(3):242–54.

[143] Roett MA, Evans P. Ovarian cancer: an overview. *Am Fam Physician*. 2009 Sep 15;80(6):609–16.

[144] Jia Y, Sun S, Gao X, Cui X. Expression levels of TUBB3, ERCC1 and P-gp in ovarian cancer tissues and adjacent normal tissues and their clinical significance. *J BUON*. 2018 Oct;23(5):1390–5.

[145] Zheng W, Li M, Lin Y, Zhan X. Encapsulation of verapamil and doxorubicin by MPEG-PLA to reverse drug resistance in ovarian cancer. *Biomedicine & Pharmacotherapy*. 2018 Dec;108:565–73.

[146] García-Carrasco M, Mendoza-Pinto C, Macias Díaz S, Vera-Recabarren M, Vázquez de Lara L, Méndez Martínez S, et al., P-glycoprotein in autoimmune rheumatic diseases. *Autoimmunity Reviews.* 2015 Jul;14(7):594–600.

[147] Picchianti-Diamanti A, Rosado M, Scarsella M, Laganà B, D'Amelio R. P-Glycoprotein and Drug Resistance in Systemic Autoimmune Diseases. *International Journal of Molecular Sciences.* 2014 Mar 20;15(3):4965–76.

[148] Tan EM, Cohen AS, Fries JF, Masi AT, McShane DJ, Rothfield NF, et al., The 1982 revised criteria for the classification of systemic lupus erythematosus. *Arthritis Rheum.* 1982 Nov;25(11):1271–7.

[149] Meaden ER, Hoggard PG, Khoo SH, Back DJ. Determination of P-gp and MRP1 expression and function in peripheral blood mononuclear cells *in vivo*. *J Immunol Methods.* 2002 Apr 1;262(1–2):159–65.

[150] Zhang B, Shi Y, Lei TC. Detection of active P-glycoprotein in systemic lupus erythematosus patients with poor disease control. *Experimental and Therapeutic Medicine.* 2012 Oct;4(4):705–10.

[151] Kansal A, Tripathi D, Rai MK, Agarwal V. Persistent expression and function of P-glycoprotein on peripheral blood lymphocytes identifies corticosteroid resistance in patients with systemic lupus erythematosus. *Clinical Rheumatology.* 2016 Feb;35(2):341–9.

[152] Perez-Guerrero EE, Gamez-Nava JI, Muñoz-Valle JF, Cardona-Muñoz EG, Bonilla-Lara D, Fajardo-Robledo NS, et al., Serum levels of P-glycoprotein and persistence of disease activity despite treatment in patients with systemic lupus erythematosus. *Clinical and Experimental Medicine*. 2018 Feb;18(1):109–17.

[153] Ragab SM, Soliman MA. P-glycoprotein-1 functional activity in CD5+CD7+ and CD20+ lymphocytes in systemic lupus erythematosus children: relation to disease activity, complications and steroid response. *Egypt J Immunol.* 2013;20(2):101–15.

[154] Qin K, Chen K, Zhao W, Zhao X, Luo J, Wang Q, et al., Methotrexate Combined with 4-Hydroperoxycyclophosphamide Downregulates Multidrug-Resistance P-Glycoprotein Expression Induced by

Methotrexate in Rheumatoid Arthritis Fibroblast-Like Synoviocytes via the JAK2/STAT3 Pathway. *J Immunol Res.* 2018;2018:3619320.

[155] Maillefert JF, Maynadie M, Tebib JG, Aho S, Walker P, Chatard C, et al., Expression of the multidrug resistance glycoprotein 170 in the peripheral blood lymphocytes of rheumatoid arthritis patients. The percentage of lymphocytes expressing glycoprotein 170 is increased in patients treated with prednisolone. *Br J Rheumatol.* 1996 May;35(5):430–5.

[156] Yudoh K, Matsuno H, Nakazawa F, Yonezawa T, Kimura T. Increased expression of multidrug resistance of P-glycoprotein on Th1 cells correlates with drug resistance in rheumatoid arthritis. *Arthritis Rheum.* 1999 Sep;42(9):2014–5.

[157] Hider SL, Owen A, Hartkoorn R, Khoo S, Back D, Silman AJ, et al., Down regulation of multidrug resistance protein-1 expression in patients with early rheumatoid arthritis exposed to methotrexate as a first disease-modifying antirheumatic drug. *Ann Rheum Dis.* 2006 Oct;65(10):1390–3.

[158] van der Heijden JW, Dijkmans BAC, Scheper RJ, Jansen G. Drug Insight: resistance to methotrexate and other disease-modifying antirheumatic drugs--from bench to bedside. *Nat Clin Pract Rheumatol.* 2007 Jan;3(1):26–34.

[159] Suzuki K, Saito K, Tsujimura S, Nakayamada S, Yamaoka K, Sawamukai N, et al., Tacrolimus, a calcineurin inhibitor, overcomes treatment unresponsiveness mediated by P-glycoprotein on lymphocytes in refractory rheumatoid arthritis. *J Rheumatol.* 2010 Mar;37(3):512–20.

[160] Diamanti AP, Rosado M, Germano V, Scarsella M, Giorda E, Podestà E, et al., Reversion of resistance to immunosuppressive agents in three patients with psoriatic arthritis by cyclosporine A: modulation of P-glycoprotein function. *Clin Immunol.* 2011 Jan;138(1):9–13.

[161] Perez-Guerrero EE, Gonzalez-Lopez L, Muñoz-Valle JF, Vasquez-Jimenez JC, Ramirez-Villafaña M, Sanchez-Rodriguez EN, et al., Serum P-glycoprotein level: a potential biomarker of DMARD failure

in patients with rheumatoid arthritis. *Inflammopharmacology*. 2018 Sep 12;
[162] Cree IA, Charlton P. Molecular chess? Hallmarks of anti-cancer drug resistance. *BMC Cancer*. 2017 Jan 5;17(1):10.
[163] Cree IA, Knight L, Di Nicolantonio F, Sharma S, Gulliford T. Chemosensitization of solid tumors by modulation of resistance mechanisms. *Curr Opin Investig Drugs*. 2002 Apr;3(4):634–40.
[164] Di Pietro A, Dayan G, Conseil G, Steinfels E, Krell T, Trompier D, et al., P-glycoprotein-mediated resistance to chemotherapy in cancer cells: using recombinant cytosolic domains to establish structure-function relationships. *Braz J Med Biol Res*. 1999 Aug;32(8):925–39.
[165] Dano K. Active outward transport of daunomycin in resistant Ehrlich ascites tumor cells. *Biochim Biophys Acta*. 1973 Oct 25;323(3):466–83.
[166] uliano RL, Ling V. A surface glycoprotein modulating drug permeability in Chinese hamster ovary cell mutants. *Biochim Biophys Acta*. 1976 Nov 11;455(1):152–62.
[167] Lehne G. P-glycoprotein as a drug target in the treatment of multidrug resistant cancer. *Curr Drug Targets*. 2000 Jul;1(1):85–99.
[168] Duan B, Huang C, Bai J, Zhang YL, Wang X, Yang J, et al., Multidrug Resistance in Hepatocellular Carcinoma. In: Tirnitz-Parker JEE, editor. *Hepatocellular Carcinoma* [Internet]. Brisbane (AU): Codon Publications; 2019 [cited 2020 Nov 5]. Available from: http://www.ncbi.nlm.nih.gov/books/NBK549189/
[169] Wu J, Lin N, Li F, Zhang G, He S, Zhu Y, et al., Induction of P-glycoprotein expression and activity by Aconitum alkaloids: Implication for clinical drug–drug interactions. *Scientific Reports*. 2016 May 3;6(1):25343.
[170] Kantharidis P, El-Osta A, deSilva M, Wall DM, Hu XF, Slater A, et al., Altered methylation of the human MDR1 promoter is associated with acquired multidrug resistance. *Clin Cancer Res*. 1997 Nov;3(11):2025–32.
[171] Garcia-Manero G, Bueso-Ramos C, Daniel J, Williamson J, Kantarjian HM, Issa JPJ. DNA methylation patterns at relapse in adult

acute lymphocytic leukemia. *Clin Cancer Res.* 2002 Jun;8(6):1897–903.

[172] Desiderato L, Davey MW, Piper AA. Demethylation of the human MDR1 5' region accompanies activation of P-glycoprotein expression in a HL60 multidrug resistant subline. *Somat Cell Mol Genet.* 1997 Nov;23(6):391–400.

[173] Siddiqui A, Kerb R, Weale ME, Brinkmann U, Smith A, Goldstein DB, et al., Association of multidrug resistance in epilepsy with a polymorphism in the drug-transporter gene ABCB1. *N Engl J Med.* 2003 Apr 10;348(15):1442–8.

[174] Zawadzka I, Jeleń A, Pietrzak J, Żebrowska-Nawrocka M, Michalska K, Szmajda-Krygier D, et al., The impact of ABCB1 gene polymorphism and its expression on non-small-cell lung cancer development, progression and therapy – preliminary report. *Scientific Reports.* 2020 Apr 10;10(1):6188.

[175] Teng YN, Wang YH, Wu TS, Hung HY, Hung CC. Zhankuic Acids A, B and C from Taiwanofungus Camphoratus Act as Cytotoxicity Enhancers by Regulating P-Glycoprotein in Multi-Drug Resistant Cancer Cells. *Biomolecules.* 2019 Nov 21;9(12).

[176] Dong J, Zhai B, Sun W, Hu F, Cheng H, Xu J. Activation of phosphatidylinositol 3-kinase/AKT/snail signaling pathway contributes to epithelial-mesenchymal transition-induced multi-drug resistance to sorafenib in hepatocellular carcinoma cells. *PLoS One* [Internet]. 2017 Sep 21 [cited 2020 Nov 5];12(9). Available from: https://www.ncbi.nlm.nih.gov/pmc/articles/PMC5608310/

[177] Li J, Duan B, Guo Y, Zhou R, Sun J, Bie B, et al., Baicalein sensitizes hepatocellular carcinoma cells to 5-FU and Epirubicin by activating apoptosis and ameliorating P-glycoprotein activity. *Biomedicine & Pharmacotherapy*. 2018 Feb 1;98:806–12.

[178] Kong J, Qiu Y, Li Y, Zhang H, Wang W. TGF-β1 elevates P-gp and BCRP in hepatocellular carcinoma through HOTAIR/miR-145 axis. *Biopharm Drug Dispos.* 2019 Feb;40(2):70–80.

[179] Warmann S, Göhring G, Teichmann B, Geerlings H, Pietsch T, Fuchs J. P-glycoprotein modulation improves in vitro chemosensitivity in

malignant pediatric liver tumors. *Anticancer Res.* 2003 Dec;23(6C):4607–11.

[180] Yuan Z, Shi X, Qiu Y, Jia T, Yuan X, Zou Y, et al., Reversal of P-gp-mediated multidrug resistance in colon cancer by cinobufagin. *Oncology Reports.* 2017 Mar 1;37(3):1815–25.

[181] Assema D, Berckel B. Blood-Brain Barrier ABC-transporter P-glycoprotein in Alzheimer's Disease: Still a Suspect? *Current Pharmaceutical Design*. 2016 Nov 30;22(38):5808–16.

[182] Bartels AL, Willemsen ATM, Kortekaas R, de Jong BM, de Vries R, de Klerk O, et al., Decreased blood–brain barrier P-glycoprotein function in the progression of Parkinson's disease, PSP and MSA. *Journal of Neural Transmission*. 2008 Jul;115(7):1001–9.

[183] Prajoko YW, Aryandono T. The Effect of P-Glycoprotein (P-gp), Nuclear Factor-Kappa B (Nf-κb), and Aldehyde Dehydrogenase-1 (ALDH-1) Expression on Metastases, Recurrence and Survival in Advanced Breast Cancer Patients. *Asian Pac J Cancer Prev.* 2019 May 25;20(5):1511–8.

In: An Introduction to P-Glycoprotein ISBN: 978-1-53619-488-3
Editors: M. Wahajuddin et al.

Chapter 3

P-GP PATHOPHYSIOLOGY: POST-TRANSLATIONAL MODIFICATION AND AFFECTING SIGNALING CASCADES

Sree-Pooja Varahachalam[1,*], Jaspreet Kaur[2,*], Minitha Jacob[3], Behnaz Lahooti[1], Tanya Chhibber[1], Alexis Hyman[3], Abhijeet Joshi[2,†] and Rahul Dev Jayant[1,≠]

[1]Department of Pharmaceutical Sciences, JH School of Pharmacy, Texas Tech University Health Science Center, Amarillo, TX, US
[2]Department for Biosciences and Biomedical Engineering, Indian Institute of Technology Indore, Indore, Madhya Pradesh, India
[3]JH School of Pharmacy, Texas Tech University Health Science Center, Abilene, TX, US

---

* Equal contribution.
† Corresponding Author's Email: abhijeet.joshi@iiti.ac.in.
≠ Corresponding Author's Email: rahuldev.jayant@gmail.com

Abstract

The PTMs (Post-translational modifications) play a pivotal role in regulating various biological functions, e.g., protein stability and its localization, and regulation of different enzymatic activity. Post-translational changes have been shown to modulate a wide range of molecular pathways along with the functional expression of the drug transporter. These modifications usually occur by adding residues of solvent-accessible amino acids to functional groups (phosphorylation), small proteins (ubiquitination), sugar chains (glycosylation) or lipids (palmitoylation). This chapter highlights the role of drug transporter, its function and importance of post-translational modifications to understand their roles in drug transporter regulation and its process.

Keywords: P-gp (P-Glycoprotein), PTM (Post-translational modification), MDR (multi-drug resistance), Phosphorylation, Membrane transport

Introduction

P-gp (P-Glycoprotein) referred to as a transmembrane protein that localized in various locations within human tissues, including nervous tissue and brain tissue. It's often known as MDR1 (multi-drug resistance protein 1), functioning as a localized transport protein by which it actively exports drugs out of the cell [1]. MDR1 has a diverse tissue distribution, being confined in several origins as the colon lining, contain endothelial cells of the (BBB) blood-brain barrier, bile and pancreatic ducts, kidney tubules, adrenal gland, small intestine and in many other tissues comprising of heart, skeletal muscles, lungs, spleen etc. Also, owing to its nature, this protein is a novel protective barrier mechanism that cells use against incompatible or toxic substances to prevent damage or injury to tissues [1]. A broad spectrum of lipophilic molecules is known to express substrate specificity towards P-gp. The mechanism behind P-gp to transport drugs out is an idea that is still in investigation. Over recent years, two proposals have made on P-gp mechanism of action: (1) the flippase or 'flip flop' mechanism and (2) 'vacuum cleaner' process. It also has not been found that these mechanisms are mutually exclusive.

P-gp as a Lipid Flippase

P-gp is a constructive translocase protein which acts upon delivering its substrates from direction embodied inside to outside the cell membrane. A molecule must be in a specific location within the bilayer and reach to the outer leaflet [1]. After which the substrate either diffusely moves into through extracellular space or revert into the inner leaflet, causing a flip-flop activity. The flippase mechanism of P-gp works similarly to other flippase activity in the body, requiring ATP hydrolysis and good substrate-binding affinity [1]. This activity allows for substrates to turn out to the extracellular space (Figure 1). Due to this, substrates in this medium found to be more energetically beneficial rather than through hydration transferring into the aqueous phase.

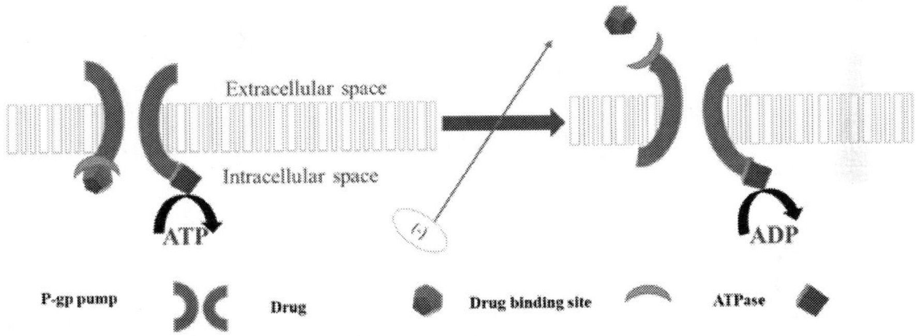

Figure 1. Diagrammatically representing flippase or 'flip flop' mechanism used by P-gp for transportation of drugs.

P-gp as a Vacuum Cleaner

It is strongly evident, in the vacuum cleaner proposed idea, MDR1 causes drug efflux to the extracellular space directly from within the cell membrane [1]. A molecule or drug will translocate to the inner leaflet to gain access to the P-gp substrate-binding pocket which then it is pushed to the extracellular aqueous medium. This mechanism also requires ATP by hydrolysis to provide the driving force for the delivery process [1]. The transporter 'vacuum' from the cell manages harmful compounds removal by eliminating it through the body's system (Figure 2).

The physiological significance of P-gp is still under some conjecture. The primary reason that concludes is the exporting of substances in vivo from the cytoplasm to the extracellular matrix. Several internal P-gp substrates that have an affinity for the protein are platelet-activating factors (PAFs), steroid hormones, bile acids, and bilirubin [2]. In the removal of these substrates through excretion, P-gp plays an indispensable role.

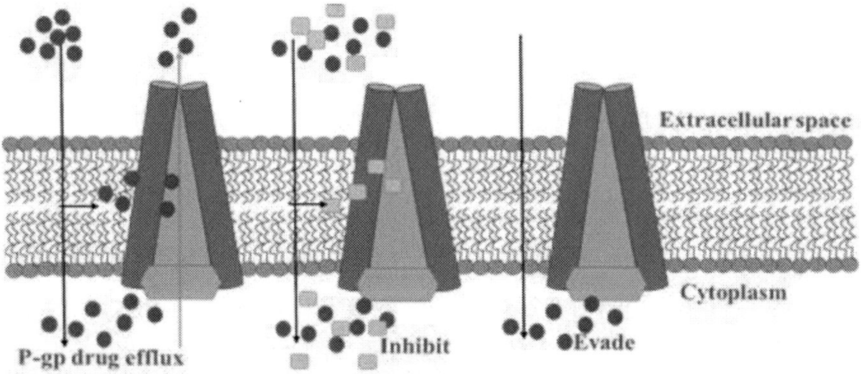

Figure 2. Diagrammatic representation of P-gp (tertiary V-shaped structure) mediated drug efflux mechanism acting as a transporter vacuum.

This mechanism has shown responsibility to the biosynthesis of lipids in the Golgi apparatus. It also plays a significant part in contributing a protective mechanism to the blood-brain barrier by preventing any brain injury or damage. [2]. Since the human brain is susceptible to specific compounds, so the P-gp is naturally used as a critical element to be a defense against disease. The protein's mode of action has also been counterintuitive when it comes to drug administration, distribution, absorption, and elimination (ADME) characteristics. The protein's protective nature stops the intake of xenobiotics from entering into the human cell, which can cause a decrease in drug effectiveness, enhanced drug elimination, and limited drug distribution [2]. A variety of inhibiting P-gp substrates have been used to counteract the effect by changing ATP supply in the body or by manipulating the cell membrane to increase drug permeability (Table 1)[3]. The inhibitory substrates acting are digoxin, doxorubicin, fexofenadine, quinidine, irinotecan, paclitaxel, and others [2].

Effect of P-gp in Pathology

Several reports suggest P-gp transporter to have some significance in disease pathology. MDR1 has contributed to the cause and development of some diseases such as cancers, tumours, immune-mediating inflammatory disorders, and brain diseases such as major depressive disorder and Alzheimer's [4]. Though despite considering P-gp transporter as an essential and selective element in several types of tissues, it is not perfect in its design. Many reports state P-gp is still prone to changes in function and amount of membrane expression.

The clinical significance of this protein has yet to be discovered due to its discovery in vitro rather than in vivo. Several defenses that this protein does possess include protection from xenobiotic aggression, removal of cytotoxic substrates, and transport of nutrients, ions, and peptides [4]. P-gp affects the absorption of oral drugs by removing drug molecules that have already been absorbed previously at the site of the lining of the intestines. Another mechanism in the BBB, P-gp behaves to reduce nervous system side effects or limit drug permeability. In the liver and kidneys, the protein contributes to their function of eliminating drugs from the system. While there is evidence that exists to show P-gp being utilized for the good of the human body, nearby changes (change in pH, thermodynamic or kinetic conditions, etc.) can cause transporter alterations [4]. Modifications consisting of changes in P-gp have not had any effect on other molecules in tissues but can ultimately affect the surrounding environment.

Recent investigations have focused on P-gp overexpression and increased function concerning tumours/cancers due to multi-drug resistance.

The in vitro studies express, P-gp strong expression is directly associated with highly cancerous or tumour cells. It is, however, unclear if protein overexpression can cause the cells to turn cancerous or vice versa. P-gp expression, however, also increases in the later stages of cancer/tumours, which implies the protein to be involved in tumour progression. The preliminary step of cancer metastasis is when original epithelial cancer cells transition into mesenchymal cells. These cells become highly mobile, which allows them to spread to distant organs. A study states, in the breast cancer cells, the upregulation of P-gp mRNA and protein resulted in resistance to a chemotherapeutic drug, doxorubicin [5]. Yano K, Tomono T, Ogihara T's article indicated that cancer transcriptional factor-induced P-gp expression and efflux colorectal cancer cells in response to chemotherapy treatment [5]. An increased function has been a proposed factor in cancer progression in recent years. Lung cancer cells obtained drug resistance without protein expression changes but instead with an increase in efflux activity [5]. Both of these conditions lead to the idea that chemotherapeutics have limited permeability, reduced binding to their desired active site, and thus provide lowered effectiveness for treatment.

Other proposed ideas that have led to disease pathology is P-gp down-regulation or reduced function. When efflux is reduced in tissues, clearance of substances and drugs from inside the cell becomes inefficient. The protein is unable to effectively serve its protective role in regulating the passage of compounds by eliminating out of the cell section. While studying the BBB research, it has indicated that when the protein is down-regulated, or the clearance rate is reduced, there is improper removal of cellular by-products. With inappropriate regulation, abnormal accumulation of cellular products concentrates in the brain. This overproduction can cause cell death and disease pathogenesis [6]. Again, it is not well understood if modifications in the environment the cause of P-gp down expression or reduced function or if the protein's alterations are the cause of the change in the tissue environment.

Pathophysiology of Various Diseases Related to P-gp

P-glycoprotein has been the most studied and well-characterized multi-drug resistant receptor transporter due to its high expression in cancer cells and its resistance to chemotherapy. Despite the protective nature in healthy cells, P-gp capabilities involve efflux of drug molecules exiting cancer cells leading to lowered chemotherapy effectiveness. One study provided 118 compounds on cancer cell lines in which more than almost 95% of the compounds had an inverse correlation between P-gp expression and drug sensitivity [7]. Some cancers, such as melanoma and renal cancer, show to have high P-gp expression from the beginning. At the same time, other solid tumours induce the protein's expression as a response to cancer drugs. During protein upregulation in the tumour's environment, there are several triggers, including inflammatory stressors, intrinsic cancer genomic instability and epigenetic mechanisms [7]. These triggers cause genes (oncogenes) that generally are the 'gate-keepers' against cancer instead tend to malfunction while promoting P-gp on the cell membrane. It has also been reported that transcriptional factors of cancer cells promote the transition of epithelial cells to mesenchymal cells and again induce P-gp expression [2]. Propositions of increased protein activity have also been showcased in lung cancer cells that acquired MDR but had an increase in efflux activity versus expression due to activation of a specific transcription factor, Snail [2]. It is not entirely sure this is the primary mechanism that P-gp enhancement aids in tumour progression. However, initial treatment with chemotherapy drugs has also played a role in inducing P-gp expression and activity (Table 1). These drug molecules seem to be ideal substrates for the protein transporter to remove them from inside the cancer cell while also "informing" the cell to adapt to its new conditions to survive. Alterations in p-gp genes are also considered to play a role because of instability in mRNA secondary structure [2]. This results in change in membrane insertion and structural orientation producing a variety of substrate affinity.

P-glycoprotein has also faced a role in pathology in the gastrointestinal (GI) system. The GI is continuously up against numerous foreign or potentially harmful substances which lead to changes in intestinal microbiota, mucosal immune responses, disrupt tissue composition, and impair tissue regeneration [8]. P-gp expression and function in the GI vary depending on the location of the tract it is located. The protein can be modulated by internal and external factors such as the intestinal cells activity and material from the surrounding environment. One such case is with ulcerative colitis which exhibits acute intestinal inflammation and leading an immune response to an inflammatory signaling protein, tumour necrosis factor-alpha (TNF-α) [8]. Increased TNF-α in the mucosa suppresses transcription and formation of the P-gp transporter, thus impairing xenobiotic efflux. TNF-α expression prevents the P-gp role in limiting tissue invasion from common bacteria such as Listeria monocytogenes (responsible for Listeriosis/Listeria) or Salmonella typhimurium (responsible for Salmonella) [8]. Overall, with impaired P-gp pump activity, the gut microbiome develops a lower threshold for microbiome imbalances and pro-inflammatory conditions.

Alzheimer's disease (AD) has become the most frequent root of dementia in the ageing population. Research has shown that an accumulation of protein material called beta-amyloid plaques in the brain contribute to the pathogenesis of AD. Due to plaque accumulation, the brain goes through what is called oxidative stress, which promotes the progression of Alzheimer's [6]. Two conclusions as to why these plaques accumulate are (1) the overproduction of beta-amyloid peptide in the brain and (2) the elimination of the peptide out the brain through transporters [6]. Different types of neurons in the central nervous system have multiple transporters, including P-glycoprotein and in high numbers. This transporter has become very important in exporting internal compounds and toxic agents, making P-gp a powerful gate-keeper for the brain. Few studies state that oxidative stress leading as a signal transduction intermediate promoting cell survival, which causes increased MDR1 expression. Despite this phenomenon, experiments have also demonstrated that if enough amyloid-beta plaques are assembled in the blood-brain barrier, this can induce P-gp degradation and reduction [9]. This degradation was proposed to be caused by the ubiquitin-proteasome pathway, which involves tagging protein with -Ub (ubiquitin) resulting in the degradation of the tagged protein. Amyloid-beta protein in the early stages of AD triggers this ubiquitination and degradation process, which leads to the reduction of P-gp expression and activity level [9]. The amyloid-beta accumulation in the brain capillaries, compromising the BBB integrity, and further causing neuronal damage and AD progression. The overall modulator of P-gp in pathology is still very complex and not well understood. While numerous experiments have been conducted, all existing studies have only been conducted *in vitro* and have yet to be observed similarly *in vivo*. However, future studies have shown promise in understanding P-gp's role in normal conditions and in malignancy.

Table 1. Chemotherapeutic drugs role in inducing P-gp expression and activity. These drug molecules are acting as ideal substrates for P-gp transporter [3]

MDR transporter inhibitory agents	P-gp substrates	MDR drugs interacting P-gp
Verapamil (Calcium channel blocker)	Cortisol (Steroid Hormone)	Daunorubicin
Azodipine (Calcium channel blocker)	IL-2	Epirubicin
Cyclosporin A (immuno-suppressive agent)	-	Mitomycin C
Flupentixol	INF-γ	Etoposide
FK 506	-	Paclitaxel
Nifedipin	Aldosterone (Steroid Hormone)	Doxorubicin
Progestron	Sphingolipids	Teniposide
Megestrol acetate	-	Vinblastine
Quinine	IL-4	Mitoxantrone
Tamoxifen	-	Vincristine
PSC 833	-	Actinomycin D
280-446	-	Topotecan

Signaling Transduction

The existence of many P-gp Inhibitors and several signal transduction routes provided has generated problems to assess the most appropriate therapy for MDR (multi-drug resistance) mediated by P-gp [10]. The pathways for signaling transduction are regulated by the signaling linking of agents to membrane proteins, causing cytoplasmic protein activation, which ultimately activates transcription factors [10]. Various signaling pathways and transcriptional factors (Figure 4) [11], including the Ras-mediated pathway, Pka or Camp pathway, are known to show expression in P-gp mediated MDR [12-14]. MDR is typically induced by overexpression of specific ATP-dependent efflux transporter pumps in the cancer patients non-responsive to chemotherapy. These pumps reside on the cytosol side of the cell membrane, leading to increase drug efflux from the resistant cell. Several experiments utilizing a wide variety of tumor cell lines and chemotherapeutic drugs have shown that ABC family cell transportation proteins help the movement of drugs across and their intracellular aggregation to successful concentrations in the cell membrane [15]. P-gp is capable of transporting both cytotoxic and amphiphilic, benign or cationic substances, and is found in tissues including the ingestion, synthesis and action of substances and environmental toxins [10]. High levels of P-gp are associated with decreased drug accumulation intracellularly, and the MDR phenotype, P-gp acts as a barrier, dropping intracellular chemical dosage concentration toward concentration gradients through active efflux [16, 17].

The drug molecule is expected to be able to cohere to a particular site within P-gp and via ATP hydrolysis is subsequently excreted out of the cell. Consequently, P-gp inhibitors can provide effective treatment for MDR [18]. P-gp is encoded by the gene ABCB1 in humans and is considered to be the result of an internal replication of the primordial series [19]. The P-gp evolution is controlled both by the stage of protein synthesis and by alternative processing, indicating that transcription interactions at the genetic level may play an intermediate role in the modification from Promoter-related P-gp region to Essential Transcription Machinery. Several experiments report P-gp behavior may be explicitly affected by its genetic expression, regulated by drug-responsive activation of ABCB1 [20]. However, search results support an acquired model of P-gp expression involving activation of ABCB1 but still little is understood about the process involved. Investigations were analyzing the signal cross-talk in transcriptional control of gene ABCB1's depicts ABCB1 is a Ras/Raf signaling pathway target [20, 21].

Possible best-described signal transduction mechanism in cell biology is Ras/ MAPK, known initially as an extracellular signal-regulated kinase (ERK). It has analyzed that cytotoxic anticancer drugs cause tension trajectories via the MAPK / MAPK kinase system (MAPKK) consisting of three consecutive kinases [12]. Specifications MAPK pathway inhibitors crucially decreased lifespan. MDR cancer cells (ABCB1 / Pgp), Suggesting that pathways activate the over-expression of ABCB1 / Pgp is Phenotype specific to MDR [22, 23]. Comprising as one of the members of the MAPK family is JNK (referred to as c-Jun NH2-terminal kinase) which binds and phosphorylate the transcription factor c-Jun's NH2-terminal activation domain. There is evidence that JNK will modulate the MDR phenotype expression [24-26]. In P-gp associated variants obtained from human cervical carcinoma cell line KB-3JNK, JNK is present in heavily active form. This presence demonstrates JNK expression may be a significant feature of cellular reaction to many anticancer drugs and help in the production of the MDR phenotype [27]. The upregulation of the MAP3K1 gene activates JNK selectively in the human cell line, subsequently resulting in increased levels of the ABCB1 mRNA and P-gp protein [28]. Various reports have been conducted, which says that the JNK signaling route may be Employed in the management of ABCB1 operations and P-gp [26, 29].

In the production of the ABCB1 / P-gp induced MDR phenotype, the functions of cAMP-dependent PKA and its activator cAMP were extensively studied. It is observed that by adenylyl cyclase, from ATP, the cAMP synthesis occurs and will rapidly break down by cAMP phosphodiesterase through hydrolysis to 5′-monophosphate adenosine (5′-AMP) [30]. Numbers of extracellular signals lead to CAMP-dependent PKA-related Activation Proteins, which could trigger the Multi specific MDR1 [13]. Activation of ABCB1 takes place in primary rat through a Camp dependent PKA pathway Hepatocytes, indicating that the ABCB1 / Pgp expression is modulated by cAMP / PKA phosphatase activity [14]. CAMP and PKA are both considered to influence MAPK58 and PI3K / Akt59 signaling [31, 32]. The mechanism of PI3 K signaling is known to affect drug resistance. While K-Ras induced MDR may need PI3 K activation, initial studies indicate that impediment of PI3 K signaling single-handed does not effectively treat ABCB1 / P-gp mediated MDR in vitro [33]. Control of the ABCB1 / P-gp-induced MDR phenotype is implicated in numerous signal inducing transduction mechanisms, various TF (transcription factors) and molecular processes. Progress in understanding the pathways that control the expression of ABCB1 has provided prospective targets for novel therapeutic intervention [10].

Pathway of P-gp Intracellular Trafficking

Intracellular trafficking pathways and the involvement of various Rab proteins of P-gp depending upon cell polarisation and primary culture choice, cell culture choice, and cell culture line or neoplasm. The accumulation of P-gp within the cell and increased levels of the chemotherapeutic drug are led by the disruption of P-gp trafficking into the plasma membrane. The trafficking comprises of a possible approach to resolving P-gp-mediated MDR in cancer. Studies of polarized as well as non-polarized cells by confocal microscopy found P-gp location in the plasma membrane and the endoplasmic reticulum (ER) of a cell, Golgi apparatus, multiple endosomes, and lysosomes [34]. For newly synthesized proteins, the ER acts as entry point leading to the secretory pathway. Folding factor and molecular chaperons were found in the ER lumen [35]. P-gp is synthesized and is correlated with calnexin and Hsc70 (comprised of 150 kDa core-glycosylated intermediate protein) during folding.

Golgi has a subsequent role in glycolipid biosynthesis. Misfolded P-gp can be degenrated quickly with proteasome-mediated degradation [36-38]. For further glycosylation, Hsc70 transfers to the Golgi (comprised of a 170 kDa mature protein) after sufficient folding in the ER although the P-gp movement from ER to Golgi is not apparent [39-41]. Current newly active proteins are, however, obtained by the cis-Golgi network from the ER, which is likely analogous to the ER-Golgi intermediate compartment. In contrast, post-translational changes exist in the trans-Golgi network (TGN)

[42]. Membrane proteins can use n glycan chains as sorting determinants that may arise with P-gp [43]. In distinct possible outcomes, membrane proteins which are at infancy can be passed to the plasma membrane, [44]. The co-localization of P-gp with EEA1 and Rab5 positively happens at early endosomes in non-polarized human cancer cells, suggesting that the endosomal pathway includes P-gp implementation to the plasma membrane.

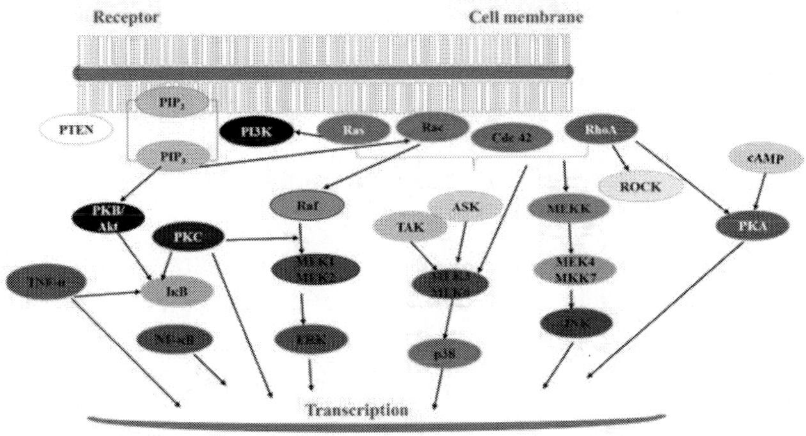

Figure 4. Signal transduction pathway and transcriptional mechanism in cancer cells [11].

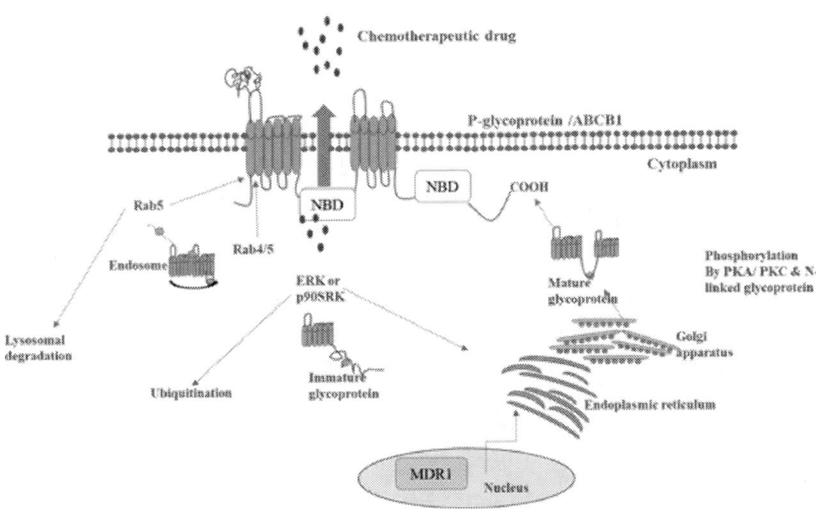

Figure 5. Regulation of P-gp/ABCB1/MDR in cancer cells [47].

Further, through an intracellular endosome pool, P-gp can directly or indirectly transfer to the apical domain in both non-polarized and polarized cells [45]. For the study of protein trafficking and endocytosis, inhibitors such as Concanamycin A, Brefeldin A and destruxin B, mycophenolic acid, a GTP synthesis inhibitor, were used [46]. P-gp traffic disruption can deliver a new method for overcoming and restricting MDR in cancer as studies are expected to scrutinize unique drug efficient-therapeutic sites. To consider the intracellular cycling and regulatory targets of P-gp molecular and cellular pathways [34].

Post-translational Moifications of Transporters

Post-translational modifications modulate the functional expression of drug transporters through a wide variety of molecular processes. These modifications may occur by the incorporation of a small protein (e.g., ubiquitination), a functional group (e.g., phosphorylation), or lipids (e.g., palmitoylation), sugar chains (e.g., glycosylation), on residues of amino acids that are accessible by solvent (Figure 6) [48]. The phosphorylation of proteins requires inserting a terminal phosphate Group on the side chains of predominantly serine and threonine residues of free hydroxyl and, to a lesser degree, on tyrosine residues [48]. It was shown that P-gp binds to tubulins with a high binding affinity to two regions in the Serine-enriched linker-domain. Still, it is unclear if the status of serine phosphorylation is crucial to the interaction [49].

The process of N-glycosylation is the mechanism of adding extracellular asparagine residues through enzymes to an oligosaccharide and is often demonstrated by the motif N-X-S / T, where X acts as any amino acid except proline (P) or aspartic acid. Phosphorylation by Pim-1 selectively modulates mature P-gp glycoform. This process appears to be able to facilitate the complete glycosylation of immature P-gp glycoforms and to facilitate surface translocation [48]. Pim-1 inhibitors are hypothesized to enhance drug tolerance To inhibit the maturation of the glycan chain of P-gp and to reduce the breakdown of the infant protein of P-gp [50]. In the first MSD also referred as multi-spanning domain, the extracellular loop of the second Multidrug resistance-associated Protein 4 (MRP4; ABCC4) represents two N-glycosylation sites [48]. Combining investigations with MRPs show that N-glycosylation may impair binding affinity and overall transport processes, but further explanations are required to decide whether this regulatory process is due to minor conformation changes or by more composite tools such as PTM cross-talk [48]. A changeable modification found on the ε-amino group of intracellular lysine is lysine acetylation. As a complex PTM response to changes in a complicated process, it has been implicated, and changed sites can be conserved between organisms [48]. Lundby and co-worker's proteomics results show that several ABC transporters can be acetylated; but for others, the functional importance remains unclear [51].

Palmitoylation implies the enzymatic attachment of an unbound Cys (cysteine) remained adjacent to the protein-lipid interface of C16 saturated fatty acid and palmitic acid [52, 53]. There are different signaling pathways, including lipid modifications such as palmitoylation, to efficiently target transporters to the plasma membrane [48]. In cholesterol efflux regulatory protein, there are four total cysteine residues palmitoylated in the C1110 and C1111 linker region-, C3 and C23 in the N-terminal region. ABCG1 is palmitoylated with, C150, C26, C311, C390, and C402 in its N-terminal domain. On the contrary, ABCA1, where several residues of palmitoylation are considered essential to expression, ABCG1 seems to have a functional role in C311 [48]. For the signaling and eventual degradation, the pathway of ubiquitin-proteasome is a physiological process via the proteasome of non-stable proteins. Ub (Ubiquitin), is an 8kDa polypeptide which is small in size and is covalently bound to available residues of lysine. For the degradative destiny of internalized ABC transporters, ubiquitination is always a mandatory step. In vitro, degradation of P-gp is facilitated by restricting of MAPK pathways in cancer cell lines and mediated by the ubiquitin-proteasome course, leading to increased resistance to chemotherapy [48]. It is to be noted that E2 ligase, which indirectly interacts with P-gp along with E3 ligase, was not immunopurified and was detected by MALDI-TOF analysis [48]. Although regulation of signaling pathways is quickly interfaced as a crucial functional facet for homeostatic processes functional integrity, there is still little evidence of effects on proteins affect from transporters. Also, the fate of the carrier after a post-translational occurrence does not necessarily lead to drastic impacts, such as deterioration.

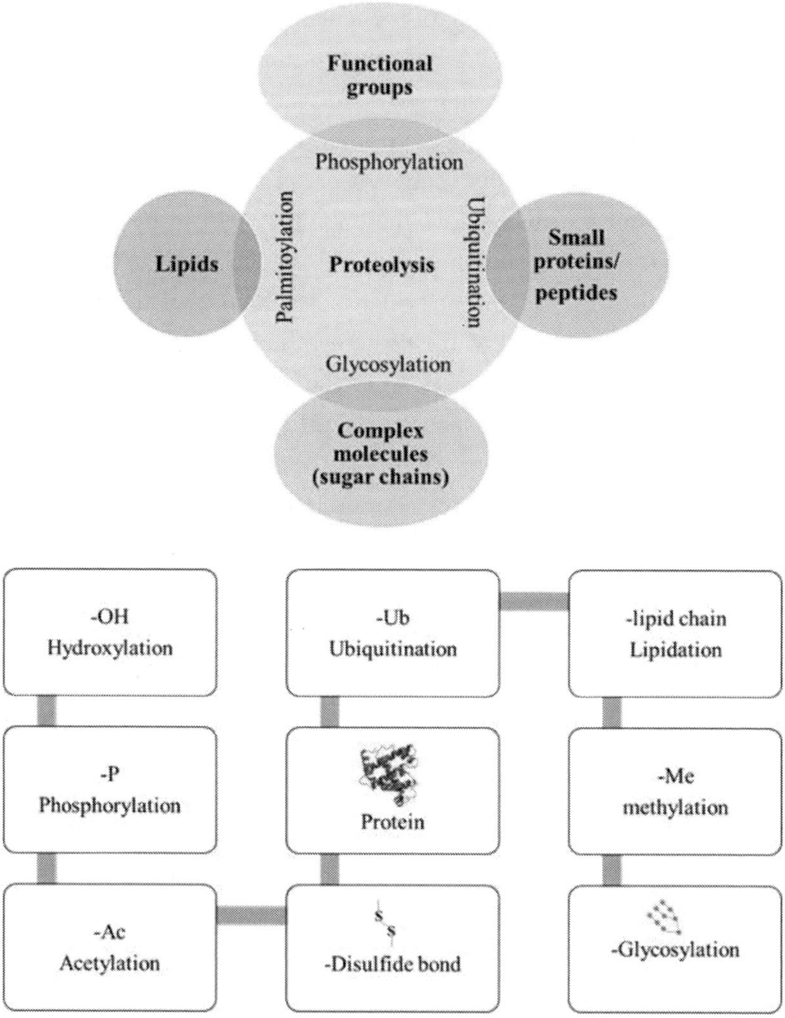

Figure 6. Strategies and types of post-translational modifications.

Conclusion

Multi-drug resistance as an outcome is reported to be a complex mechanism comprising of profound strategies in the treatment of cancer patients. P-gp is, however, most focused and studied out of many resistance mechanisms. The success as therapeutic modulator remains in the circumference of P-gp expression level and its tool in the tumour activity. Many studies suggest the expression of P-gp involves signaling pathways at cellular levels associated with transcriptional factors. These can be enzymes such as ubiquitinated enzymes, chaperons and kinases, which overall regulate the activity of cells towards chemotherapeutic drugs influencing sensitivity and function of P-glycoprotein. The reduced sensitivity to drugs/ therapy is subjected to a variety of processes such as the increase in drug efflux, transduction signaling, reduced drug uptake, DNA repairing and increased expression of plasma membrane drug efflux pumps. The modulation during drug binding sites towards P-gp has a unique pattern for each drug. Since ABC transporter are involved in MDR and P-gp remains the prominent member referred to as ATP-binding cassette (ABC transporter), it facilitates the efflux of almost all the drugs. This transporter plays an essential role in absorption of particular drug, distribution and removal procedure.

Nevertheless, transporter expression, as well as function, influences the development or deterioration of several diseases. Therefore, the P-gp transporter has shown some significance as MDR1 has contributed to the cause and consequence of some diseases such as cancers, tumours, immune-mediating inflammatory disorders, and brain diseases such as major depressive disorder and Alzheimer's in disease pathology. Due to its nature, this protein is a novel protective barrier mechanism that cells use against incompatible and toxic substances to prevent damage or injury to tissues. Therefore, P-gp is found to be expressed in various normal cells and protects them from harmful substances, as many clinical studies are ongoing to understand the mechanism behind functional characteristics of P-gp. The protein's mode of action has also been counterintuitive when it comes to drug administration, distribution, absorption, and elimination (ADME) characteristics. The protein's protective nature stops the intake of xenobiotics from entering into the human cell, which can cause a decrease in drug effectiveness, enhanced drug elimination, and limited drug distribution. P-gp is found to be localized at the apical side of brain endothelium, limited exposure to xenobiotics since numerous substrates binds to P-gp, this protein in defense prevents them from travelling across CNS. The challenge being the down-regulation of P-gp outcome in increasing concentration of the toxic substance in CNS, leading to side-effects. So, as per reports and studies investigated, P-gp is known to be a dominant efflux transporter. The upregulation of these P-gp transporters leads to reduced effectiveness of therapies targeting site at CNS. The studies also suggest investigating transporters specificity for substrate when delivering or targeting drugs for brain-related diseases. This also concludes to regulate transporter behavioural mechanism and expression of a particular drug and disease specificity in overcoming P-gp mediated therapy resistance or MDR. Therefore, to overcome MDR P-gp substrate, inhibitory agents are identified which regulates signaling pathways, localization, stability, degradation, expression and activity of P-gp in various diseases. These studies perhaps, will provide the clinical guidance against chemoresistance. The expression and function of P-gp are regulated by multiple factors including polymorphism, the interaction of the drug with cellular background, genetics and more importantly, disease pathology. P-gp mediates cellular drug efflux and uptake depending upon expression and function, which as a result of this regulates and optimize treatment response against pathologies. The investigations in the field of proteomics and pharmacokinetic modelling with changes in transporter expression levels will impact the pharmacokinetics of drugs and its treatment strategies.

REFERENCES

[1] Sharom, F. J., Complex interplay between the P-glycoprotein multidrug efflux pump and the membrane: its role in modulating protein function. *Frontiers in oncology,* 2014. 4: p. 41.

[2] Dewanjee, S., et al., Natural products as alternative choices for P-glycoprotein (P-gp) inhibition. *Molecules*, 2017. 22(6): p. 871.

[3] Gustav, L., P-glycoprotein as a Drug Target in the Treatment of Multidrug Resistant Cancer. *Current Drug Targets,* 2000. 1(1): p. 85-99.

[4] Atilano-Roque, A., et al., Effect of disease pathologies on transporter expression and function. *The Journal of Clinical Pharmacology*, 2016. 56: p. S205-S221.

[5] Yano, K., T. Tomono, and T. Ogihara, Advances in studies of P-glycoprotein and its expression regulators. *Biological and Pharmaceutical Bulletin*, 2018. 41(1): p. 11-19.

[6] Sita, G., et al., *P-glycoprotein (ABCB1) and oxidative stress: Focus on Alzheimer's disease*. Oxidative Medicine and Cellular Longevity, 2017. 2017.

[7] Robinson, K. and V. Tiriveedhi, Perplexing Role of P-Glycoprotein in Tumor Microenvironment. *Frontiers in Oncology*, 2020. 10: p. 265.

[8] Cario, E., P-glycoprotein multidrug transporter in inflammatory bowel diseases: More questions than answers. *World journal of gastroenterology*, 2017. 23(9): p. 1513.

[9] Chai, A. B., et al., P-glycoprotein: a role in the export of amyloid-β in Alzheimer's disease? *The FEBS journal*, 2020. 287(4): p. 612-625.

[10] Sui, H., Z. Fan, and Q. Li, Signal transduction pathways and transcriptional mechanisms of ABCB1/Pgp-mediated multiple drug resistance in human cancer cells. *Journal of International Medical Research*, 2012. 40(2): p. 426-435.

[11] Sui, H., Z.-Z. Fan, and Q. Li, Signal Transduction Pathways and Transcriptional Mechanisms of ABCB1/Pgp-mediated Multiple Drug Resistance in Human Cancer Cells. *Journal of International Medical Research*, 2012. 40: p. 426 - 435.

[12] Nakagami, H., et al., A mitogen-activated protein kinase kinase kinase mediates reactive oxygen species homeostasis in Arabidopsis. *Journal of Biological Chemistry*, 2006. 281(50): p. 38697-38704.

[13] Rohlff, C. and R. I. Glazer, Regulation of multidrug resistance through the cAMP and EGF signalling pathways. *Cellular signalling*, 1995. 7(5): p. 431-443.

[14] Ziemann, C., et al., The role of prostaglandin E receptor-dependent signaling via cAMP in Mdr1b gene activation in primary rat hepatocyte cultures. *Journal of Pharmacology and Experimental Therapeutics*, 2006. 317(1): p. 378-386.

[15] Ozben, T., Mechanisms and strategies to overcome multiple drug resistance in cancer. *FEBS letters*, 2006. 580(12): p. 2903-2909.

[16] De Vries, E. F., et al., Can celecoxib affect P-glycoprotein-mediated drug efflux? A microPET study. *Nuclear medicine and biology*, 2008. 35(4): p. 459-466.

[17] Stavrovskaya, A., Cellular mechanisms of multidrug resistance of tumor cells. *Biochemistry c/c of Biokhimiia*, 2000. 65(1): p. 95-106.

[18] Klappe, K., et al., Lipid dependence of ABC transporter localization and function. *Chemistry and Physics of Lipids*, 2009. 161(2): p. 57-64.

[19] Chen, C.-j., et al., Internal duplication and homology with bacterial transport proteins in the mdr1 (P-glycoprotein) gene from multidrug-resistant human cells. *Cell*, 1986. 47(3): p. 381-389.

[20] Vasconcelos, F. C., et al., Variation of MDR proteins expression and activity levels according to clinical status and evolution of CML patients. *Cytometry Part B: Clinical Cytometry*, 2011. 80(3): p. 158-166.

[21] Miltenberger, R. J., et al., v-Raf activates transcription of growth-responsive promoters via GC-rich sequences that bind the transcription factor Sp1. Cell Growth & Differentiation: *the Molecular Biology Journal of the American Association for Cancer Research,* 1995. 6(5): p. 549-556.

[22] Duraj, J., et al., Flavonoid quercetin, but not apigenin or luteolin, induced apoptosis in human myeloid leukemia cells and their resistant variants. *Neoplasma*, 2005. 52(4): p. 273.

[23] Kisucka, J., et al., Reversal effect of specific inhibitors of extracellular-signal regulated protein kinase pathway on P-

glycoprotein mediated vincristine resistance of L1210 cells. *General physiology and biophysics*, 2001. 20(4): p. 439-444.
[24] Weston, C. R. and R. J. Davis, Signaling specificity--a complex affair. *Science*, 2001. 292(5526): p. 2439-2440.
[25] Lagadinou, E., et al., c-Jun N-terminal kinase activation failure is a new mechanism of anthracycline resistance in acute myeloid leukemia. *Leukemia*, 2008. 22(10): p. 1899-1908.
[26] Bark, H. and C.-H. Choi, PSC833, cyclosporine analogue, downregulates MDR1 expression by activating JNK/c-Jun/AP-1 and suppressing NF-κB. *Cancer chemotherapy and pharmacology*, 2010. 65(6): p. 1131-1136.
[27] Osborn, M. T. and T. C. Chambers, Role of the stress-activated/c-Jun NH2-terminal protein kinase pathway in the cellular response to adriamycin and other chemotherapeutic drugs. *Journal of Biological Chemistry*, 1996. 271(48): p. 30950-30955.
[28] Comerford, K. M., E. P. Cummins, and C. T. Taylor, c-Jun NH2-Terminal Kinase Activation Contributes to Hypoxia-Inducible Factor 1α–Dependent P-Glycoprotein Expression in Hypoxia. *Cancer research*, 2004. 64(24): p. 9057-9061.
[29] Sui, H., et al., COX-2 contributes to P-glycoprotein-mediated multidrug resistance via phosphorylation of c-Jun at Ser63/73 in colorectal cancer. *Carcinogenesis*, 2011. 32(5): p. 667-675.
[30] Merkle, D. and R. Hoffmann, Roles of cAMP and cAMP-dependent protein kinase in the progression of prostate cancer: cross-talk with the androgen receptor. *Cellular signalling*, 2011. 23(3): p. 507-515.
[31] Misra, U. K. and S. V. Pizzo, Epac1-induced cellular proliferation in prostate cancer cells is mediated by B-Raf/ERK and mTOR signaling cascades. *Journal of cellular biochemistry*, 2009. 108(4): p. 998-1011.
[32] Leone, V., et al., PGE2 inhibits apoptosis in human adenocarcinoma Caco-2 cell line through Ras-PI3K association and cAMP-dependent kinase A activation. *American Journal of Physiology-Gastrointestinal and Liver Physiology*, 2007. 293(4): p. G673-G681.
[33] Lee, J. T., et al., *Roles of the RAF/MEK/ERK and PI3K/PTEN/AKT pathways in malignant transformation and drug resistance.*

[34] Fu, D. and I. M. Arias, Intracellular trafficking of P-glycoprotein. *The International Journal of Biochemistry & Cell Biology*, 2012. 44(3): p. 461-464.

[35] High, S., et al., Glycoprotein folding in the endoplasmic reticulum: a tale of three chaperones? *FEBS Letters*, 2000. 476(1-2): p. 38-41.

[36] Horwich, A. L., Protein folding in the cell: an inside story. *Nature Medicine*, 2011. 17(10): p. 1211-1216.

[37] Loo, T. W. and D. M. Clarke, Correction of Defective Protein Kinesis of Human P-glycoprotein Mutants by Substrates and Modulators. *Journal of Biological Chemistry*, 1997. 272(2): p. 709-712.

[38] Goldberg, A. L., Protein degradation and protection against misfolded or damaged proteins. *Nature*, 2003. 426(6968): p. 895-899.

[39] Molinari, A., et al., P-glycoprotein expression in the Golgi apparatus of multidrug-resistant cells. *International Journal of Cancer*, 1994. 59(6): p. 789-795.

[40] Tanaka, A. R., et al., The ABCA1 Q597R mutant undergoes trafficking from the ER upon ER stress. *Biochemical and Biophysical Research Communications,* 2008. 369(4): p. 1174-1178.

[41] Ameen, N., M. Silvis, and N. A. Bradbury, Endocytic trafficking of CFTR in health and disease. *Journal of Cystic Fibrosis*, 2007. 6(1): p. 1-14.

[42] Presley, J. F., et al., ER-to-Golgi transport visualized in living cells. *Nature*, 1997. 389(6646): p. 81-85.

[43] Mohamed, L. A., J. N. Keller, and A. Kaddoumi, Role of P-glycoprotein in mediating rivastigmine effect on amyloid-β brain load and related pathology in Alzheimer's disease mouse model. *Biochimica et Biophysica Acta (BBA) - Molecular Basis of Disease*, 2016. 1862(4): p. 778-787.

[44] Kipp, H. and I.M. Arias, Newly Synthesized Canalicular ABC Transporters Are Directly Targeted from the Golgi to the Hepatocyte Apical Domain in Rat Liver. Journal of Biological Chemistry, 2000. 275(21): p. 15917-15925.

[45] Fu, D. and B. D. Roufogalis, Actin disruption inhibits endosomal traffic of P-glycoprotein-EGFP and resistance to daunorubicin

accumulation. *American Journal of Physiology-Cell Physiology*, 2007. 292(4): p. C1543-C1552.

[46] Fu, D. and I. Arias, Intracellular trafficking of P-glycoprotein. *The international journal of biochemistry & cell biology*, 2011. 44: p. 461-4.

[47] Katayama, K., K. Noguchi, and Y. Sugimoto, Regulations of P-Glycoprotein/ABCB1/MDR1 in Human Cancer Cells. *New Journal of Science*, 2014. 2014: p. 476974.

[48] Czuba, L. C., K. M. Hillgren, and P. W. Swaan, Post-translational modifications of transporters. *Pharmacology & Therapeutics*, 2018. 192: p. 88-99.

[49] Georges, E., The P-Glycoprotein (ABCB1) Linker Domain Encodes High-Affinity Binding Sequences to α- and β-Tubulins. *Biochemistry*, 2007. 46(25): p. 7337-7342.

[50] Xie, Y., et al., Pim-1 kinase protects P-glycoprotein from degradation and enables its glycosylation and cell surface expression. *Molecular Pharmacology*, 2010: p. mol.109.061713.

[51] Lundby, A., et al., Proteomic analysis of lysine acetylation sites in rat tissues reveals organ specificity and subcellular patterns. *Cell reports*, 2012. 2(2): p. 419-431.

[52] Guan, X. and C. A. Fierke, Understanding protein palmitoylation: Biological significance and enzymology. *Science China Chemistry*, 2011. 54(12): p. 1888-1897.

[53] Dietrich, L. E. P. and C. Ungermann, On the mechanism of protein palmitoylation. *EMBO reports*, 2004. 5(11): p. 1053-1057.

In: An Introduction to P-Glycoprotein ISBN: 978-1-53619-488-3
Editors: M. Wahajuddin et al.

Chapter 4

Mechanistic Comprehension towards the Role of P-Glycoprotein in Limiting the Pharmacokinetic and Pharmacological Efficacy of Drugs

Swati Chaturvedi[1,2], Nazneen Sultana[1], Mamunur Rashid[1], Divya Chauhan[1], Zaiba Naseem[3], Ravindra Varma Alluri[4] and M. Wahajuddin[1,2,*]

[1]Pharmaceutics and Pharmacokinetics Division,
CSIR - Central Drug Research Institute, Lucknow, India
[2]Academy of Scientific and Innovative Research (AcSIR),
Ghaziabad, India
[3]Faculty of Pharmacy, Integral University,
Lucknow, Uttar Pradesh, India
[4]Systems Medicine, Clinical Pharmacology and Safety Sciences,
R&D AstraZeneca, Cambridge, UK

---

* Corresponding Author's Email: wahajuddin@gmail.com.

ABSTRACT

P-glycoprotein (P-gp), a well explored efflux transporter associated with multidrug resistance is expressed at the cellular membrane of all major drug eliminating organs. Several structurally diverse endogenous molecules and xenobiotics are substrates for P-gp. Due to its importance in limiting the pharmacokinetic and therapeutic response of a drugs, P-gp has been considered as crucial facet during the early phase of drug discovery and development programmes. Functional modulation of P-gp determines the drug to be a pharmacologically active and successful candidate molecule in future. Further, the relative contribution of P-gp against number of diseases and disorders has appended it as a powerful tool towards the pre-clinical and clinical management for any health infirmity. Due to its role in modulating drug disposition or altering bioavailability, P-gp transporter have gained interest of researchers to target it for drug development process. This could be accomplished either by non-competitive or competitive inhibition of P-gp transporter thereby regulating the bioavailability of drug and consequently the optimal concentration could reach the target site. Moreover, P-gp has also been reported to be involved in potential drug-drug interaction i.e., the pharmacokinetic interaction of two active moieties that directly proportionate the hindrance in their pharmacological and toxicological effect. The present chapter will review the recent literature focusing on the basic, structural, functional and pathophysiological role of P-gp and targeted drugs during pre-clinical and clinical drug discovery and development process.

Keywords: P-glycoprotein, transporter, pharmacokinetic, pharmacodynamics, drug-drug interaction, herb-drug interaction

INTRODUCTION AND BACKGROUND

Adenosine triphosphate (ATP) binding cassette (ABC) transporters comprise an extremely diverse class of membrane proteins, that utilizes energy derived from ATP hydrolysis to efflux substrates across biological membranes. P-glycoprotein (P-gp), also commonly referred to as ATP-binding cassette sub-family B member 1 (ABCB1) or multidrug resistance 1 (MDR1) protein is the foremost characterized efflux transporter associated with multidrug resistance (MDR) in humans. P-gp was first identified in cancer cells and its expression is correlated with MDR in different cancer types (Ref). Apart from cancerous cells, P-gp is expressed in all major drug eliminating organs such as the intestine (apical membrane of enterocytes), liver (bile canaliculi of hepatocytes), kidney (apical surface of proximal convoluted tubular cells) and blood brain barrier (BBB) (apical surface of endothelial cells) (Schinkel 1999). Additionally P-gp is also expressed in several other organs and tissues such as lungs, heart, testis, adrenals, prostrate, skin, spleen and skeletal muscle (Thiebut et al. 1987). Due to its ubiquitous expression, P-gp plays a protective role against the entry of xenobiotics into the body. For orally administered drugs, P-gp can limit bioavailability of its substrates, thereby leading to sub-optimal exposures and pharmacological efficacy. Additionally P-gp can also impact distribution, metabolism and elimination of drug molecules (Lin, 2003). Therefore, modulation of P-gp needs to be carefully considered as it can lead to desirable (increased exposures and efficacy) or undesirable (toxicity) effects.

In the present chapter the authors have discussed the structure and function of P-gp, its pharmacokinetic and pharmacological relevance including the drug-drug interactions.

Structure and Function of P-gp

P-gp is a 170 kDa molecular weight transmembrane glycoprotein consisting of 1276-1280 amino acids, encoded by MDR1 gene. The most commonly accepted model of P-gp consists of two pseudo-symmetric halves, each half containing a hydrophilic nucleotide binding domain (NBD) and six hydrophobic transmembrane domains (TMD) which includes 10-15 kDa of N-terminal glycosylation N-linked glycosylation (NLG) is a complicated biosynthetic method that regulates the maturation of proteins via the secretory pathway. This co-translational modification is regulated with the aid of a series of enzymatic reactions, which effects in the transfer of a core glycan from the lipid carrier to a protein substrate (Galban, Galbán et al. 2010). The N and C-terminal are organized into 6 transmembrane domains (TMD) being hydrophobic in nature and a hydrophilic nucleotide binding domain that are joined by a 60 amino acid. The two ATP binding domains of P-gp are known as nucleotide-binding folds (NBFs), located in the cytoplasm to transport the substrates across the membranes (Li, Yuan et al. 2010, Mollazadeh, Sahebkar et al. 2018). These pumps are mostly unidirectional containing three regions: Walker A, B, and signature C motifs. Among these, signature C motifs is thought to accelerate ATP hydrolysis and the transduction of the energy of ATP hydrolysis to the conformational changes in the membrane. Contrasting to ATP-bindings sites that are present at Walker A motifs, P-gp had substrate binding sites throughout the transmembrane domains. The major drug-binding sites resides in TM6 and TM12 and TM1, TM4, TM10, and TM11. Amino acids attached to TM1 forms binding pocket that plays a pivotal role in determining the suitable P-gp substrate size and glycoside residues attached to TM 2 and TM 3 determines the P-gp substrate specificity. Other TM2/11 domains ensures that the drug-binding pocket must be enclosed at the cytoplasmic side of P-gp. Additionally, intracellular loops and even ATP binding domains also had the drug binding sites (Kim and Chen 2018).

P-GP AND DRUG PHARMACOKINETICS/BIOAVAILABILITY

Pharmacokinetics is the study of the time course of drug absorption, distribution, metabolism and excretion. It concerns the relationship of these processes to the intensity and time course of pharmacologic response (efficacy and toxicity) of drugs (Leveque and Jehl 1995). The first step, i.e., the rate and extent of oral absorption is largely dependent on solubility, permeability and dissolution properties of drug molecules. However, P-gp expressed on the apical membrane of enterocytes can also limit oral absorption of its substrates by actively pumping drug molecules from cytosol back into intestinal lumen (Figure 1), thereby reducing portal bioavailability. For dual substrates, P-gp and CYP3A4 interplay can influence the amount of drug metabolized during intestinal first-pass (Ito,

Kusuhara et al. 1999). In a recent research, the interplay between P-gp and CYP3A4 drug-drug interaction has been investigated using precision-cut intestinal slices (PCIS) of human jejunum, ileum and colon treated with different P-gp inhibitors and dual substrate such as quinidine at different regions (Li, de Graaf et al. 2017). Additionally, P-gp also mediates elimination of drugs via active biliary and renal secretion (Figure 1). Similarly, P-gp plays an important role in distribution of drugs to central nervous system (Doan, Humphreys et al. 2002). For instance, P-gp expressed at the apical membrane of BBB limits the amount of drug entering into the brain, there by playing a protective role. Hence, for CNS active drugs, it is important to dial out efflux liability to ensure adequate CNS exposures. Due to P-gp's central role in modulating drug pharmacokinetics and toxicity, inhibition or induction of P-gp is an important aspect to be considered during drug development and clinical trials. In the sections below, studies demonstrating the role of P-gp in oral drug absorption, distribution and clearance of drugs are discussed.

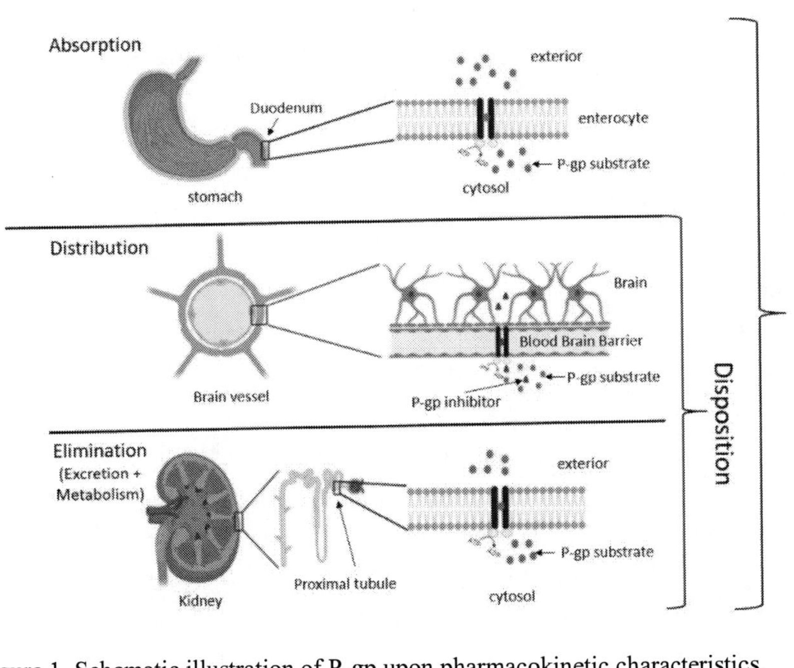

Figure 1. Schematic illustration of P-gp upon pharmacokinetic characteristics.

EFFECT OF P-GP ON DRUG ABSORPTION

P-glycoprotein (P-gp) is highly expressed in both intestinal epithelial cells and endothelial cells of brain capillaries, and functions as an efflux transporter in both organs. The impact of P-gp on intestinal absorption and brain uptake of drugs is quantitatively very different (Yano, Tomono et al. 2018). P-glycoprotein exports structurally and pharmacologically diverse hydrophobic compounds such as anti-cancer agents, immunosuppressive agents, steroid hormones, calcium channel blockers, β-blockers and cardiac glycosides. Substrates of P-gp can identified by conducting bidirectional permeability assays in cells expressing P-gp such as the Caco-2 and MDCKII-MDR1 cells. For example, the transport and efflux of vinblastine and docetaxel was demonstrated using Caco-2 cells (Takanaga, Ohnishi et al. 1998). The basolateral to apical (B to A) transport of both the drugs was found to be 10-20 fold high as compared to apical to basolateral membrane (A to B). Similar results were evidenced when cyclosporine transport was evaluated using Caco-2 cells. Further, the bidirectional permeability of vinblastine, docetaxel, cyclosporine and small peptides was reduced to unity in the presence of P-gp inhibitors (Hunter, Hirst et al. 1993, Wils, Phung-Ba et al. 1994). Recently, group of researchers also demonstrated the use of an using chamber system with porcine intestine as a surrogate device for scrutinizing the intestinal absorption of drugs (Arnold, Thorens et al. 2019).

Although P-gp expression and activity has been reported to gradually increase in the small intestine from the proximal to the distal regions (Mouly and Paine 2003) thereby increased absorption of some drugs from the distal (ileum and jejunum) part of intestine has been observed (Stephens, O'Neill et al. 2001, Kilic, Batu et al. 2004) but there are also reports demonstrating just the opposite with respect to the absorption of some drugs (Yigitaslan, Erol et al. 2016). For example, the absorption of cyclosporine and tacrolimus in rats was found to be significantly increased when co-administered with P-gp inhibitors (verapamil) as evaluated through *in vitro* and *in vivo* experiments (Yigitaslan, Erol et al. 2016). In this study, the researchers have identified that the ideal absorption of tacrolimus was highly increased when co administered with P-gp inhibitor (rifampicin) but no difference was perceived at ileum and jejunum regions of small intestine for cyclosporine when co-administered with verapamil/rifampicin suggesting the localization of P-gp varies across the small intestine and hence the plasma concentration of the drugs also get altered. This is also one the most important facet in attributing to the consequences of drug-drug interactions. Some of the recently updated alterations of therapeutically active molecules and drugs are listed in Table 1. Furthermore, the phytotherapeutically active drugs also fall into the category of P-gp modulation. The co-administration of herbal constituents also affects the absorption of other herbal or synthetic molecules leading to drug-herb and herb-herb interactions. For example, *Rhizoma Atractylodis Macrocephalae* extract reduced the absorption rate of strychnine and brucine by enhancing the P-gp activity in Caco-2 cell line and everted intestinal sac model (Barthe, Bessouet et al. 1998) and in situ single-pass intestinal perfusion model (Lü, Jiang et al. 2020). Induction or inhibition of P-gp can alter the area under the curve (AUC), maximum plasma concentration (C_{max}), and absolute bioavailability of drugs. For instance, the intestinal absorption of berberine, an herbal supplement having multi-therapeutic benefits, was found to be significantly increased through inhibition of intestinal P-gp transporter. The metabolism of berberine was also decreased thereby elevating the berberine levels in plasma after 50mg/kg oral administration to rats without significant cytotoxicity (Kwon, Lim et al. 2020).

Although appreciable efforts have been made to investigate the role of P-gp *in vitro*, the direct evidence for the involvement of P-gp in drug absorption was derived from *in vivo* studies using the Mdr1a knockout mice. Recently, researchers have attempted to generate MDR1-knockout induced pluripotent cell line using genome editing technology (Negoro, Kawai et al. 2020). Furthermore, it was also shown that the oral absorption of paclitaxel and consequently the plasma AUC were increased by 2- and 6-fold in the Mdr1a knockout mice, compared to wild-type, after intravenous and oral drug administration, respectively (Chen, Liu et al. 2003). An advantage of using the *in vivo* Mdr1a knockout mice model is that it permits examining

Table 1. Altered pharmacokinetic characteristics due to P-glycoprotein transporter modulation

P-gp modulator	T_{max}	Bioavailability/ AUC	Dose	Drug Interacted	Inference	Reference
Synthetic Drugs						
Lc478	15-30 (min)	234%	20 mg/kg	Docetaxel	Bioavailability ↑	(Han, Kim et al. 2020)
Verapamil	-	-	25 mg/kg	Cyclosporin	Plasma concentration↑	(Yigitaslan, Erol et al.)
Rifampicin	-	-	250 mg/kg	Cyclosporin	Plasma concentration↓	(Yigitaslan, Erol et al.)
Verapamil	-	-	25 mg/kg	Tacrolimus	Plasma concentration↑	(Yigitaslan, Erol et al.)
Rifampicin	-	-	250 mg/kg	Tacrolimus	Plasma concentration↓	(Yigitaslan, Erol et al.)
Oxypeucedanin	104.60 ± 11.68 (min)	463.90 ± 47.29 (μg·h/l)	8 mg/kg	Docetaxel	Auc ↑by1.21 folds	(Dong, Liao et al. 2018)
Resveratrol	0.91 ± 0.13 (h)	2555.31 ± 704.04 (ng.h/ml)	50 mg/kg	Fexofenadine	Auc ↑	(Bedada, Yellu et al. 2016)
Fostamatinib	1.0 (h)	18.3(ng.h/ml)	0.25 mg BID	Digoxin	Plasma concentration↑by1.7 fold	(Martin, Gillen et al. 2015)
Coumarin derivative (LL-348)	4.0 ± 1.6, 3.0 ± 0.0, 0.5 ± 0.0 (h)	2783 ± 328, 3076 ± 386, 7428 ± 2127(ng.h/ml)	0.5, 2, 5 mg/kg	Paclitaxel	Auc ↑	(Lee, Chae et al. 2014)
Verapamil	2.2 ± 0.45, 2.4 ± 0.55, 2.6 ± 0.89 (h)	1817 ± 363, 1355 ± 307, 2275 ± 841 (ng.h/ml)	0.5, 2, 5 mg/kg	Paclitaxel	Auc ↑	(Lee, Chae et al. 2014)
HZ08	-	5.5 ± 0.2, (h μg /ml)	4 mg/kg	Adriamycin	No significant effect in Auc	(Zhang, Feng et al. 2015)

P-gp modulator	T_{max}	Bioavailability/ AUC	Dose	Drug Interacted	Inference	Reference
Verapamil	-	9.4 ± 1.1(h μg /ml)	4 mg/kg	Adriamycin	Auc ↑	(Zhang, Feng et al. 2015)
HM30181	2.5, 4.5, 2.5 (h)	98.7 ± 37.9, 100.7 ± 37.6, 79.7 ± 38.4 (μg·h/l)	15, 60, 180 mg	Loperamide	Auc ↑	(Kim, Lee et al. 2014)
Bosutinib	3.99 (h)	1186 (ng·h/ml)	100 mg	Dabigatran	No significant effect	(Hsyu, Pignataro et al. 2017)
PSC833 (valspodar)	-	298 ± 37(ng·h/ml)	10 mg/kg	Sunitinib	Bioavailability ↑ by 1.8 fold	(Kunimatsu, Mizuno et al. 2013)
Zosuquidar	2.0 ± 0.0 2.5 ± 0.6 (h)	969 ± 749, 2140 ± 2706 (ng·h/ml)	10, 100 mg/kg	Aliskiren	Auc ↑ by 8.3 fold	[11]
Cyclosporin A	2.5 ± 0.6, 4.0 ± 1.2, 6.0 ± 1.2 (h)	1799 ± 1312, 4285 ± 2880, 3601 ± 1056(ng·h/ml)	10, 30, 100 mg/kg	Aliskiren	Auc ↑ by 42.1 fold	(Tsukimoto, Ohashi et al. 2015)
Efonidipine	0.63 ± 0.1, 0.61 ± 0.12 (h)	593 ± 101, 763 ± 145(ng·h/ml)	1 and 3 mg/kg	Repaglinide	Auc ↑	(Li, Choi et al. 2012)
Simvastatin	0.24 ± 0.05, 0.24 ± 0.05(h)	328 ± 62, 392 ± 74(ng·h/ml)	0.3 and 1.0 mg/kg	Diltiazem	Auc ↑	(Choi, Choi et al. 2011)
Simvastatin	0.44 ± 0.1, 0.43 ± 0.1 (h)	301 ± 57, 325 ± 62 (ng·h/ml)	0.3 and 1.0 mg/kg	Desacetyldiltiazem	Auc ↑	(Choi, Choi et al. 2011)
Baicalein	0.25, 0.25 (h)	12 587 ± 126, 706 ± 165, 805 ± 178 (ng·h/ml)	0.4, 2 and 8 mg/kg	Nimodipine	Auc ↑	(Cho, Choi et al. 2011)
Nifedipine	0.71 ± 0.1, 0.79 ± 0.1 (h)	631 ± 114, 812 ± 154(ng·h/ml)	1 and 3 mg/kg	Repaglinide	Auc ↑ significantly	(Choi, Choi et al. 2013)
Venetoclax	2.0 (h)	36.7(ng·h/ml)	100mg	Digoxin	Auc ↑ by 9%	(Chiney, Menon et al. 2018)
Barnidipine	0.5-4 (h)	1.76 ± 0.35 1.93 ± 0.28 (ng·h/ml)	1 and 10 mg/kg	Talinolol	Bioavailability ↑	(Ozturk, Ozturk et al. 2017)
Nifedipine	0.71 ± 0.19(h)	7012 ± 1192(ng·h/ml)	0.8 mg/kg	Atorvastatin	Auc ↑ significantly	(Lee, Choi et al. 2015)

Table 1. (Continued)

P-gp modulator	T_{max}	Bioavailability/ AUC	Dose	Drug Interacted	Inference	Reference
Nifedipine	0.64 ± 0.14(h)	8496 ± 1444(ng·h/ml)	0.8 mg/kg	Fluvastatin	Auc ↑ significantly	(Lee, Choi et al. 2015)
Nifedipine	0.71 ± 0.19 (h)	7217 ± 1469(ng·h/ml)	0.8 mg/kg	Pravastatin	Auc ↑ significantly	(Lee, Choi et al. 2015)
Nifedipine	0.64 ± 0.14 (h)	9008 ± 1802(ng·h/ml)	0.8 mg/kg	Simvastatin	Auc ↑ significantly	(Lee, Choi et al. 2015)
Rifampin	2.00 (h)	33.1 (μmh)	600 mg	Doravirine	No significant effect in Auc	(Yee, Khalilieh et al. 2017)
Natural Products						
Quinidine	3.0 (h)	139.2 ± 56.0(ug.h/L)	600 mg	Loperamide	Auc ↑	(Kim, Lee et al. 2014)
Diosmin	0.92 ± 0.13 (h)	1934.21 ± 598.71 (ng.h/ml)	50 mg/kg	Fexofenadine	Bioavailability ↑	(Neerati and Kumar Bedada 2015)
Piperine	-	651.03 (ng.h/ml)	10 mg/kg	Doxorubicin	No significant effect in Auc	(Kim, Shin et al. 2018)
Capsaicin	-	661.02 (ng.h/ml)	5 mg/kg	Doxorubicin	No significant effect in Auc	(Kim, Shin et al. 2018)
[6]-Gingerol	-	579.44 (ng.h/ml)	5 mg/kg	Doxorubicin	No significant effect in Auc	(Kim, Shin et al. 2018)
Capsaicin	5.3 ± 2.4, 7.8 ± 2.6, 6.7 ± 2.0 (h)	88.2 ± 18.0, 112.9 ± 31.9, 129.2 ± 14.0 (ug.h/ml)	0.3, 1, 3 mg/kg	Cyclosporin	Bioavailability ↑	(jia Zhai, Shi et al. 2013)
Piperine	1.2 ± 0.6(h)	7750 ± 2080 (ng/h/ml)	20 mg/kg	Fexofenadine	Auc ↑ by 180% to 190%	(Jin and Han 2010)
Quinidine	36 (h)	34(ng/h/ml)	600 mg	Naloxegol	Auc ↑ by 1.4 fold	(Bui, She et al. 2016)

P-gp modulator	**T_{max}**	**Bioavailability/ AUC**	**Dose**	**Drug Interacted**	**Inference**	**Reference**
Sinapic acid	2.0 (h)	54.24 ± 1.193 (ug.h/ml)	20 mg/kg	Carbamazepine	Auc ↑ by 57.18%	(Raish, Ahmad et al. 2019)
Quercetin	0.25, 0.25, 0.25 (h)	244 ± 63.2, 344 ± 98.6, 439 ± 107.3 (ng·h/ml)	0.6, 3 or 15 mg/kg	Doxorubicin	Auc ↑	(Choi, Piao et al. 2011)
Dengzhan Shengmai capsule (Erigeron breviscapus + Panax ginseng + Ophiopogon japonicas + Schisandra chinensis)	0.8 ± 0.2(h)	2.0 ± 0.2(ng/ml.h)	97.2 mg/kg	Clopidogrel	Auc ↑	(Chen, Zhao et al. 2016)
Schisandra Lignans Extract	7.50 ± 1.00 to 11.34 ± 2.74 (h)	9045 ± 2203 to 24127 ± 3845 (ng/ml.h)	500 mg/kg	Ginsenosides	Auc ↑	(Liang, Zhou et al. 2014)
Glycyrrhizin	2.4 ± 32.2 (h)	2,218.3 ± 724.3(ng/ml.h)	75 mg	Talinolol	No significant alteration in Auc	(Yan, Fang et al. 2013)
Gallic acid	2 ± 0.8 (h)	440.96 ± 0.04(ug.h/ml)	50 mg/kg	Linagliptin	Auc ↑ 2.45-fold	(Shaik and Vanapatla 2019)
Ellagic acid	2 ± 0.8 (h)	391.14 ± 0.02(ug.h/ml)	50 mg/kg	Linagliptin	Auc ↑ 1.2-fold	(Shaik and Vanapatla 2019)

the intestinal excretion by interrupting the bile flow via gallbladder cannulation. Hence, with the continued studies on paclitaxel using the cannulated mice, it was shown that 11% of the dose was excreted in the intestinal lumen within 90 min after intravenous administration of the drug in to Mdr1a wild-type mice. Interestingly, only 2.5% of the dose was excreted in the intestinal lumen of Mdr1a knockout gallbladder cannulated mice (Brinkmann 2002, Lagas, Vlaming et al. 2006). Mechanistically, biliary and urinary excretions were the main pathways examined. In another clinical study, it was shown that intestinal P-gp level is a potential determinant of cyclosporine oral dose in living donor liver transplant patients. Similarly, duodenal P-gp mRNA levels were inversely correlated with AUC and C_{max} of oral talinolol in healthy human subjects. Unlike the direct evidence derived from Mdr1a knockout mice, the involvement of MDR1 in drug absorption is extremely difficult to prove in human. Thus, the vast majority of studies conducted to examine the role of MDR1 in drug absorption in human often derive their conclusions based on the use of pharmacological inhibitors against P-gp. Therefore, these studies can only provide a qualitative but not quantitative assessment of the role of P-gp in drug absorption. Moreover, the absence of a specific P-gp inhibitor makes it more difficult to estimate the quantitative contribution of P-gp in drug absorption, since many of the P-gp inhibitors are CYP3A4 and other efflux transporters inhibitors. It is worth mentioning that, even in healthy volunteers who might be administered drugs which are P-gp substrates, the intra- and inter-patients variations in AUC and C_{max} could be attributed to genetic polymorphisms of the P-gp and various disease states which might influence the P-gp efflux capacity (Lo and Burckart 1999, Masuda, Goto et al. 2003).

Effect of P-gp Upon Drug Distribution

Numerous studies have investigated the role of P-gp on drug absorption, metabolism and excretion, however, its role in drug distribution has not been well explored. Although, the stage of drug distribution plays a critical role during examination of drug response directly affecting the pharmacokinetics and pharmacodynamics relationship of a drug. This might be due to the scarcity of useful experimental tools to examine the role of distribution in drug disposition. Drug distribution has been an important facet in determining drug disposition, especially when referring to the barriers present in the body such as brain (blood brain barrier) and in females during pregnancy (placental barrier). Similar to the non-identical characteristics of the brain with other organs, the connecting link between mother and fetus; placenta is also a barrier with unique traits like blood brain barrier. Both the placenta and blood brain barrier expresses the P-gp at their membranes that further restricts the entry of many xenobiotics, harmful and large sized molecules in to the brain and fetus. Number of times, many beneficial substances are also unable to cross the both the barriers due to their substrate specificity towards P-gp that effluxes the molecules outwards, and sometimes, the harmful substances being lipophilic in nature also enters the brain and fetus causing toxicity to the brain and fetus. Despite of the hydrophilic nature, a molecule is further unable to penetrate the blood brain barrier due to the presence of P-gp at the endothelial membrane of blood brain barrier.

Along with the Lipinski's rule of five, the presence and absence of efflux transporters at the membrane and the physicochemical properties of drug are interlinked to each other in order to penetrate the barriers altering its pharmacokinetic and pharmacodynamics properties. The central nervous system acting drugs that are P-gp substrates are the most affected with the efflux transporters. Taking an example of loperamide, a potent opiate drug is a P-gp substrate due to which its distribution to brain is limited. In a recent research it has been reported that the P-gp (Mdr1a) knockdown rats shows the enhancement in penetration of loperamide across blood brain barrier (Huang, Li et al. 2015) consequently increasing the therapeutic efficacy of the drug. Similarly, the presence of P-gp at an another barrier that is brain-ocular barrier has also been seen hindering the entry of loperamide into the ocular tissues from systemic circulation (Tatke, Janga et al. 2018). Correspondingly, in other studies, drugs like domeperidone (a dopaminergic antagonist), a P-gp substrate and an antipsychotic drug, had limited entry in to brain thus failed to show its therapeutic activity effectively (Swain, Orzechowski et al. 2013) (Ela, Härtter et al. 2004). The investigation related to pharmacokinetics parameters have also been performed by many researchers using *in vitro* (cell line) and *in vivo* (animal) models.

The application of MDCK-Mdr1a transfected cell line is the most widely employed cell line for studying the blood brain barrier permeability of a drug thereby predicting the human brain penetration potency of lead compounds (Feng, Doran et al. 2018). Recently, novel amino-1,4-oxazine and its derivatives were discovered as BACE 1 inhibitors, examining the activity using MDCK-Mdr1a cell lines for penetration efficacy (Veenstra, Rueeger et al. 2018). Moreover, in a recent study, a P-gp transfected LLC-PK1 cell line was transfected with P-gp and validated for the prediction of rat and human unbound brain to plasma ratio of novel central nervous system acting drug during its early discovery programme (Nicolaï, Chapy et al. 2020). Many studies have been performed using the Mdr1a knockout rats and mice, e.g., brain concentration of fexofenadine was found to be 9 fold increase in knockout mice as compared to wild type mice (Zhao, Kalvass et al. 2009). Similar studies on HIV protease inhibitors showed that brain concentrations and brain to plasma ratios of indinavir, nelfinavir, and saquinavir are significantly increased in Mdr1a knockout mice compared to wild-type (Robillard, Chan et al. 2014, Agrawal, Rowe et al. 2019).

Further, P-gp is also known to be involved in the uptake and efflux of many xenobiotics from the placenta as mentioned earlier. P-gp being the dominant among all other efflux transporters has been shown to be expressed in the human placenta from the first trimester until delivery (Liu and Liu 2019). (Afrouzian et al.) with his colleagues have identified the role of efflux transporters in bio-disposition of pravastatin across placenta obtained from pre-clampsiatic patients (Afrouzian, Al-Lahham et al. 2018). An exhaustive updated literatures with respect to the expression and function of P-gp in the placenta and fetus has been updated in a recent review by Han et al. (Han, Gao et al. 2018). Recent studies also demonstrated the utilization of positron emission tomography (PET) ligand (e.g., verapamil) for assessing the changes in P-gp function and expression across blood brain barrier using rat as animal model (Syvänen, Luurtsema et al. 2011).

Moreover, considering the placental barrier, studies are performed using the cultured human placenta choriocarcinoma epithelial cells as the ethical and moral constraints would not allow the clinical trial on pregnant women. The activity and expression of P-gp at the placental barrier was identified by investigating the distribution of vinblastine, vincristine, and digoxin across the cells (Bai, Sun et al. 2016). The concentration of these drugs was found to be higher at A side than B side but when co-exposed with cyclosporine the transportation of these drugs was reversed, thereby increasing the concentration at B side than A side. Hence, the presence of P-gp at placental barrier prevents the entry of harmful substances and other xenobiotics across the placenta. Furthermore, in a recent study, the maternal and fetal concentration of nor buprenorphine, an active metabolite of buprenorphine (prescribed during pregnancy for opiate addiction) was quantified for any toxicity to fetal using P-gp knockdown mice. The conjugated metabolite was found to be 3-7 times greater in fetal are under the curve than the maternal are under the curve. Hence, it may be concluded that P-gp plays an important role in determining entry of compounds across placental barrier (Liao, Gao et al. 2017).

EFFECT OF P-GP UPON DRUG METABOLISM

Drug metabolism is the phenomenon which involves the enzymatic conversion of drugs into metabolites by cytochromes, UGTs and other enzymes present in liver. Liver has been the main site for drug metabolism due to the presence of several drug metabolizing enzymes, although small intestine, kidneys and few other organs also play a role in metabolism of some drugs (Gibson and Skett 2013). There are various types of cytochrome P450 enzymes involved in metabolism of most of the drugs but CYP3A4 is the main hepatic and intestinal metabolic enzyme that contributes to the metabolism of majority of endogenous and exogenous chemical entities. Furthermore, the presence of P-gp in small intestine also bestow towards the drug metabolism by synergistically increasing or decreasing the drug absorption at the site along with CYP3A4 (Meyer 1996). Although, the

CYP3A4 is distributed uniformly throughout the liver, its expression varies along the length of small intestine with decrease in concentration starting from proximal to distal parts of the intestine (Ref).

P-gp is present at the luminal membrane of the hepatic and renal tubular cells facing the bile duct and renal tubular lumen. Hence, it could be said that the interaction of P-gp occurs post cellular uptake, distribution and metabolism of drugs in both liver and kidney (Figure 2). The interplay between P-gp and CYP3A4 is also responsible for many food drug interactions (Nebert and Dalton 2006). For example, co-administration of grapefruit juice with CYP3A4 and P-gp substrates. The exposure of grapefruit juice did not alter the activity of hepatic CYP3A4, while the activity of intestinal CYP3A4 was reduced as evaluated using triazolam was as a surrogate marker for CYP3A4 activity (Culm-Merdek, von Moltke et al. 2006). Similarly for cyclosporine, it was found that P-gp (not CYP3A4) at intestine reduces the bioavailability of cyclosporine (Lown, Mayo et al. 1997). Plasma-concentration/time profiles of cyclosporine was examined in volunteers who were exposed either with grapefruit or Seville orange juice. CYP3A4 activity was found to be decreased in the patients administered with grapefruit juice but not affected with Seville orange juice exposure. Also, the AUC (area under the curve) and C_{max} (maximum concentration) of cyclosporine was found to be significantly enhanced by the administration of grapefruit juice but not by Seville orange juice (De Castro, Mertens-Talcott et al. 2007). Further, the intake of grapefruit juice also increased the oral bioavailability of midazolam (Kawaguchi-Suzuki, Nasiri-Kenari et al. 2017), felodipine (Amadi and Peters 2017), and saquinavir (Crawford 2017) without affecting hepatic elimination of these drugs. Therefore, by using grapefruit juice as an inhibitor of both CYP3A4 and P-gp, researchers were able to determine oral bioavailability of drugs that are substrates for both CYP3A4 and P-gp by comparing the oral AUC before and after the ingestion of grape fruit juice (Crawford 2017, Bailey 2019). Number of investigations have investigated the interplay between P-gp transporter and CYP3A4 enzyme. The metabolite of indinavir, a P-gp and CYP3A4 substrate drug was found to be higher at the apical side of Caco-2 cells than the basolateral membrane of cells (Calitz, Gouws et al. 2015). These results were also confirmed in a study under *in vivo* conditions. The intestinal first pass metabolism of indinavir was found to be significantly increased from 6 to 34% when administered to rats exposed to dexamethasone (Zhao, Zou et al. 2017). Dexamethasone is known to enhance the enzymatic activity of CYP3A4 and transporter P-gp. It therefore suggests that both P-gp and CYP3A4 acts synergistically and are responsible for reduction in oral bioavailability of indinavir (Hochman, Chiba et al. 2001). Similar results were obtained with cyclosporine when exposed to Caco-2 cells. The bioavailability of loperamide, a dual substrate, was found to be increased at low doses in portal vein-cannulated P-gp–competent and P-gp–deficient mice by minimizing the intestinal first pass metabolism of drug (Dufek, Knight et al. 2013).

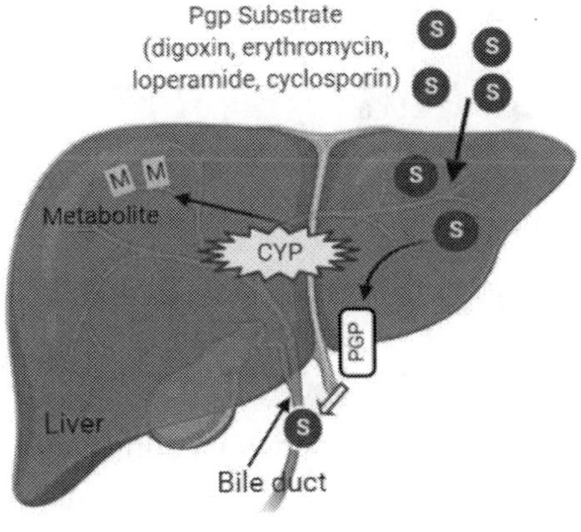

Figure 2. Effect of P-gp upon drug metabolism in liver.

Moreover, the interplay between intestinal P-gp and CYP3A4 also plays an important role behind the drug metabolism or bioavailability as investigated by Cummins et al. 2002 using N-methyl piperazine-Phe-homoPhe-vinylsulfone phenyl (K77, a cysteine protease inhibitor; P-gp and CYP3A4 substrate) and felodipine (CYP3A4 substrate only) were measured across CYP3A4- transfected Caco-2 cells in the presence of an inhibitor of and not CYP3A4, GG918 (Cummins, Jacobsen et al. 2002) (Figure 3).

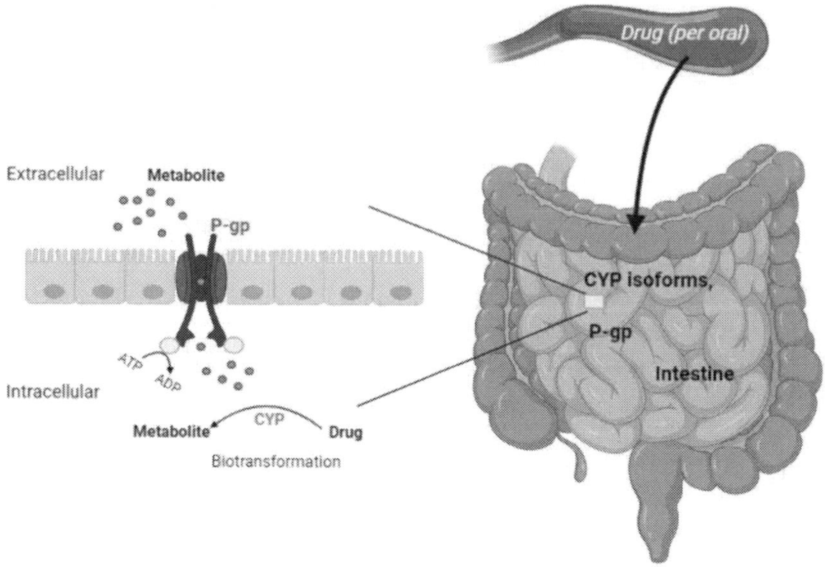

Figure 3. Diagrammatic representation of P-gp and CYP interplay.

The plausible involvement of P-gp along with CYP3A4 was also affirmed by other studies in which the Caco-2 cells were transfected with CYP3A4. The cells were further treated with P-gp inhibitor LY335979 and saquinavir. The metabolite of saquinavir was found to be increased which is regulated by CYP3A4. Therefore, it could be suggested that both CYP3A4 and P-gp play an interconnecting role during drug metabolism (Wang, Pal et al. 2012). Thus, by inhibiting P-gp activity, the metabolite will readily accumulate inside the cells as the metabolite itself is a P-gp substrate. Interestingly, a direct link between CYP3A4 and P-gp was scrutinized in gut wall of humans. In this study, the small intestine was perfused with quinidine using multi-luminal perfusion catheter in eight healthy volunteers. It was shown that the dose-corrected plasma quinidine AUC from 0 to 3 h was negatively correlated with both intestinal P-gp and CYP3A4 contents. In addition, dose-corrected intraluminal quinidine concentrations were positively correlated with intestinal P-gp expression (Mouly, Paine et al. 2004). The interplay hypothesis has been also shown to be valid in liver. (Lau et al.) Demonstrated through elegant experiments that, in an isolated perfused rat liver model, digoxin CYP3A-mediated metabolism increased in animals treated with quinidine, the P-gp inhibitor, compared with control animals. It was concluded that through inhibiting the biliary secretion of digoxin, quinidine increases the digoxin metabolism by prolonging its exposure to hepatic CYP3A (Jain and Sisodia 2019). Theoretically, the interplay between P-gp and CYP3A4 is an attractive subject to investigate. However, studies carried out to prove that the synergism between CYP3A4 and P-gp occurs at the transcriptional regulation level have failed (ref). Therefore, the functional interaction between both CYP3A4 and P-gp warrants further studies.

EFFECT OF P-GP UPON DRUG ELIMINATION

The unchanged form of drugs and their metabolites are eliminated from the body via liver/kidneys. During excretion through bile duct, the drug moves along the concentration gradient from basolateral to apical membrane. P-gp present at the apical membrane of the hepatocytes actively pumps its substrates into the bile. Similarly, renal uptake also takes place during renal excretion at the basolateral membrane of kidney and drugs are pump into the urine by the P-gp expressed at luminal membrane of epithelial cells in kidney, resulting in elimination of drug from the body (Akamine, Yasui-Furukori et al. 2019). It was firstly demonstrated using *in vitro* experimental conditions through canalicular membrane vesicles for the transport of drugs like daunomycin, doxorubicin and vincristine. Inhibition of P-gp (by verapamil exposure) decreases the transport of daunomycin suggesting contribution of P-gp transporter in the biliary excretion of drug (Kwon, Kamath et al. 1996).

Further, elimination of vincristine and doxorubicin was observed through biliary excretion in the perfused rat liver (Booth, Brouwer et al. 1998). Importance of P-gp in the biliary excretion process can also be concluded from the data obtained from metabolism study of digoxin in mice using Mdr1a receptors. It was observed that the digoxin is excreted in urine and bile mainly as non-metabolized drug. Since digoxin has narrow therapeutic window it can lead to unexpected side effects with modest alteration in the biliary or renal clearance. Furthermore, the biliary clearance of digoxin has been raised to 3-fold in the Mdr1a knockout mice, indicating the importance of the P-gp in the biliary excretion process. Besides digoxin, similar result was observed with other drugs such as vecuronium, doxorubicin and vinblastine, wherein the biliary clearance was enhanced to 3-to 5-times in Mdr1a mice when compared to knockout (Lin 2003). Taking an example of rat model, pretreatment of dexamethasone, a P-gp inducer, increased the biliary clearance of rhodamine-123 to 8-fold (Yumoto, Murakami et al. 2001) In human models, evaluation of P-gp role in biliary excretion is limited due the complicated extraction process of human bile. A clinical study showed partial reduction in the systemic digoxin exposure due to enhances digoxin biliary excretion (Greiner, Eichelbaum et al. 1999). In contrast, biliary excretion of doxorubicin and digoxin was significantly decreased when P-gp was inhibited by quinidine and GF120918 (Annaert, Turncliff et al. 2001). Contradictory to one step biliary excretion, the renal excretion involve more than one step, namely glomerular filtration, secretion from renal tubular and renal tubular lumen reabsorption. Hence the renal clearance (CLR) can be related to these three process by the following equation:

$$CLR = fu.GFR + CLs - CLR_A$$

where CLR, fu, GFR, CLs, and CLA_A refers: renal clearance, fraction of unbound drug in plasma, glomerular filtration rate, reabsorption clearance, secretion clearance (Lin 2003). Reabsorption and secretion are active processes while GFR is a passive process in which different transporters are involved. Role of P-gp in tubular secretion can be determined by the in-vitro systems. For Instant, the two extensively used models to study renal P-gp function are the porcine kidney epithelial cells (LLC-PK1) and the Madin-Darby canine kidney (MDCK) transfected by human MDR1 gene. Identification of P-gp inhibitors and substrates is done by bidirectional transport studies and the recommended cells by the United States Food and Drug Administration (USFDA) guidance for this studies are MDR1-MDCK, MDR1- LLC-PK1, or Caco-2 (Zhang, Zhang et al. 2008). The study has shown that the transport of vinblastine, digoxin, and cyclosporin from B-to-A trans-epithelial is greater than A-to-B trans-epithelial in LLC-PK1 cell line. In the similar way, the B-to-A transport of vinblastine was observed to be 6-times higher than the A-to-B trans-epithelial transport in MDCK cell line. Apart from this technique, another extensively used in-vitro method used for the identification of P-gp role in the renal tubular secretion is isolated perfused kidney. By conjugating the equation 2 with the result obtained from this technique, one can determine the step by step involvement of each process in the overall renal clearance process. For example, the CLR/(f_u.GFR) of the administered drug more than unity refers to tubular secretion of the drug whereas, CLR/(fu.GFR) less than unity indicates the tubular lumen reabsorption of drug. Based on this approach, active secretion of digoxin was observed from the isolated perfused kidney of rat. Further addition of verapamil and quinidine cause the inhibition of digoxin tubular secretion. The renal clearance of digoxin was compared in Mdr1a wild-type mice and knockout and it showed 3-times higher digoxin renal clearance in Mdr1a wild-type mice than the knockout mice (Horio, Chin et al. 1989, Yamazaki, Neway et al. 2001, Chu, Bleasby et al. 2007). Whereas in contradictory to digoxin, non-metabolized doxorubicin showed higher renal clearance in Mdr1 knockout mice when compared to Mdr1a wild type. Similar results were noticed with three other basic compounds namely; azidoprocainamide, tributyltrimethylammonium and vecuronium (Smit, Schinkel et al. 1998). The cause of confliction in data could be due to the interference of other transport systems in the renal clearance of doxorubicin, azidoprocainamide, tributyltrimethylammonium and vecuronium by elevating the compensatory mechanism to the loss of Mdr1.

Pathophysiology Behind P-gp and Drug Interaction

The P-gp has been reported to modulate the multidrug resistance phenomenon of majority of anticancer, anti-tubercular, and anti-bacterial drugs etc. The reversal of this process involves multi signaling pathways as reported in previous literatures. Studies have been performed suggesting the possible involvement of many intercellular molecules like NFκβ/PI3K/Akt (Wang, Jia et al. 2016, Muthusamy, Gunaseelan et al. 2019), Nrf2 (Lou, Guo et al. 2019), JNK, RAGE/ NFκβ (Xie, Yu et al. 2017, Choi, Lee et al. 2019), Rafl/AP1 (Wang, Lv et al. 2017) etc and their modulation. Moreover, flavonoids have also been reported to alter the P-gp activity through modulation of upstream and downstream molecules of Wnt pathway (Mohana, Ganesan et al. 2018). An exhaustive list of some of the drugs altering the cascade mechanism behind P-gp (Figure 4) and pharmacological drug-drug interaction is incorporated in Table 2.

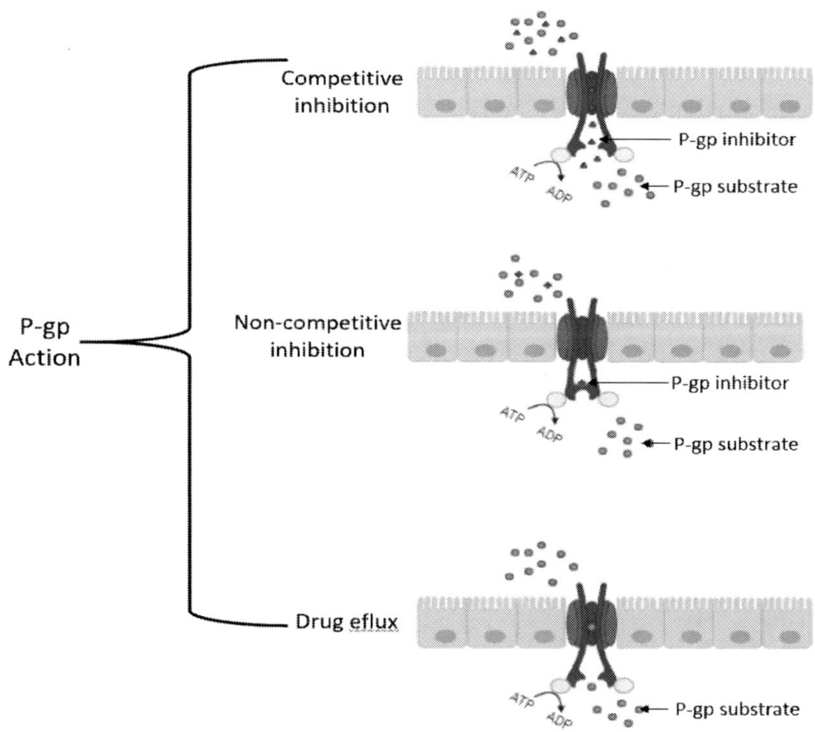

Figure 4. Schematic Representation of P-gp mediated mechanism of action.

Table 2. P-gp mediated pharmacodynamic properties of synthetic/herbal drugs

P-gp modulator	Signaling pathway	Drug	Disease	Outcome	Reference
HZ08	Atpase inhibition	Adriamycin	Tumor	Synergistic effect	(Zhang, Feng et al. 2015)
Efonidipine	Inhibition of CYP3A4 and P-gp efflux pump	Repaglinide	Diabetes	Significant hypoglycemic effect on oral administration	(Li, Choi et al. 2012)
Gambogic acid	Down-regulation of P-gp function	Adriamycin	Lung cancer	Synergistic effect	(Wang, Yang et al. 2014)
Verapamil	P-gp mediated efflux inhibition	Paclitaxel	Cancer	Synergistic effect	(Wang, Zhang et al. 2011)
Verapamil	ATP-dependent efflux pump inhibition	Ursolic acid	Skin cancer	Synergistic effect	(Junco, Mancha et al. 2013)
Sinapine	Suppression of FGFR4-FRS2α-ERK1/2 signaling pathway	Doxorubicin	Tumor	Synergistic effect	(Guo, An et al. 2014)
Tariquidar	Inhibition of P-gp efflux pump	Paclitaxel	Ovarian cancer	Synergistic effect	(Zhang, Sriraman et al. 2016, Li, Guan et al. 2017)
Saikosaponin D	Inhibited P-gp-mediated drug efflux	Adriamycin	Breast cancer	Synergistic effect	(Li, Guan et al. 2017)
Novel compound 160a (Quinoline derivative)	Inhibited P-gp-mediated drug efflux	Doxorubicin	Cancer	Synergistic effect	(Zhou, Chung et al. 2019)
Taxifolin	P-gp atpase stimulation	Doxorubicin	Cancer	Synergistic effect	(Shebley, Sandhu et al. 2018)
Ferulic acid	PI3K/Akt/NF-κb signaling pathway	Doxorubicin	Cancer	Synergistic effect	(Muthusamy, Gunaseelan et al. 2019)
Hyperin	Block P-gp efflux pump function	Vincristine	Colon cancer	Synergistic effect	(Wang, Zhang et al. 2018)
Nilotinib	Blocked FBS-induced ERK1 and p38 MAPK activation	Doxorubicin	Colon cancer	Synergistic effect	(Villar, Vögler et al. 2012)

Conclusion and Future Perspectives

P-glycoprotein is one of the main transporter responsible for effluxing a wide variety of substrates, thereby influencing absorption and disposition of several drugs. Hence the role of P-gp in influencing the plasma, tissue pharmacokinetics and pharmacodynamics of drugs is actively investigated during drug discovery and development using several *in vitro* and *in vivo* models. Additionally, drug-drug interactions (victim and perpetrator) caused due to modulation (e.g., inhibition or induction) of P-gp by co administered drugs/herbs are carefully considered/studied during clinical trials. Few studies have indicated that P-gp and CYP3A4 can enhance/reduce extraction of drugs during intestinal first-pass. More studies are needed to gain additional understanding on the interplay. Positron emission tomography (PET) studies are increasingly used to study distribution of P-gp substrates into various organs such as the brain in pre-clinical species and humans. Further refinements are needed in this area to gain cellular/sub-cellular level of spatial resolution. Additionally, in silico models such as physiologically based pharmacokinetic (PBPK) models are increasingly used to investigate the role of P-gp in absorption and drug-drug interactions (DDIs) and are submitted to regulatory agencies. PBPK models can also be valuable tools to investigate the interplay using data generated from *in vitro* systems. However, much validation is needed to increase confidence in the predictive accuracy of PBPK models for transporter based interactions.

Acknowledgments

The authors are thankful to Director, CSIR-CDRI for continuous encouragement and support. Swati Chaturvedi acknowledges CSIR, India, for providing the research fellowship.

Conflict of Interest

The authors declare that there are no conflicts of interest.

References

Afrouzian, M., R. Al-Lahham, S. Patrikeeva, M. Xu, V. Fokina, W. G. Fischer, S. Z. Abdel-Rahman, M. Costantine, M. S. Ahmed and T. Nanovskaya (2018). "Role of the efflux transporters BCRP and MRP1 in human placental bio-disposition of pravastatin." *Biochemical pharmacology* 156: 467-478.

Agrawal, N., J. Rowe, J. Lan, Q. Yu, C. A. Hrycyna and J. Chmielewski (2019). "Potential Tools for Eradicating HIV Reservoirs in the Brain: Development of Trojan Horse Prodrugs for the Inhibition of P-Glycoprotein with Anti-HIV-1 Activity." *Journal of medicinal chemistry* 63(5): 2131-2138.

Akamine, Y., N. Yasui-Furukori and T. Uno (2019). "Drug-drug interactions of P-gp substrates unrelated to CYP metabolism." *Current drug metabolism* 20(2): 124-129.

Amadi, C. and E. E. Peters (2017). "Fruit/vegetable–drug interactions: Pharmacokinetic Assay with a CYP3A4 Substrate." *World Journal of Pharmaceutical Research* 6(4): 213-224.

Annaert, P. P., R. Z. Turncliff, C. L. Booth, D. R. Thakker and K. L. Brouwer (2001). "P-glycoprotein-mediated in vitro biliary excretion in sandwich-cultured rat hepatocytes." *Drug metabolism and disposition* 29(10): 1277-1283.

Arnold, Y. E., J. Thorens, S. Bernard and Y. N. Kalia (2019). "Drug transport across porcine intestine using an Ussing chamber system: regional differences and the effect of P-glycoprotein and CYP3A4 activity on drug absorption." *Pharmaceutics* 11(3): 139.

Bai, M. r., D. l. Sun and C. h. Zheng (2016). "Expression and Regulation of Drug Transporters in Placenta." *Yao xue xue bao= Acta pharmaceutica Sinica* 51(6): 879-885.

Bailey, D. (2019). "*Drug administration and grapefruit.*" Compendium of pharmaceuticals and specialties. Ottawa, Ontario, Canada: Canadian Pharmacists Association: L11-L46.

Barthe, L., M. Bessouet, J. Woodley and G. Houin (1998). "The improved everted gut sac: a simple method to study intestinal P-glycoprotein." *International Journal of Pharmaceutics* 173(1-2): 255-258.

Bedada, S. K., N. R. Yellu and P. Neerati (2016). "Effect of resveratrol on the pharmacokinetics of fexofenadine in rats: Involvement of P-glycoprotein inhibition." *Pharmacological Reports* 68(2): 338-343.

Booth, C. L., K. R. Brouwer and K. L. Brouwer (1998). "Effect of multidrug resistance modulators on the hepatobiliary disposition of doxorubicin in the isolated perfused rat liver." *Cancer research* 58(16): 3641-3648.

Brinkmann, U. (2002). Functional polymorphisms of the human multidrug resistance (MDR1) gene: correlation with P glycoprotein expression and activity in vivo. *Novartis Foundation Symposium*, Wiley Online Library.

Bui, K., F. She, D. Zhou, K. Butler, N. Al-Huniti and M. Sostek (2016). "The effect of quinidine, a strong P-glycoprotein inhibitor, on the pharmacokinetics and central nervous system distribution of naloxegol." *Journal of Clinical Pharmacology* 56(4): 497-505.

Calitz, C., C. Gouws, J. Viljoen, J. Steenekamp, L. Wiesner, E. Abay and J. Hamman (2015). "Herb-drug pharmacokinetic interactions: transport and metabolism of indinavir in the presence of selected herbal products." *Molecules* 20(12): 22113-22127.

Chen, C., X. Liu and B. J. Smith (2003). "Utility of Mdr1-gene deficient mice in assessing the impact of P-glycoprotein on pharmacokinetics and pharmacodynamics in drug discovery and development." *Current drug metabolism* 4(4): 272-291.

Chen, X., Z. Zhao, Y. Chen, X. Gou, Z. Zhou, G. Zhong, Y. Cai, M. Huang and J. Jin (2016). "Mechanistic understanding of the effect of Dengzhan

Shengmai capsule on the pharmacokinetics of clopidogrel in rats." *Journal of Ethnopharmacology* 192: 362-369.

Chiney, M. S., R. M. Menon, O. F. Bueno, B. Tong and A. H. Salem (2018). "Clinical evaluation of P-glycoprotein inhibition by venetoclax: a drug interaction study with digoxin." *Xenobiotica* 48(9): 904-910.

Cho, Y. A., J. S. Choi and J. P. Burm (2011). "Effects of the antioxidant baicalein on the pharmacokinetics of nimodipine in rats: A possible role of P-glycoprotein and CYP3A4 inhibition by baicalein." *Pharmacological Reports* 63(4): 1066-1073.

Choi, D. H., J. S. Choi, C. Li and J. S. Choi (2011). "Effects of simvastatin on the pharmacokinetics of diltiazem and its main metabolite, desacetyldiltiazem, after oral and intravenous administration in rats: Possible role of P-glycoprotein and CYP3A4 inhibition by simvastatin." *Pharmacological Reports* 63(6): 1574-1582.

Choi, H., E. H. Lee, M. Han, S. H. An and J. Park (2019). "Diminished Expression of P-glycoprotein Using Focused Ultrasound Is Associated with JNK-Dependent Signaling Pathway in Cerebral Blood Vessels." *Frontiers in Neuroscience* 13: 1350.

Choi, J. S., I. Choi and D. H. Choi (2013). "Effects of nifedipine on the pharmacokinetics of repaglinide in rats: Possible role of CYP3A4 and P-glycoprotein inhibition by nifedipine." *Pharmacological Reports* 65(5): 1422-1430.

Choi, J. S., Y. J. Piao and K. W. Kang (2011). "Effects of quercetin on the bioavailability of doxorubicin in rats: Role of CYP3A4 and P-gp inhibition by quercetin." *Archives of Pharmacal Research* 34(4): 607-613.

Chu, X.-Y., K. Bleasby, J. Yabut, X. Cai, G. H. Chan, M. J. Hafey, S. Xu, A. J. Bergman, M. P. Braun and D. C. Dean (2007). "Transport of the dipeptidyl peptidase-4 inhibitor sitagliptin by human organic anion transporter 3, organic anion transporting polypeptide 4C1, and multidrug resistance P-glycoprotein." *Journal of Pharmacology and Experimental Therapeutics* 321(2): 673-683.

Crawford, D. (2017). "Food-drug interactions: The grapefruit effect." *Nursing made Incredibly Easy* 15(2): 49-54.

Culm-Merdek, K. E., L. L. von Moltke, L. Gan, K. A. Horan, R. Reynolds, J. S. Harmatz, M. H. Court and D. J. Greenblatt (2006). "Effect of extended exposure to grapefruit juice on cytochrome P450 3A activity in humans: comparison with ritonavir." *Clinical Pharmacology & Therapeutics* 79(3): 243-254.

Cummins, C. L., W. Jacobsen and L. Z. Benet (2002). "Unmasking the dynamic interplay between intestinal P-glycoprotein and CYP3A4." *Journal of Pharmacology and Experimental Therapeutics* 300(3): 1036-1045.

De Castro, W. V., S. Mertens-Talcott, H. Derendorf and V. Butterweck (2007). "Grapefruit juice–drug interactions: Grapefruit juice and its components inhibit P-glycoprotein (ABCB1) mediated transport of talinolol in Caco-2 cells." *Journal of pharmaceutical sciences* 96(10): 2808-2817.

Doan, K. M. M., J. E. Humphreys, L. O. Webster, S. A. Wring, L. J. Shampine, C. J. Serabjit-Singh, K. K. Adkison and J. W. Polli (2002). "Passive permeability and P-glycoprotein-mediated efflux differentiate central nervous system (CNS) and non-CNS marketed drugs." *Journal of Pharmacology and Experimental Therapeutics* 303(3): 1029-1037.

Dong, W., Z. G. Liao, G. W. Zhao, X. J. Guan, J. Zhang, X. L. Liang and M. Yang (2018). "Reversal effect of oxypeucedanin on p-glycoprotein-mediated drug transport." *Molecules* 23(8).

Dufek, M. B., B. M. Knight, A. S. Bridges and D. R. Thakker (2013). "P-glycoprotein increases portal bioavailability of loperamide in mouse by reducing first-pass intestinal metabolism." *Drug Metabolism and Disposition* 41(3): 642-650.

Ela, A. A. E., S. Härtter, U. Schmitt, C. Hiemke, H. Spahn-Langguth and P. Langguth (2004). "Identification of P-glycoprotein substrates and inhibitors among psychoactive compounds—implications for pharmacokinetics of selected substrates." *Journal of Pharmacy and Pharmacology* 56(8): 967-975.

Feng, B., A. C. Doran, L. Di, M. A. West, S. M. Osgood, J. Y. Mancuso, C. L. Shaffer, L. Tremaine and J. Liras (2018). "Prediction of human brain penetration of P-glycoprotein and breast cancer resistance protein substrates using in vitro transporter studies and animal models." *Journal of Pharmaceutical Sciences* 107(8): 2225-2235.

Galban, C. J., S. Galbán, M. E. Van Dort, G. D. Luker, M. S. Bhojani, A. Rehemtulla and B. D. Ross (2010). Applications of molecular imaging. *Progress in molecular biology and translational science*, Elsevier. 95: 237-298.

Gibson, G. G. and P. Skett (2013). *Introduction to drug metabolism*, Springer.

Greiner, B., M. Eichelbaum, P. Fritz, H.-P. Kreichgauer, O. Von Richter, J. Zundler and H. K. Kroemer (1999). "The role of intestinal P-glycoprotein in the interaction of digoxin and rifampin." *The Journal of clinical investigation* 104(2): 147-153.

Guo, Y., H. An, L. Feng, Q. Liu, S. Wang and T. Zhang (2014). "Sinapine as an active compound for inhibiting the proliferation of Caco-2 cells via downregulation of P-glycoprotein." *Food and Chemical Toxicology* 67: 187-192.

Han, L. W., C. Gao and Q. Mao (2018). "An update on expression and function of P-gp/ABCB1 and BCRP/ABCG2 in the placenta and fetus." *Expert opinion on drug metabolism & toxicology* 14(8): 817-829.

Han, S. Y., E. S. Kim, B. H. You, H. S. Chae, Q. Lu, Y. W. Chin, H. C. Ahn, S. J. Chung, K. Lee and Y. H. Choi (2020). "Effect of treatment period with LC478, a disubstituted adamantayl derivative, on P-glycoprotein inhibition: its application to increase docetaxel absorption in rats." *Xenobiotica* 50(7): 863-874.

Hochman, J. H., M. Chiba, M. Yamazaki, C. Tang and J. H. Lin (2001). "P-glycoprotein-mediated efflux of indinavir metabolites in Caco-2 cells expressing cytochrome P450 3A4." *Journal of Pharmacology and Experimental Therapeutics* 298(1): 323-330.

Horio, M., K.-V. Chin, S. J. Currier, S. Goldenberg, C. Williams, I. Pastan, M. M. Gottesman and J. Handler (1989). "Transepithelial transport of drugs by the multidrug transporter in cultured Madin-Darby canine kidney cell epithelia." *Journal of Biological Chemistry* 264(25): 14880-14884.

Hsyu, P. H., D. S. Pignataro and K. Matschke (2017). "Effect of bosutinib on the absorption of dabigatran etexilate mesylate, a P-glycoprotein substrate, in healthy subjects." *European Journal of Clinical Pharmacology* 73(1): 57-63.

Huang, L., X. Li, J. Roberts, B. Janosky and M.-H. J. Lin (2015). "Differential role of P-glycoprotein and breast cancer resistance protein in drug distribution into brain, CSF and peripheral nerve tissues in rats." *Xenobiotica* 45(6): 547-555.

Hunter, J., B. H. Hirst and N. L. Simmons (1993). "Drug absorption limited by P-glycoprotein-mediated secretory drug transport in human intestinal epithelial Caco-2 cell layers." *Pharmaceutical research* 10(5): 743-749.

Ito, K., H. Kusuhara and Y. Sugiyama (1999). "Effects of intestinal CYP3A4 and P-glycoprotein on oral drug absorption—theoretical approach." *Pharmaceutical research* 16(2): 225-231.

Jain, A. and J. Sisodia (2019). "*Quinidine*."

jia Zhai, X., F. Shi, F. Chen and Y. ning Lu (2013). "Capsaicin pretreatment increased the bioavailability of cyclosporin in rats: Involvement of P-glycoprotein and CYP 3A inhibition." *Food and Chemical Toxicology* 62: 323-328.

Jin, M. J. and H. K. Han (2010). "Effect of piperine, a major component of black pepper, on the intestinal absorption of fexofenadine and its implication on food-drug interaction." *Journal of Food Science* 75(3): H93--H96.

Junco, J. J., A. Mancha, G. Malik, S. J. Wei, D. J. Kim, H. Liang and T. J. Slaga (2013). "Resveratrol and P-glycoprotein inhibitors enhance the anti-skin cancer effects of ursolic acid." *Molecular Cancer Research* 11(12): 1521-1529.

Kawaguchi-Suzuki, M., N. Nasiri-Kenari, J. Shuster, F. G. Gmitter Jr, P. Cancalon, F. de Oliveria, J. Kight, E. M. Handberg, C. J. Pepine and R. F. Frye (2017). "Effect of Low-Furanocoumarin Hybrid Grapefruit Juice Consumption on Midazolam Pharmacokinetics." *The Journal of Clinical Pharmacology* 57(3): 305-311.

Kilic, F. S., O. Batu, B. a. Sirmagul, E. Yildirim and K. Erol (2004). "Intestinal absorption of digoxin and interaction with nimodipine in rats." *Polish journal of pharmacology* 56(1): 137-144.

Kim, T. E., H. Lee, K. S. Lim, S. Lee, S. H. Yoon, K. M. Park, H. Han, S. G. Shin, I. J. Jang, K. S. Yu and J. Y. Cho (2014). "Effects of HM30181, a P-glycoprotein inhibitor, on the pharmacokinetics and pharmacodynamics of loperamide in healthy volunteers." *British Journal of Clinical Pharmacology* 78(3): 556-564.

Kim, T. H., S. Shin, S. D. Yoo and B. S. Shin (2018). "Effects of phytochemical P-glycoprotein modulators on the pharmacokinetics and tissue distribution of doxorubicin in mice." *Molecules* 23(2).

Kim, Y. and J. Chen (2018). "Molecular structure of human P-glycoprotein in the ATP-bound, outward-facing conformation." *Science* 359(6378): 915-919.

Kunimatsu, S., T. Mizuno, M. Fukudo and T. Katsura (2013). "Effect of P-glycoprotein and breast cancer resistance protein inhibition on the pharmacokinetics of sunitinib in rats." *Drug Metabolism and Disposition* 41(8): 1592-1597.

Kwon, M., D. Y. Lim, C. H. Lee, J.-H. Jeon, M.-K. Choi and I.-S. Song (2020). "Enhanced Intestinal Absorption and Pharmacokinetic Modulation of Berberine and Its Metabolites through the Inhibition of P-Glycoprotein and Intestinal Metabolism in Rats Using a Berberine Mixed Micelle Formulation." *Pharmaceutics* 12(9): 882.

Kwon, Y., A. V. Kamath and M. E. Morris (1996). "Inhibitors of P-glycoprotein-mediated daunomycin transport in rat liver canalicular membrane vesicles." *Journal of pharmaceutical sciences* 85(9): 935-939.

Lagas, J. S., M. L. Vlaming, O. van Tellingen, E. Wagenaar, R. S. Jansen, H. Rosing, J. H. Beijnen and A. H. Schinkel (2006). "Multidrug resistance protein 2 is an important determinant of paclitaxel pharmacokinetics." *Clinical Cancer Research* 12(20): 6125-6132.

Lee, C. K., J. S. Choi and D. H. Choi (2015). "Effects of HMG-CoA reductase inhibitors on the pharmacokinetics of nifedipine in rats:

Possible role of P-gp and CYP3A4 inhibition by HMG-CoA reductase inhibitors." *Pharmacological Reports* 67(1): 44-51.

Lee, K., S. W. Chae, Y. Xia, N. H. Kim, H. J. Kim, S. Rhie and H. J. Lee (2014). "Effect of coumarin derivative-mediated inhibition of P-glycoprotein on oral bioavailability and therapeutic efficacy of paclitaxel." *European Journal of Pharmacology* 723(1): 381-388.

Leveque, D. and F. Jehl (1995). "P-glycoprotein and pharmacokinetics." *Anticancer research* 15(2): 331.

Li, C., D. H. Choi and J. S. Choi (2012). "Effects of efonidipine on the pharmacokinetics and pharmacodynamics of repaglinide: Possible role of CYP3A4 and P-glycoprotein inhibition by efonidipine." *Journal of Pharmacokinetics and Pharmacodynamics* 39(1): 99-108.

Li, C., X. Guan, H. Xue, P. Wang, M. Wang and X. Gai (2017). "Reversal of P-glycoprotein-mediated multidrug resistance is induced by saikosaponin D in breast cancer MCF-7/adriamycin cells." *Pathology Research and Practice* 213(7): 848-853.

Li, M., I. A. de Graaf, E. van de Steeg, M. H. de Jager and G. M. Groothuis (2017). "The consequence of regional gradients of P-gp and CYP3A4 for drug-drug interactions by P-gp inhibitors and the P-gp/CYP3A4 interplay in the human intestine ex vivo." *Toxicology in Vitro* 40: 26-33.

Li, Y., H. Yuan, K. Yang, W. Xu, W. Tang and X. Li (2010). "The structure and functions of P-glycoprotein." *Current medicinal chemistry* 17(8): 786-800.

Liang, Y., Y. Zhou, J. Zhang, T. Rao, L. Zhou, R. Xing, Q. Wang, H. Fu, K. Hao, L. Xie and G. Wang (2014). "Pharmacokinetic compatibility of ginsenosides and Schisandra lignans in Shengmai-san: From the perspective of P-glycoprotein." *PLoS ONE* 9(6): e98717-e98717.

Liao, M. Z., C. Gao, L. M. Shireman, B. Phillips, L. J. Risler, N. K. Neradugomma, P. Choudhari, B. Prasad, D. D. Shen and Q. Mao (2017). "P-gp/ABCB1 exerts differential impacts on brain and fetal exposure to norbuprenorphine." *Pharmacological research* 119: 61-71.

Lin, J. (2003). "yamazaki, M. Role of P-glycoprotein in pharmacokinetics: clinical implications." *Clin Pharmacokinet* 42(1): 59-98.

Liu, L. and X. Liu (2019). Contributions of drug transporters to blood-placental barrier. *Drug Transporters in Drug Disposition, Effects and Toxicity*, Springer: 505-548.

Lo, A. and G. J. Burckart (1999). "P-glycoprotein and drug therapy in organ transplantation." *The Journal of Clinical Pharmacology* 39(10): 995-1005.

Lou, Y., Z. Guo, Y. Zhu, G. Zhang, Y. Wang, X. Qi, L. Lu, Z. Liu and J. Wu (2019). "Astragali radix and its main bioactive compounds activate the Nrf2-mediated signaling pathway to induce P-glycoprotein and breast cancer resistance protein." *Journal of ethnopharmacology* 228: 82-91.

Lown, K. S., R. R. Mayo, A. B. Leichtman, H. l. Hsiao, D. K. Turgeon, P. Schmiedlin-Ren, M. B. Brown, W. Guo, S. J. Rossi and L. Z. Benet (1997). "Role of intestinal P-glycoprotein (mdr1) in interpatient variation in the oral bioavailability of cyclosporine." *Clinical pharmacology & therapeutics* 62(3): 248-260.

Lü, D., Q. Jiang, J. Zhang, R. Zeng, Z. Liao and X. Liang (2020). "Effect of Baizhu (Rhizoma Atractylodis Macrocephalae) extract on intestinal absorption of brucine and strychnine in vitro and in situ." *Journal of Traditional Chinese Medicine= Chung i tsa Chih Ying wen pan* 40(4): 562-570.

Martin, P., M. Gillen, D. Millson, S. Oliver, C. Brealey, R. Elsby, M. Baluom, D. Lau and T. Mant (2015). "Effects of Fostamatinib on the Pharmacokinetics of Digoxin (a P-Glycoprotein Substrate): Results from in Vitro and Phase i Clinical Studies." *Clinical Therapeutics* 37(12): 2811-2822.

Masuda, S., M. Goto, T. Kiuchi, S. Uemoto, T. Kodawara, H. Saito, K. Tanaka and K.-i. Inui (2003). "Enhanced expression of enterocyte P-glycoprotein depresses cyclosporine bioavailability in a recipient of living donor liver transplantation." *Liver transplantation* 9(10): 1108-1113.

Meyer, U. A. (1996). "Overview of enzymes of drug metabolism." *Journal of pharmacokinetics and biopharmaceutics* 24(5): 449-459.

Mohana, S., M. Ganesan, N. R. Prasad, D. Ananthakrishnan and D. Velmurugan (2018). "Flavonoids modulate multidrug resistance through wnt signaling in P-glycoprotein overexpressing cell lines." *BMC cancer* 18(1): 1-11.

Mollazadeh, S., A. Sahebkar, F. Hadizadeh, J. Behravan and S. Arabzadeh (2018). "Structural and functional aspects of P-glycoprotein and its inhibitors." *Life sciences* 214: 118-123.

Mouly, S. and M. F. Paine (2003). "P-glycoprotein increases from proximal to distal regions of human small intestine." *Pharmaceutical research* 20(10): 1595-1599.

Mouly, S. J., M. F. Paine and P. B. Watkins (2004). "Contributions of CYP3A4, P-glycoprotein, and serum protein binding to the intestinal first-pass extraction of saquinavir." *Journal of Pharmacology and Experimental Therapeutics* 308(3): 941-948.

Muthusamy, G., S. Gunaseelan and N. R. Prasad (2019). "Ferulic acid reverses P-glycoprotein-mediated multidrug resistance via inhibition of PI3K/Akt/NF-$κ$B signaling pathway." *Journal of Nutritional Biochemistry* 63: 62-71.

Muthusamy, G., S. Gunaseelan and N. R. Prasad (2019). "Ferulic acid reverses P-glycoprotein-mediated multidrug resistance via inhibition of PI3K/Akt/NF-κB signaling pathway." *The Journal of nutritional biochemistry* 63: 62-71.

Nebert, D. W. and T. P. Dalton (2006). "The role of cytochrome P450 enzymes in endogenous signalling pathways and environmental carcinogenesis." *Nature Reviews Cancer* 6(12): 947-960.

Neerati, P. and S. Kumar Bedada (2015). "Effect of diosmin on the intestinal absorption and pharmacokinetics of fexofenadine in rats." *Pharmacological Reports* 67(2): 339-344.

Negoro, R., K. Kawai, M. Ichikawa, S. Deguchi, K. Takayama and H. Mizuguchi (2020). "Establishment of MDR1-knockout human induced pluripotent stem cell line." *Drug Metabolism and Pharmacokinetics*.

Nicolaï, J., H. Chapy, E. Gillent, K. Saunders, A.-L. Ungell, J.-M. Nicolas and H. Chanteux (2020). "Impact of In Vitro Passive Permeability in a P-gp-transfected LLC-PK1 Model on the Prediction of the Rat and

Human Unbound Brain-to-Plasma Concentration Ratio." *Pharmaceutical Research* 37(9): 1-17.

Ozturk, N., D. Ozturk, Z. Pala-Kara and A. Okyar (2017). "Pharmacokinetics of talinolol is modified by barnidipine: Implication of P-glycoprotein modulation." *Pharmazie* 72(1): 29-34.

Raish, M., A. Ahmad, M. A. Ansari, K. M. Alkharfy, A. Ahad, F. I. Al-Jenoobi, A. M. Al-Mohizea, A. Khan and N. Ali (2019). "Effects of sinapic acid on hepatic cytochrome P450 3A2, 2C11, and intestinal P-glycoprotein on the pharmacokinetics of oral carbamazepine in rats: Potential food/herb-drug interaction." *Epilepsy Research* 153: 14-18.

Robillard, K. R., G. N. Chan, G. Zhang, C. la Porte, W. Cameron and R. Bendayan (2014). "Role of P-glycoprotein in the distribution of the HIV protease inhibitor atazanavir in the brain and male genital tract." *Antimicrobial agents and chemotherapy* 58(3): 1713-1722.

Schinkel, A. H. (1999). "P-Glycoprotein, a gatekeeper in the blood–brain barrier." *Advanced drug delivery reviews* 36(2-3): 179-194.

Shaik, M. and S. R. Vanapatla (2019). "Enhanced oral bioavailability of linagliptin by the influence of gallic acid and ellagic acid in male Wistar albino rats: Involvement of p-glycoprotein inhibition." *Drug Metabolism and Personalized Therapy* 34(2).

Shebley, M., P. Sandhu, A. Emami Riedmaier, M. Jamei, R. Narayanan, A. Patel, S. A. Peters, V. P. Reddy, M. Zheng, L. de Zwart, M. Beneton, F. Bouzom, J. Chen, Y. Chen, Y. Cleary, C. Collins, G. L. Dickinson, N. Djebli, H. J. Einolf, I. Gardner, F. Huth, F. Kazmi, F. Khalil, J. Lin, A. Odinecs, C. Patel, H. Rong, E. Schuck, P. Sharma, S. P. Wu, Y. Xu, S. Yamazaki, K. Yoshida and M. Rowland (2018). "Physiologically Based Pharmacokinetic Model Qualification and Reporting Procedures for Regulatory Submissions: A Consortium Perspective." *Clin Pharmacol Ther* 104(1): 88-110.

Smit, J. W., A. H. Schinkel, B. Weert and D. K. Meijer (1998). "Hepatobiliary and intestinal clearance of amphiphilic cationic drugs in mice in which both mdr1a and mdr1b genes have been disrupted." *British journal of pharmacology* 124(2): 416-424.

Stephens, R. H., C. A. O'Neill, A. Warhurst, G. L. Carlson, M. Rowland and G. Warhurst (2001). "Kinetic profiling of P-glycoprotein-mediated drug efflux in rat and human intestinal epithelia." *Journal of Pharmacology and Experimental Therapeutics* 296(2): 584-591.

Swain, M., K. Orzechowski, H. Swaim, Y. Jones, M. Robl, C. Tinaza, M. Myers, M. Jhingory, L. Buckely and V. Lancaster (2013). "P-gp substrate-induced neurotoxicity in an Abcb1a knock-in/Abcb1b knock-out mouse model with a mutated canine ABCB1 targeted insertion." *Research in veterinary science* 94(3): 656-661.

Syvänen, S., G. Luurtsema, C. F. Molthoff, A. D. Windhorst, M. C. Huisman, A. A. Lammertsma, R. A. Voskuyl and E. C. de Lange (2011). "(R)-[11 C] Verapamil PET studies to assess changes in P-glycoprotein expression and functionality in rat blood-brain barrier after exposure to kainate-induced status epilepticus." *BMC medical imaging* 11(1): 1.

Takanaga, H., A. Ohnishi, H. Matsuo and Y. SAWADA (1998). "Inhibition of vinblastine efflux mediated by P-glycoprotein by grapefruit juice components in caco-2 cells." *Biological and Pharmaceutical Bulletin* 21(10): 1062-1066.

Tatke, A., K. Y. Janga, B. Avula, X. Wang, M. M. Jablonski, I. A. Khan and S. Majumdar (2018). "P-glycoprotein Restricts ocular penetration of loperamide across the blood-ocular barriers: a comparative study in Mdr1a knock-out and wild type Sprague Dawley rats." *AAPS PharmSciTech* 19(4): 1662-1671.

Tsukimoto, M., R. Ohashi, N. Torimoto, Y. Togo, T. Suzuki, T. Maeda and Y. Kagawa (2015). "Effects of the inhibition of intestinal P-glycoprotein on aliskiren pharmacokinetics in cynomolgus monkeys." *Biopharmaceutics and Drug Disposition* 36(1): 15-33.

Veenstra, S. J., H. Rueeger, M. Voegtle, R. Lueoend, P. Holzer, K. Hurth, M. Tintelnot-Blomley, M. Frederiksen, J.-M. Rondeau and L. Jacobson (2018). "Discovery of amino-1, 4-oxazines as potent BACE-1 inhibitors." *Bioorganic & medicinal chemistry letters* 28(12): 2195-2200.

Villar, V. H., O. Vögler, J. Martínez-Serra, R. Ramos, S. Calabuig-Fariñas, A. Gutiérrez, F. Barceló, J. Martín-Broto and R. Alemany (2012).

"Nilotinib counteracts P-glycoprotein-mediated multidrug resistance and synergizes the antitumoral effect of doxorubicin in soft tissue sarcomas." *PLoS ONE* 7(5).

Wang, F., P. Lv, Y. Gu, L. Li, X. Ge and G. Guo (2017). "Galectin-1 knockdown improves drug sensitivity of breast cancer by reducing P-glycoprotein expression through inhibiting the Raf-1/AP-1 signaling pathway." *Oncotarget* 8(15): 25097.

Wang, F., D. Zhang, Q. Zhang, Y. Chen, D. Zheng, L. Hao, C. Duan, L. Jia, G. Liu and Y. Liu (2011). "Synergistic effect of folate-mediated targeting and verapamil-mediated P-gp inhibition with paclitaxel - polymer micelles to overcome multi-drug resistance." *Biomaterials* 32(35): 9444-9456.

Wang, H., X.-H. Jia, J.-R. Chen, J.-Y. Wang and Y.-J. Li (2016). "Osthole shows the potential to overcome P-glycoprotein-mediated multidrug resistance in human myelogenous leukemia K562/ADM cells by inhibiting the PI3K/Akt signaling pathway." *Oncology reports* 35(6): 3659-3668.

Wang, L.-H., J.-Y. Yang, S.-N. Yang, Y. Li, G.-F. Ping, Y. Hou, W. Cui, Z.-Z. Wang, W. Xiao and C.-F. Wu (2014). "Suppression of NF-κB Signaling and P-glycoprotein Function by Gambogic Acid Synergistically Potentiates Adriamycin -induced Apoptosis in Lung Cancer." *Current Cancer Drug Targets* 14(1): 91-103.

Wang, L. M., M. Y. Zhang, Q. S. Zhu, C. F. Lu and X. Bai (2018). "Hyperin enhances the sensitivity of HCT8/VCR colon cancer cell line to vincristine by down-regulating P-glycoprotein." *Clinical Laboratory* 64(3): 269-275.

Wang, Z., D. Pal and A. K. Mitra (2012). "Stereoselective evasion of P-glycoprotein, cytochrome P450 3A, and hydrolases by peptide prodrug modification of saquinavir." *Journal of pharmaceutical sciences* 101(9): 3199-3213.

Wils, P., V. Phung-Ba, A. Warnery, D. Lechardeur, S. Raeissi, I. J. Hidalgo and D. Scherman (1994). "Polarized transport of docetaxel and vinblastine mediated by P-glycoprotein in human intestinal epithelial cell monolayers." *Biochemical pharmacology* 48(7): 1528-1530.

Xie, Y., N. Yu, Y. Chen, K. Zhang, H. Y. Ma and Q. Di (2017). "HMGB1 regulates P-glycoprotein expression in status epilepticus rat brains via the RAGE/NF-κB signaling pathway." *Molecular Medicine Reports* 16(2): 1691-1700.

Yamazaki, M., W. E. Neway, T. Ohe, I.-W. Chen, J. F. Rowe, J. H. Hochman, M. Chiba and J. H. Lin (2001). "In vitro substrate identification studies for p-glycoprotein-mediated transport: species difference and predictability of in vivo results." *Journal of Pharmacology and Experimental Therapeutics* 296(3): 723-735.

Yan, M., P. F. Fang, H. D. Li, P. Xu, Y. P. Liu, F. Wang, H. L. Cai and Q. Y. Tan (2013). "Lack of effect of continuous glycyrrhizin administration on the pharmacokinetics of the P-glycoprotein substrate talinolol in healthy volunteers." *European Journal of Clinical Pharmacology* 69(3): 515-521.

Yano, K., T. Tomono and T. Ogihara (2018). "Advances in studies of P-glycoprotein and its expression regulators." *Biological and Pharmaceutical Bulletin* 41(1): 11-19.

Yee, K. L., S. G. Khalilieh, R. I. Sanchez, R. Liu, M. S. Anderson, H. Manthos, T. Judge, J. Brejda and J. R. Butterton (2017). "The Effect of Single and Multiple Doses of Rifampin on the Pharmacokinetics of Doravirine in Healthy Subjects." *Clinical Drug Investigation* 37(7): 659-667.

Yigitaslan, S., K. Erol, C. C. A. i. C. And and undefined "*The effect of P-glycoprotein inhibition and activation on the absorption and serum levels of cyclosporine and tacrolimus in rats*." advances.umed.wroc.pl.

Yigitaslan, S., K. Erol and C. Cengelli (2016). "The effect of P-glycoprotein inhibition and activation on the absorption and serum levels of cyclosporine and tacrolimus in rats." *Advances in Clinical and Experimental Medicine* 25(2): 237-242.

Yumoto, R., T. Murakami, M. Sanemasa, R. Nasu, J. Nagai and M. Takano (2001). "Pharmacokinetic interaction of cytochrome P450 3A-related compounds with rhodamine 123, a P-glycoprotein substrate, in rats pretreated with dexamethasone." *Drug metabolism and disposition* 29(2): 145-151.

Zhang, L., Y. Zhang, J. M. Strong, K. Reynolds and S.-M. Huang (2008). "A regulatory viewpoint on transporter-based drug interactions." *Xenobiotica* 38(7-8): 709-724.

Zhang, Y., Y. Feng, K. N. Darshika, B. Zhang, Y. Hu, W. Fang, Y. Li and W. Huang (2015). "The effect of multidrug resistance modulator HZ08 on pharmacodynamics and pharmacokinetics of adriamycin in xenograft-nude mice." *European Journal of Pharmaceutical Sciences* 66: 109-117.

Zhang, Y., S. K. Sriraman, H. A. Kenny, E. Luther, V. Torchilin and E. Lengyel (2016). "Reversal of chemoresistance in ovarian cancer by co-delivery of a P-glycoprotein inhibitor and paclitaxel in a liposomal platform." *Molecular Cancer Therapeutics* 15(10): 2282-2293.

Zhao, Q., Y. Zou, C. Huang, P. Lan, J. Zheng and S. Ou (2017). "Formation of a hydroxymethylfurfural–cysteine adduct and its absorption and cytotoxicity in Caco-2 Cells." *Journal of agricultural and food chemistry* 65(45): 9902-9908.

Zhao, R., J. C. Kalvass, S. B. Yanni, A. S. Bridges and G. M. Pollack (2009). "Fexofenadine brain exposure and the influence of blood-brain barrier P-glycoprotein after fexofenadine and terfenadine administration." *Drug metabolism and disposition* 37(3): 529-535.

Zhou, Y., P. Y. Chung, J. Y. W. Ma, A. K. Y. Lam, S. Law, K. W. Chan, A. S. C. Chan, X. Li, K. H. Lam, C. H. Chui and J. C. O. Tang (2019). "Development of a novel quinoline derivative as a P-glycoprotein inhibitor to reverse multidrug resistance in cancer cells." *Biology* 8(4).

In: An Introduction to P-Glycoprotein ISBN: 978-1-53619-488-3
Editors: M. Wahajuddin et al.

Chapter 5

P-GLYCOPROTEIN, A BIOLOGICAL AND MEDICINAL CHEMISTRY/RADIOCHEMISTRY POINT OF VIEW

***Carmen Abate**, *Nicola Antonio Colabufo*† and *Marialessandra Contino*≠**
Dipartimento di Farmacia-Scienze del Farmaco,
Università degli Studi di Bari, Bari, Italy

ABSTRACT

P-glycoprotein is an important transporter belonging to ATP-Binding Cassette pumps (ABC-B1). This transporter plays a fundamental role in several degenerative diseases such as Alzheimer's, Parkinson's and other forms of dementia, as well as in tumors. This transporter is localized at the blood brain barrier (BBB) where it is involved in the efflux of endogenous and exogenous compounds and it is overexpressed in several tumor cell lines determining Multi Drug Resistance (MDR). In this chapter, we will

* Corresponding Author's Email: carmen.abate@uniba.it.
† Corresponding Author's Email: nicolaantonio.colabufo@uniba.it.
≠ Corresponding Author's Email: marialessandra.contino@uniba.it.

examine the *in vitro* biological assays useful to establish the P-gp interactive mechanisms of a ligand and its potential in terms of therapy and diagnosis. In addition, examples of Structure Activity Relationship (SAR) studies of P-gp modulators will be described. Moreover, P-gp imaging by PET with different radioligands (^{11}C and ^{18}F -radiolabelled) will be herein discussed. Finally, the difficulty in the definition of a pharmacophore for the design of substrates, modulators and inhibitors is also critically approached in this chapter.

Keywords: P-glycoprotein, ATP-Binding Cassette pumps (ABC-B1), degenerative diseases, Multi Drug Resistance (MDR), radioligands, radiolabeled

Introduction

ABC transporter superfamily is the most important family of transmembrane proteins comprising seven subfamilies and enclosing about fifty transport proteins. These pumps efflux various endogenous and exogenous compounds across cell membranes and their role is fundamental for the neurophysiology of the Central Nervous System (CNS), where their alteration in terms of activity and expression seems to be linked to several pathologies such as Alzheimer's, Parkinson's, and epilepsy. In addition, these pumps are involved in Ocular disease, in Chronic Rhinosinusitis, and mainly in several forms of MultiDrug Resistance (MDR) in cancer where their expression and activity is largely increased with consequent reduction of the bioavailability of the drug in tumour cells [1-3].

P-glycoprotein (P-gp) is an ABC pump belonging to the ABC-B subfamily known as ABCB1 transporter, and to date it is largely studied in terms of binding sites, and in its role and localization because these details allow to defining how the pump is involved in physiological/pathological pathways. It is a 170 KDa protein crossing the lipid bilayer of the cell membrane with six Trans Membrane Domains (TMD) as a single chain. At the cytoplasmic side, it presents two sites for linking ATP (Nucleotide Binding Domains, NBDs). For each cycle P-gp employs the first ATP for a conformational change of the Trans Membrane helix to efflux a wide range of substrates, and the second ATP to set back the pump to the initial active state [4-8]. At the CNS level, P-gp effluxes several drugs as well as endogenous compounds from metabolism, and among the latters, several studies also report β-amyloid and α-synuclein, that are validated biomarkers for Alzheimer's and Parkinson's diseases, respectively [9-12].

Considering the crucial role of P-gp in several physio-pathological states, "old drugs" such as veramapil, loperamid, cyclosporine, elacridar, tariquidar, metoclopramide, as well as novel compounds have been studied [13-16] with the aim to identify the pharmacophores for substrates, inhibitors and modulators. Although several classes of compounds have been published, the Structure Activity Relationship (SAR) studies are useful and somehow coherent only intraclass and, all together these studies have not contributed to uniquely disclose the pharmacophore. In addition, the methodologies to study the potency and the mechanism of action for each compound by biological assays are sometimes different to univocally define a P-gp ligand, as reported in the biological chapter.

P-gp imaging by PET studies may have an important role because P-gp, but also other ABC transporters defined as "sister proteins" as the Breast Cancer Resistance Protein (BCRP) that is a P-gp monomer, and the Multidrug Resistance associated Protein 1 (MRP1) display a decreased expression and function in Alzheimer's disease [17-19] and in epilepsy [20-22], whereas in brain tumours, an increase in P-gp (but also in BCRP and MRP1) expression and function [23, 24] has been detected, as well as in multiple sclerosis [25], in schizophrenia and Creutzfeldt-Jakob disease. By contrast, in depression, P-gp expression and function is increased [26, 27].

One of the difficulties to define a pharmacophore for P-gp ligands (substrate and inhibitor) is due to the poor selectivity of several compounds that bind P-gp in the same manner as they bind BCRP. Moreover also other ABC proteins could be involved in the binding of ligands, such as ABCC1 and ABCC2 transporters, better known as MRP1 and MRP2, respectively. Moreover, some compounds display a substrate or inhibitor behavior in a dose-dependent manner [28], and sometimes the same compound may act as inhibitor on P-gp and substrate *vs* BCRP and MPRs [29]. These are some of the difficulties that led to develop only few but significant PET radiotracers. The best P-gp compounds known in the literature have been radiolabelled (several compounds as 11C-, few as 18F-radiotracers) and used in Positron Emission Tomography (PET) in animal models and in human studies and will be illustrated in the specific section: *PET ligands for P-gp*.

A Biological Point of View: The P-Gp Interacting Mechanism

As previously mentioned, the compounds identified as P-gp ligands are several and structurally unrelated because of the accommodating nature of the binding site(s) in the protein, responsible for the interaction with different types of agents classified as substrates, inhibitors, modulators and inducers/activators *vs* the pump [14, 30, 31].

Generally, substrates, inhibitors and modulators interact with the pump exerting a type of final action that can be considered as an “inhibition” or a decreased activity, since this interaction may have the inhibition of the transport of a P-gp substrate, as final effect; while an inducer or an activator leads to an increased activity of the transporter as final effect. An univocal biological assay to classify a P-gp ligand as belonging to one of the above mentioned classes of compounds is still controversial but several papers report the use of a combination of biological assays to hit the aim [32-45].

These three biological assays are: 1) the study of the inhibition of the transport of a profluorescent probe, that is a known P-gp substrate; 2) the determination of a parameter, *i.e.*, the apparent permeability ratio (P_{app}); 3) the measure of the ATP cell consumption. All these assays are performed in a cell line overexpressing P-gp [32-45].

In the first assay, the competition for the binding site of a P-gp substrate, the acethoxymethyl ester of calcein (Calcein-AM), is evaluated (Figure 1). Calein-AM is a P-gp substrate and it is not fluorescent *per se*; therefore, in a cell line overexpressing P-gp, the probe does not enter the cell. By contrast, when P-gp is blocked (by a ligand interacting with the pump, thus all the above three types of ligands), Calcein-AM enters the cell and in the cytosol it is hydrolized to the fluorescent calcein by the esterases. Calcein is not a P-gp substrate and, being hydrophilic, can not be effluxed by passive diffusion so that it remains in the cytosol of the cells showing fluorescence. The detected fluorescence is directly correlated to the entity of the P-gp block. Thus, this first assay gives information only about the existence of an interaction with the pump and about the potency of this interaction.

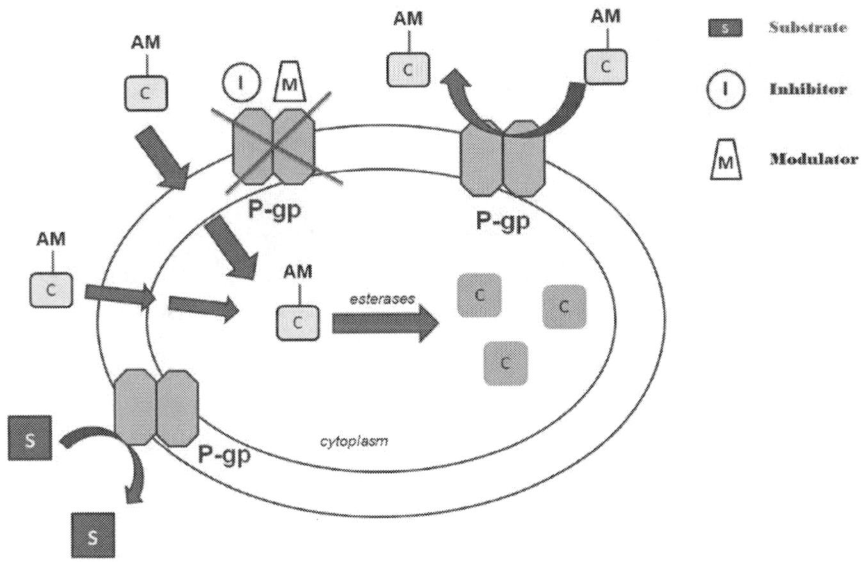

Figure 1. Calcein-AM assay.

The second assay is performed in a monolayer of cells mimicking the blood brain barrier where the P-gp is highly expressed at the apical level (Figure 2). The assay measures the ratio between two fluxes: (1) from the basolateral to apical compartments (BA), due to passive diffusion since P-gp is apically expressed; and (2) from the apical to basolateral compartment (AB), influenced by the P-gp-mediated active transport.

A BA/AB ratio < 2 means that the flux from apical to basolateral is higher than the flux from basolateral to apical, and thus no active transport is observed at the apical level where P-gp is present and the compound can overcome the membrane without any efflux. In this case the tested compound may be classified as a P-gp inhibitor.

A BA/AB > 2 means that the flux from basolateral to apical compartment is higher than the flux from apical to basolateral, and this finding means that a P-gp mediated efflux is occurring at the apical level and the compound can enter the cell membrane only by passive diffusion (at the basal level) while at the apical level it is effluxed by the pump. In this case the test compound may be classified as P-gp substrate or modulator.

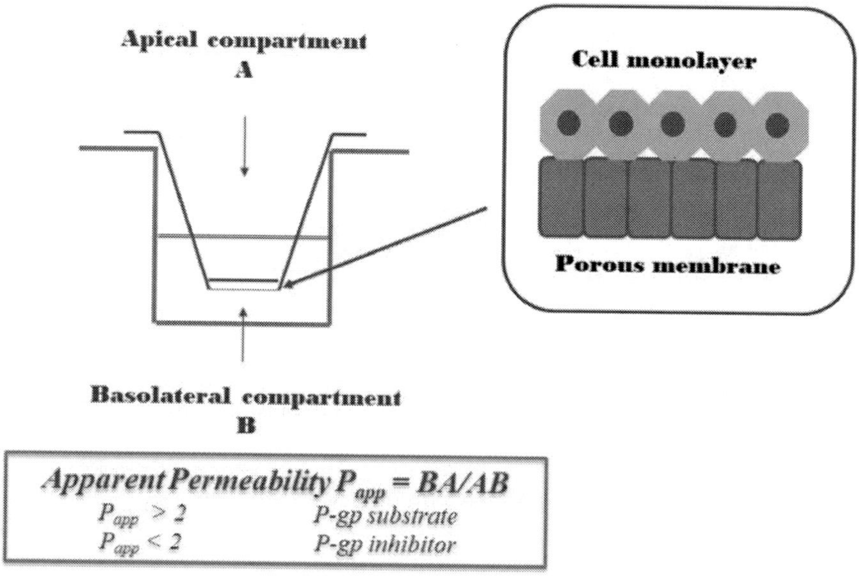

Figure 2. Determination of Apparent permeability.

The third assay, completes the second assay since only a P-gp substrate, being transported by the pump, induces an ATP cell consumption, while a P-gp inhibitor does not induce ATP consumption since it is not transported by the pump but binds the protein in its specific site.

In Table 1 the classification of P-gp ligands on the basis of the results from the three biological assays is reported. Generally, a substrate is a ligand actively transported by P-gp, thus inducing an ATP cell depletion and having a P_{app}>2; an inhibitor is not transported and thus it does not induce an ATP cell depletion and has a P_{app}< 2 (Category I). Substrates are subcategorized in Category II based on their different response to the three combined assays and are classified in nontransported (IIA) and transported substrates (IIB1-3) (Category II, Table 1).

In conclusion, the definition of the binding sites is still controversial, however, in order to simplify the classification, a substrate, to be transported through the translocation mechanism, firstly binds the substrate site on P-gp and simultaneously an ATP molecule binds the NBDs (Figure 3). The hydrolysis of this ATP molecule drives the efflux of the substrate. An inhibitor blocks the P-gp translocation, binding P-gp on the NBDs site not allowing ATP to bind the pump. A modulator is able to reduce the binding of a substrate through a negative allosteric interaction in a non competitive manner in a different site [14] (Figure 3).

Table 1. Classification of P-gp ligands in categories on the basis of the three biological assays

P-gp ligands		P_{app}	**ATP cell depletion**	**Substrate transport inhibition**
Category I				
	Unambiguous nonsubstrates	<2	No	No
	Unambiguous substrates	>2	Yes	Yes
	Inhibitors	<2	No	Yes
Category II				
IIA	*Nontransported substrates*	<2	Yes	Yes
IIB_1	*Transported substrates*	>2	No	No
IIB_2	*Transported substrates*	>2	Yes	No
IIB_3	*Transported substrates*	>2	No	Yes

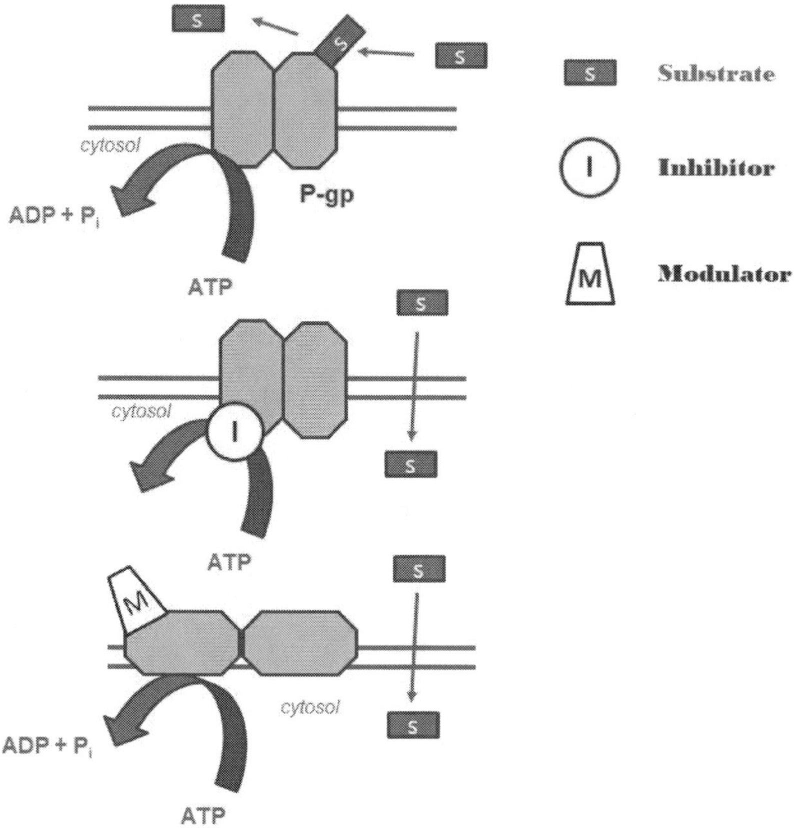

Figure 3. Different mechanisms of a P-gp substrate, inhibitor or modulator.

SUBSTRATES, INHIBITORS AND MODULATORS: THE PIVOTAL ROLE OF P-GP IN THE THERAPY AND DIAGNOSIS OF PATHOLOGICAL CONDITIONS

P-gp ligands may be used both in the oncological and in neurodegenerative fields as therapeutic agents or diagnostic tools with different potentialities.

In the diagnostic field, the use of substrates or inhibitors may give different information about the expression or the activity of the pump. A substrate, administered alone or in combination with a modulator, may be useful in the evaluation of P-gp activity, while a radiolabelled inhibitor, may be useful to detect P-gp expression. This information can be of great interest to early identify a decreased activity of the transporter, as occurs in Alzheimer's or Parkinson's diseases where P-gp is downregulated and/or not active, or an overexpression of the protein, as occurs in resistant tumours. For this purpose, great attention has attracted the development of P-gp radioligands as reported in the section *PET ligands for P-gp* reported below.

In the therapeutic field in oncology, the final effect induced by an inhibitor or a substrate is the same, restoring the cell sensitivity to antineoplastic agents, even if exerted with a different mechanism. Therefore, one of the most attempted strategies to overcome MDR in cancer therapy has been the use of a P-gp ligand acting as substrate or inhibitor, in co-administration with the antineoplastic drugs to hamper the drug efflux reversing resistance [46, 47]. However, this approach failed when translated into clinic for different reasons, as stated in the next chapter [48].

Recently, a new therapeutic strategy due to a phenomenon called collateral sensitivity (CS) has been proposed. CS occurs when a compound is able to selectively kill MDR cells but it does not exert the same effect on the drug-sensitive parental cells from which MDR cells are derived [49-53].

CS was firstly described in 1952 [50] when it was observed that drug-resistant *Escherichia coli* showed hypersensitivity to different drugs, displaying a potential weakness as a result of the drug selection process; then in 1985, CS was also observed in cells overexpressing P-gp. Four main hypotheses have been suggested as CS inducing mechanisms in MDR cells: 1) the induction of reactive oxygen species (ROS); 2) an high sensitivity to changes in energy levels; 3) the efflux of endogenous substrates pivotal in cell survival; 4) the induction of membrane perturbation. The measure of CS may be performed in vitro by a parameter defined Selectivity Ratio (SR).

The SR represents the ratio between the cytotoxicity of a compound in the parental cells and the cytotoxicity in the corresponding MDR-derived cells (SR= EC_{50} parental cells/EC_{50} MDR cells).

A SR value >1 means that the EC_{50} value obtained in the MDR cell line is lower than the EC_{50} value obtained in the parental cell counterpart (consequently, the cytotoxicity is higher in the MDR cells), and therefore the compounds exerts CS.

On the contrary, a SR value <1 means that the EC_{50} value obtained in the MDR cell line is higher than the EC_{50} value obtained in the parental cell counterpart (consequently, the cytotoxicity is higher in the parental cells), and therefore there is a resistance of the MDR line *vs* the compound (that is effluxed by the pump). A SR >2 is a typical value found for compounds classified as CS-promoting agent [49]. This new type of compounds may be really helpful to overcome MDR in cancer since they exploit the expression of the MDR proteins to lead the MDR cells to suicide.

The approach represented by CS-promoting agents is different from the co-administration strategy of P-gp inhibitors with antineoplastic drugs since this latter strategy has the aim to re-sensitize MDR cells to the antineoplastic drug by restoring its access to the MDR cells; CS-promoting agents may be used alone since these agents selectively kill MDR cells and may be in addition associated to the antineoplastic drugs to exert a synergic cytotoxicity *vs* resistant tumours.

We may define CS as a synthetic lethality, where the genetic changes responsible for the resistance *vs* a specific agent, are followed by the induction of hypersensitivity *vs* a second agent [51].

P-Glycoprotein Inducers and Activators

These classes of ligands may be considered as one single class on the basis of the final induced effect, that is the "increase" of the activity of the transporter. Anyway, there is a substantial difference between a P-gp inducer and a P-gp activator due to their different rate of action. Indeed, a P-gp inducer exerts its activity by the increase in P-gp expression with a consequent increase also in the pump activity [54]. A P-gp activator, differently from the inducer, displays the ability to increase P-gp activity without any effect on P-gp expression [55, 56]. Indeed, a P-gp activator binds P-gp leading to a conformational change, responsible for the efflux of a substrate, that is bound on a different binding site on the pump [55, 56].

For this reason, since the activation mechanism is a direct mechanism and does not involve the expression of the protein, it is a rapid process [56].

Both inducers and activators are able to increase P-gp expression and/or activity in a time- and concentration-dependent manner [57, 58] exerting their protective role by increasing the cellular efflux of toxic drugs or xenobiotics and decreasing the intracellular accumulation and, consequently, their toxicity.

The importance of inducers has been demonstrated *in vitro* and *in vivo* mainly as therapeutic detoxification approach in different type of poisonings. For instance, in the 2006, Dinis-Oliveira and coworkers demonstrated *in vivo* the efficacy of P-gp induction through dexamethasone in Paraquat poisonings [59-61]. The same effect was then observed *in vitro* for other P-gp inducers as synthetic corticosteroid in different cell models confirming P-gp induction as an effective approach against paraquat poisoning and generally validating P-gp induction strategy as an effective antidotal pathway *vs* the P-gp substrates cytotoxicity [57, 58, 62-64].

This class of compounds is under evaluation also for the treatment of neurodegenerative diseases such as AD and PD in which a P-gp decreased activity was also demonstrated for their onset [63-68].

In 2012, Abuznait and Kaddoumi demonstrated that the main pathological hallmark of Alzheimer's disease, *i.e.*, Aβ40 and Aβ42, responsible for the formation of senile plaques, were P-gp substrates [65] and this finding, together with the decreased P-gp activity observed in the disorder, suggested a pivotal role for P-gp in the etiology of the neurodegenerative disease.

Considering the observed effects endowed with P-gp inducers/ stimulators class of compounds, the "activation" of P-gp may also result in an interesting alternative strategy in the therapy of disorders caused by the accumulation or the absorption of a specific substrate as in neurodegenerative diseases.

For this purpose, recently a small molecule named MC111 [71], belonging to the MC70-derived library of compounds (see next chapter), has been proposed as a new multitarget approach for the therapy of Alzheimer disease. MC111 was able to simultaneously act as P-gp and BCRP inducer and stimulator and it was also found able to induce neurites sprouting. Therefore, new attempts now are ongoing to use also *in vivo* this new approach to re-habilitate P-gp in the diseases where it is not active as in AD and PD.

A MEDICINAL CHEMISTRY POINT OF VIEW: DEVELOPMENT OF P-GP INTERACTING COMPOUNDS

The P-gp efflux pump is characterized by a versatile drug-binding region able to host a variety of compounds. More recent models and the high-resolution crystal structure of P-gp suggest a wide and flexible drug-binding space, rather than different drug binding sites, where more molecules can be also simultaneously accommodated [31, 72-75]. The amino acids present in this plastic region, mostly hydrophobic/aromatic, next to hydrophilic and charged residues, create a number of drug binding sub-sites. P-gp ligands are hydrophobic and amphipathic molecules, that interact with the transporter mostly through hydrophobic and van der Waals interactions, with the few polar amino acids residues able to establish additional hydrogen and ionic bonds [76, 77].

In order to overcome P-gp-mediated MDR in cancer treatment, a great interest has initially driven the discovery and development of P-gp inhibitors or modulators.

Briefly, as recent updates report on the origins of the synthesis of P-gp modulators [54, 78, 79], the calcium channel blocker Verapamil (Figure 4) and the immunosuppressive agent cyclosporin A (Figure 4) were found to be MDR modulators. The two drugs, that weakly bind P-gp [80, 81], were used in early clinical trials, and needed high doses to compensate for their low affinity binding, resulting in serious side effects and toxicity. Also the antiestrogen tamoxifen, calmodulin antagonists and the antimalarial quinine [82, 83], that belong to this first generation of MDR modulators, were characterized by inconvenient pharmacokinetic, as they were substrates for other transporters and inhibitors for CYP3A4 enzyme. Therefore, the low potency and specificity and the important side effects of the early P-gp modulators prompted the production of a second generation of compounds. This second generation was developed from the structural modification of verapamil, cyclosporine (leading to valspodar) and other immunosuppressive agents such as tacrolimus. These novel compounds were more potent and with less side effects compared to the first generation, but again, they were generally endowed with the drawback of inhibiting CYP450 with related toxicity (e.g., increase to toxic concentrations of the co-administered antineoplastic agents) [84, 85]. This important limitation led to a third generation of modulators, such as elacridar and tariquidar (Figure 4), with more favorable physicochemical and pharmacokinetic properties. The initial success of these compounds was based on their more focused development based on previous SAR studies and a better knowledge about the possible modes of interaction with P-gp. Previous studies had demonstrated the importance of a hydrogen bond acceptor group, the critical role of a hydrophobic ring, an alkyl spacer and an aromatic portion (π- π interactions within the binding pocket) [86, 87]. Among the classes of compounds, tricyclic residues such as trifluoperazine, phenothiazine, phenoxazine, dibenzosuberane (zosuquidar, Figure 4), and acridones (elacridar, Figure 4) were able to confer strong P-gp inhibitory activity when linked to a protonatable *N*-atom (in particular if belonging to a tertiary amine) [86-91]. Among the basic moieties, tetrahydroisoquinoline has been widely applied as conferring strong activity at the P-gp, as in elacridar [92] and tariquidar [93], both bearing a 6,7-dimethoxy-2-phenethyl-1,2,3,4-tetrahydroisoquinoline nucleus linked to an aryl-substituted amide. Many of these compounds underwent clinical trials in co-administration with anticancer drugs. However, while this third generation of inhibitors was endowed with increased potency (EC_{50} < 100 nM), specificity for P-gp and was devoid of pharmacokinetic interactions with the co-administered anticancer drugs, all clinical trials failed [54, 78, 79].

Such failure may depend on a number of reasons and not all of them are quite clear [94, 95].

First generation	
Verapamil	Ciclosporin A
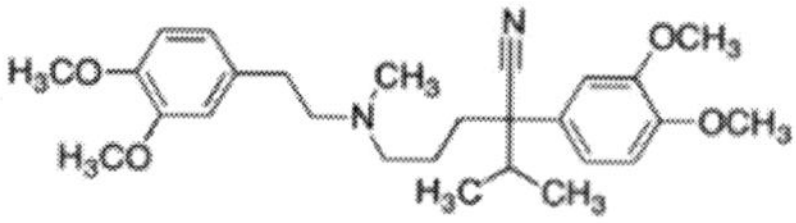	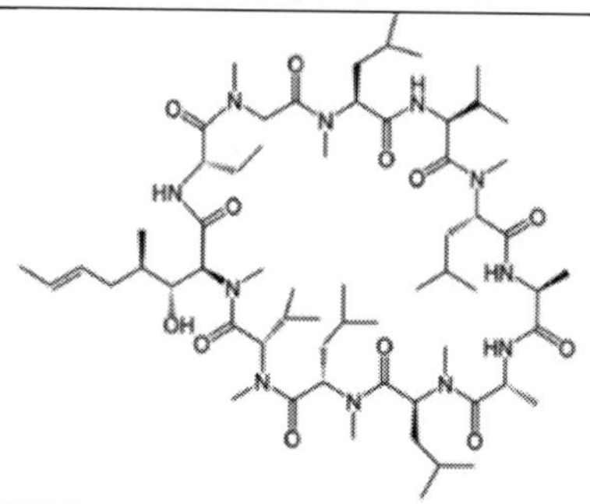
Third generation	
Elacridar	Tariquidar
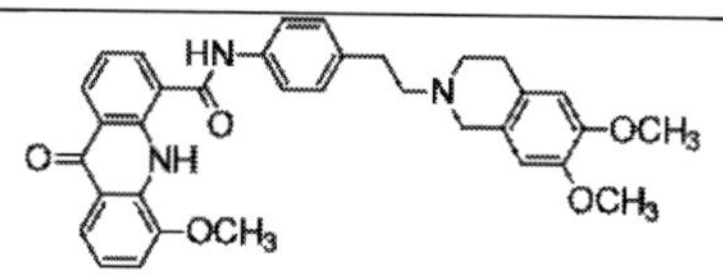	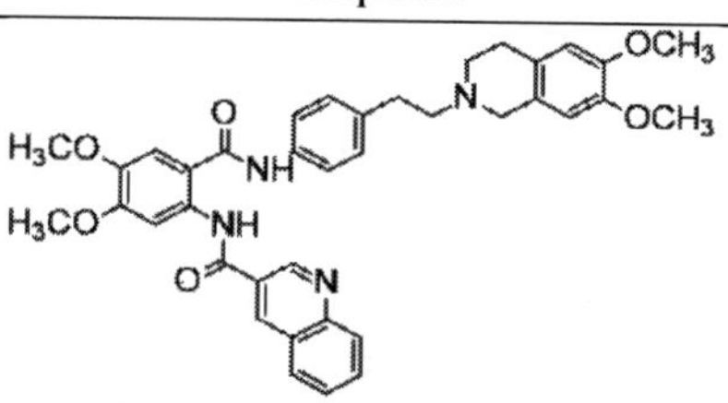
Zosuquidar	
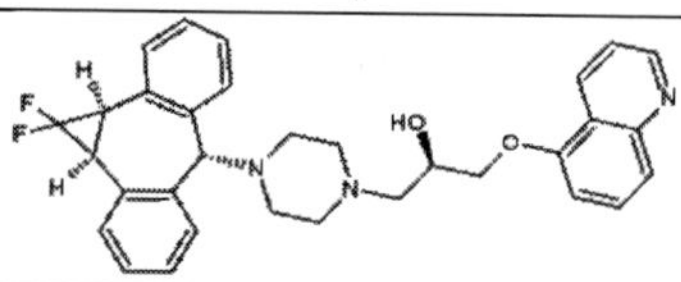	

Figure 4. Representative structures of P-gp-modulators belonging to the 1st and 3rd generations.

Despite the improvement through the generations, the P-gp affinity of the third generation inhibitors is still generally low in comparison with the affinity of the drugs that are clinically used. During the years, SAR analyses and the several computational studies undertaken, have surely contributed to the elucidation of some key interactions of P-gp with its modulators [77, 96-98]. High lipophilicity (log P value higher than 2.9), high molecular weight (more than 18 atoms) to assure hydrophobic/van der Waals interactions, and one tertiary basic amine are needed, with inhibitors generally being more lipophilic than substrates. Nevertheless, even if a better knowledge has been achieved, the P-gp drug binding sites are not well-defined in comparison with the binding sites of other drugs targets, since P-gp, for its intrinsic activity devoted to the efflux of differently structured xenobiotics, is a quite 'accommodating' protein. Additionally, the diverse conformations that the P-gp adopts through its extrusion processes make the definition of the binding pockets even more complicated. Some computational studies were focused on the prediction of the different types of activity of P-gp modulators (as substrates or inhibitors), to conveniently avoid the set of experimental assays, and for some classes of molecules good prediction scores were obtained [99-110]. However, small structural changes in the drug often lead to unlikely predictable shift in the activity (from substrate to inhibitor and *vice versa*): the flexible binding site may or may not incorporate some proximal amino acids, thus reverting the functional activity in the presence of a minimal structural change. An example is given by the indole based P-gp modulators (EC_{50} values 2.25 and 2.34 μM respectively) shown in Figure 5 in which the N-atom of the 6,7-dimethoxytetrahydroisoquinoline is amidic. The only difference in the two compounds is the position of the amide function, either in the chain or in the 6,7-dimethoxytetrahydroisoquinoline nucleus. The activity is thus shifted from P-gp substrate (depleting ATP) to P-gp inhibitor (not depleting ATP) [111]. The plasticity of the P-gp structure is further corroborated by the recently obtained structure of P-gp by cryo-electron microscopy (cryo-em), where zosuquidar (inhibitor) and paclitaxel (substrate) bind the same drug-binding pocket, driving diverse conformational changes that account for the diverse activity [73].

All of these features make the design of high affinity and specific P-gp modulators a quite challenging duty.

Importantly, the use of P-gp inhibitors interferes with P-gp in healthy cells and tissue (such as BBB and intestine), so that these compounds are characterized by an intrinsic toxicity due to the wide distribution and protecting role of the P-gp. Additionally, the co-administration of P-gp inhibitors with the anticancer agent increases the plasma concentration of the latter by competing with metabolism and excretion, increasing the toxicity of the latter.

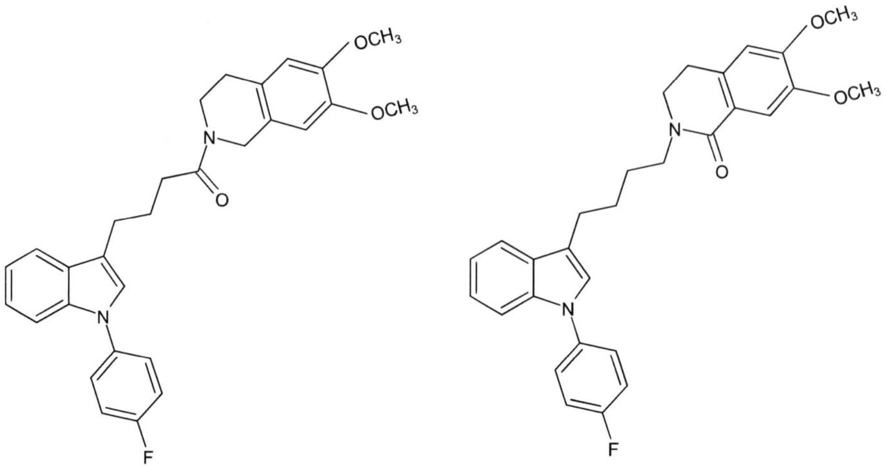

A B

Figure 5. Indole based P-gp modulators: Small structural changes address the P-gp activity.

Despite all these difficulties, MDR remains a major issue to be solved in oncology so that diverse strategies involving P-gp are under study to overcome resistance. The presence of multiple binding sites has been exploited with the development of bivalent compounds with increased activity compared to the monomer counterparts [112-114]. Targeted delivery of P-gp inhibitors to cancer cells through nanotechnologies is also under study, [115-122] in order to reduce toxicity to healthy tissues. Optimization of clinical drugs in order to avoid P-gp-mediated efflux has been adopted. Decades of research on the complex structures of natural anticancer agents have led to identify the optimal sites for modification in order to by-pass P-gp efflux. Examples are structural modifications on vinblastine, whose C20' site resulted in an optimal position for decreasing P-gp interaction [123]. The C20' fluorination have led to Vinflunine with decreased P-gp-mediated efflux compared to other vinca alkaloids and better pharmacokinetic, thus entering clinical use as second-line treatment of urothelial tumors [124-127]. Specific structural modifications to the microtubule-targeting epothilones, led to compounds such as Ixabepilone with a drastically reduced P-gp substrate activity, so that in 2007 it was approved by FDA (but not by EMA) for treating metastatic breast cancer in monotherapy or in combination with capecitabin [128-131]. Several semisynthetic analogues of taxanes have been generated leading to drugs such as cabazitaxel (approved for metastatic prostate cancer treatment) and ortataxel (under clinical trial for different tumors) with considerably increased activity in P-gp overexpressing tumors compared to paclitaxel ([132-137] www.ema.europa.eu; www.fda.gov).

Also multifunctional drugs, able to simultaneously interact with multiple targets other than P-gp have been developed and continue to be developed as a way to overcome MDR in tumors and neurodegenerative diseases. Examples are compounds that act as NO-donors, metal chelators, or that modulate sigma receptors, carbonic anhydrase XII, and BCRP [47, 71, 138-147].

Of course, the potent third generation inhibitors have furnished lead compounds in the search of potent P-gp inhibitors. Tariquidar (EC_{50} = 0.044 μM) and elacridar (EC_{50} = 0.014 μM), that are not highly P-g specific as they also bind BCRP, have inspired several SAR studies. As an example, in one of these studies, the common feature of these two third generation inhibitors, i.e., the 6,7-dimethoxy-2-phenethyl-1,2,3,4-tetrahydroisoquinoline nucleus, was kept and the benzamide function was changed by exploring different aromatic rings (in sizes, shapes and decoration with methoxy groups) [43]. The benzamide function was also replaced by the corresponding ester and alkylamine in order to evaluate how these portions of the molecules could address P-gp selectivity and mechanisms of interaction (General structure in Figure 6A). Although these compounds were less potent than the lead compounds, the small changes across the three series led to interesting differences in the activities: amide and amines were more potent than esters and were P-gp substrates (EC_{50} values ranging from 0.3 μM to 1.01 μM; category IIB3, Table 1) and inactive towards BCRP. Most of the esters (EC_{50} values ranging from 0.33 μM to 10 μM) belonged to the same category of P-gp non-transported substrate with

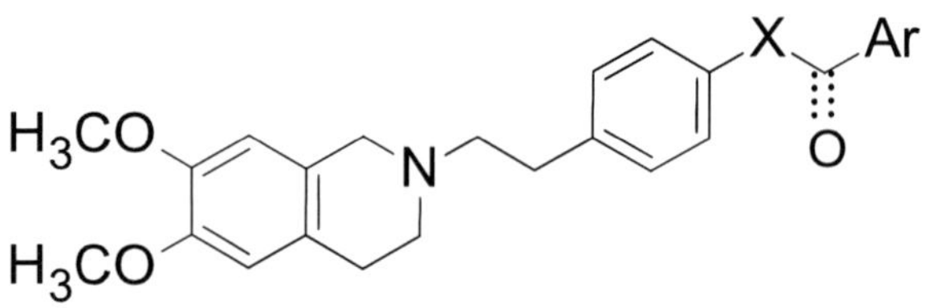

Figure 6A. General structure of novel 6,7-dimethoxy-2-phenethyl-1,2,3,4-tetrahydroisoquinoline.

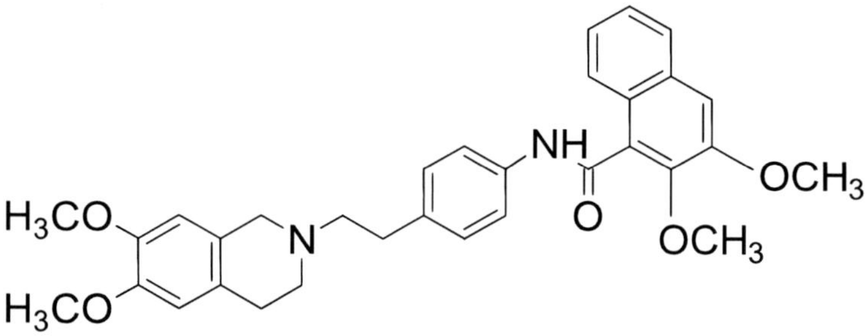

Ortho-methoxy naphthalene derivative

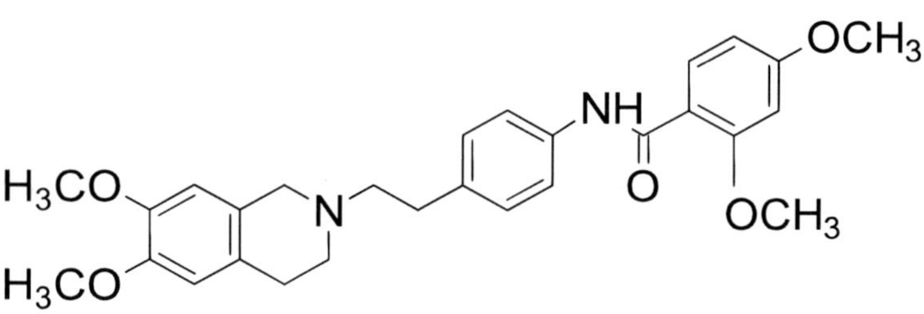

Ortho-methoxy benzene derivative

Figure 6B. Ortho-methoxy benzamides with nanomolar activity at P-gp.

the exception of one ester that was an unambiguous substrate (Category I, Table 1) and another one that was a 'pure' and highly P-gp selective inhibitor (Category I, Table 1). This is another example of how difficult is the prediction of the P-gp activity, as small changes in the structure are able to determine a complete switch in the activity (see Figure 5 as well). The interesting data obtained led to further explore these classes of compounds based on the 6,7-dimethoxy-2-phenethyl-1,2,3,4-tetrahydroisoquinoline scaffold exploring more aromatic substituents in the amide and ester series. Most of the compounds were selective for the P-gp transporter and importantly, independently from the presence of the amide or ester function. Although a clear SAR could not be obtained with these classes, the presence of an ortho-methoxy group in the amide series led to nanomolar P-gp ligands belonging to the II3B class, with the benzene (EC_{50} = 40.5 nM) and the naphthalene (EC_{50} = 47.8 nM) derivatives displaying nanomolar EC_{50} values comparable to the lead compounds tariquidar and elacridar (Figure 6B) [45].

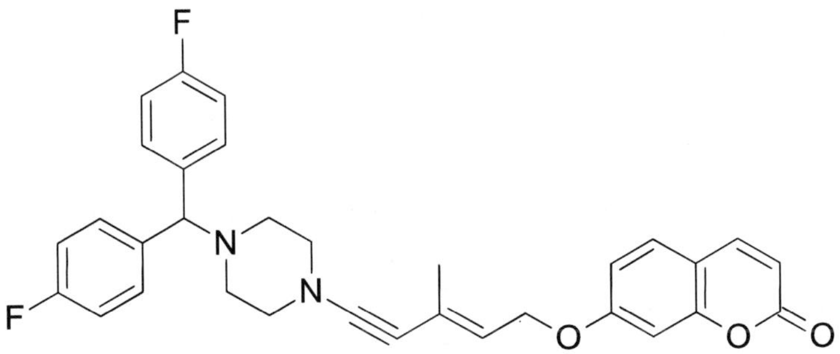

Coumarin with CS property

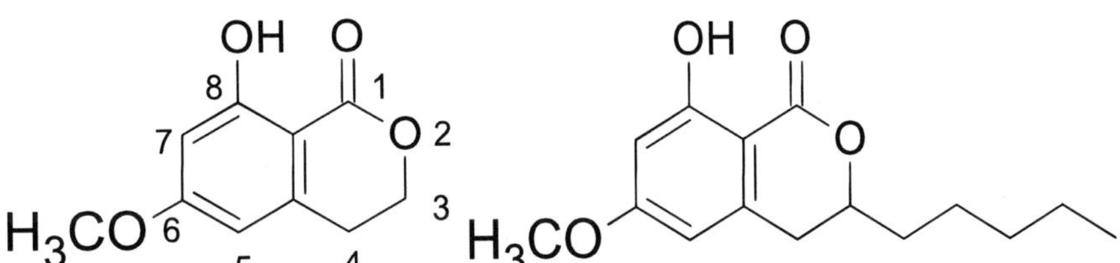

8-OH-3,4-dihydroisocoumarin and its 3-pentyl derivative

Figure 7. Coumarin and isocoumarin.

A source of P-gp modulators is given by natural food and herbal extracts that contain diverse ABC (and P-gp) transporter inhibitors, such as flavonoids, poliphenols, coumarins etc. [148, 149]. In this context, flavonoids (containing the phenylcromanone nucleus), have played an important role in furnishing P-gp inhibitors [150-152]. They have been extensively studied in their different forms (flavones, isoflavones, flavanones, flavonols, flavanols, and chalcones) to determine the structural requirements for P-gp interactions. Synthetic dimers of flavoinoids have been produced in accordance with the strategy of simultaneously binding more sites [114]. Also natural or synthetic coumarins, have been investigated with their ability to inhibit P-gp and restore anticancer drug activity with promising *in vitro* data, though in the micromolar range [153-155]. Some of these compounds such as the synthetic coumarin reported in Figure 7A seemed to be endowed with Collateral Sensitivity properties as well (see the Biology section).

Less explored than flavonoids have been isocoumarins and 3,4-dihydroisocoumarins, that are secondary metabolites contained in fungi, bacteria and plants. These compounds are endowed with several drug-like properties and an important structural versatility so that a recent study has analyzed some natural and synthetic isocoumarins [156]. Although, these compounds are active in inhibiting P-gp only in the micromolar range (doxorubicine activity in cancer cells is restored in co-administration with 50 μM of the most promising isocoumarin), SAR and molecular docking to the P-gp of the 3,4-dihydroisocoumarin derivatives have shown some important clues to improve the biological profile of these derivatives. For transporter inhibition the isocoumarin bicycle (Figure 7B) has to carry in 8-position the hydroxy group (that stabilizes the interaction with P-gp through H-bond with Y306), and in 3-position an hydrophobic carbon chain (a pentyl chain was the best, although only few compounds were analyzed in order to define the best fit). The best compounds of this small series were also able to inhibit BCRP resulting in dual inhibitors, as a pursued strategy for diverse therapeutic aims (see above). Additionally, the 3-pentyl derivative reported in Figure 7B provided hints for CS that need to be further explored (see the Biology section).

Several more classes of P-gp substrates or inhibitors have been produced and extensively reviewed [54, 75, 78, 79]. Several are under development and here follows an example of SAR studies focused on the optimization of a promising P-gp-inhibitor belonging to the biphenyl derivatives class.

Biphenyl derivatives bearing a tetrahydroisoquinoline moiety have provided a very interesting class of P-gp inhibitors. MC70 (4'-(6,7-Dimethoxy-3,4-dihydro-1*H*-isoquinolin-2-yl-methyl)-biphenyl-4-ol) is the first in class and it comes from an evolution of P-gp modulators developed starting from the sigma ligand PB28, which was characterized by a moderate P-gp inhibiting activity. SAR studies on PB28, in which the cyclohexylpiperazine basic moiety was replaced by the 6,7-dimethoxytetrahydroisoquinoline led to the P-gp inhibitors MC18 first (EC_{50} = 1.64 μM), and MC70 right afterwards (Figure 8A) [157, 158]. In particular, the biphenyl derivative MC70 (EC_{50} = 0.69 μM) emerged from a small series of analogues whose synthesis was based on the evidence that conformational restriction of the non-basic portion improved P-gp inhibition activity. This compound was extensively studied for its biological properties, showing moderate activity toward MRP1 (EC_{50} = 9.30 μM) and BRCP (EC_{50} = 73 μM). The results from MC70 prompted the authors to use it as a lead compound for its optimization, also given its moderate selectivity towards the other efflux pumps. Bioisosters, superior homologue (insertion of flexible alkyl chain between the biphenyl and the tetrahydroisoquinoline ring) and conformational restricted analogues of MC70 were still P-gp-selective and potent ligands [38]. Alkylation with flexible alkyl chains of the phenolic group in MC70 produced compounds highly potent and selective for P-gp, reaching nanomolar activity when the alkyl chain was a butyl group (EC_{50} = 5.2 nM, Figure 8B). In contrast to MC70, most of these alkyl derivatives were P-gp substrates, while the O-butyl analogue of MC70 belonged to the II3B category (non transported substrate), as the immunomodulator ciclosporin A, but importantly the MC70 derivative is devoid of immunomodulation activity [42]. Alkylation of the phenolic group in MC70 was pushed further with the decoration of the alkyl spacer (from ethyl to butyl) with a furazan (1,2,5-oxadiazoles) cycle, as furazans were previously reported to display activity at P-gp [159]. Therefore, a small library of furazan derivatives of MC70 decorated with groups with different stereoelectronic and lipophilic properties were produced as selective P-gp modulators (EC_{50} values from the sub-nanomolar to the low micromolar range) (Figure 8C) [41]. Interestingly, functionalization of the phenolic group of MC70 with these alkylfurazans substituents switched the activity from P-gp inhibitor to selective (inactive towards MRP1 and BCRP) P-gp non transported substrates (II3B category). Excellent low nanomolar/subnanomolar (EC_{50} values from 1.3 nM to 0.60 nM) activities were shown by 3-phenylsulfoxide, 3-methoxy and 3-benzyloxy furazans without a clear SAR, despite the docking study whose results are more in agreement with the wider pocket reported by Szewczyk (more accommodating for hydrophobic drugs and lipids) than the crystal from Aller [160]. The study confirmed furazans as key structures to bind with high affinity and modulate P-gp, with a versatility due to the possibility to conveniently modify the substituent on the furazan ring to modulate pharmaco -kinetic and -dynamic properties.

Because P-gp showed tolerance towards decoration of the phenolic group in MC70, isosteric substitutions were conducted by insertion of a NH group, whose acidity was increased through inclusion in a heteroarene, or through connection to an electron-withdrawing moiety (Figure 8D) [44]. The variety of changes had the aim to prevent metabolic transformations to the phenol ring, while exploring the P-gp protein space and activity through a set of compounds with different lipophilic, steric and electronic properties. Most of the derivatives were less potent than MC70, and again, a switch in the activity from moderately selective inhibitor to selective non-transported P-gp substrates (IIB3 category) was obtained with these novel MC70 derivatives. Some compounds such as the benzensulfonamide-bearing compound were as potent as MC70, and only the N-(benzenesulfonyl)benzenesulfonamide derivative displayed a considerable activity in the nanomolar range (EC_{50} = 15 nM, Figure 8D). This last compound increased the toxicity of P-gp substrates, such as doxorubicin, when used in co-administration in cancer stem cells (the hardest cells components in tumors to be defeated). Metadynamics simulation gave insights into the potent activity of the (benzenesulfonyl)benzenesulfonamide derivative in comparison with the less potent (EC_{50} = 0.87 μM) benzenesulfonamide counterpart. The hydrophobic interactions, that govern the binding to P-gp, were enriched by hydrogen bonds with a more prone-to-efflux motion for the former (in line with the highest potency).

Keeping the phenol function and the basic moiety in MC70 unchanged, the electronic properties of the biphenyl core were modulated by decoration at the 2- or 3- position on the phenol ring or at 2'- or 3'- on the benzyl ring with electron -donating or -withdrawing substituents, characterized by hydrogen bond -donor or -acceptor properties (Figure 8E) [161]. Alternatively, fluorine, nitro, methoxy and amino groups were inserted in the described positions, leading to compounds less potent than MC70 (EC_{50} ranging from 1.51 μM to 15.2 μM) but with high P-gp selectivity (inactive against MRP1 and BCRP). These MC70 derivatives also displayed a non-transported substrate activity (IIB3 category). No great differences in the potency and activity were conferred by the different substituents on the biphenyl ring, with just the nitro group determining a decrease (EC_{50} around 15 μM) when present in position 2′ and 3 of the biphenyl core (where the influence on the pKa of the phenol is stronger). On the other hand, docking studies justified the highest activity of the 2'-methoxy derivative (Figure 8E, EC_{50} = 1.51 μM), as the methoxy group at that position of the biphenyl core may engage an additional point of anchorage by interacting with Tyr953 through a molecule of water.

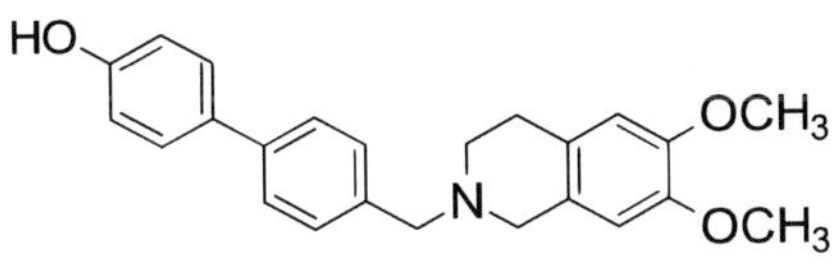

A) MC70

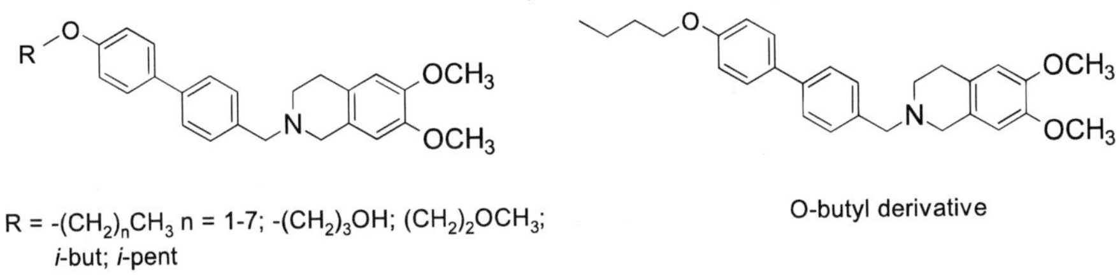

B) O-alkyl analogues general structure and the corresponding O-butyl derivative

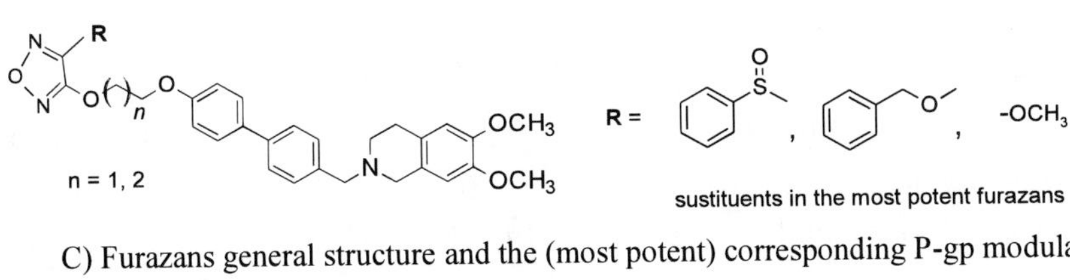

C) Furazans general structure and the (most potent) corresponding P-gp modulators.

Figure 8. (Continued)

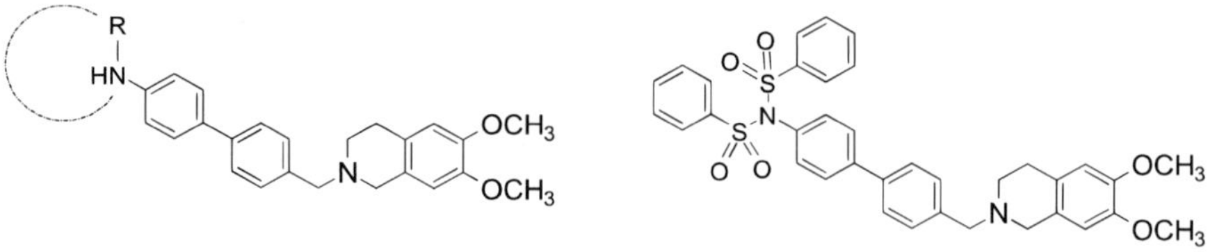

(benzensulfonyl)benzensulfonamide derivative

D) OH-replacement of MC70 with N(H) bearing groups and the benzenesulfonyl)benzenesulfonamide derivative

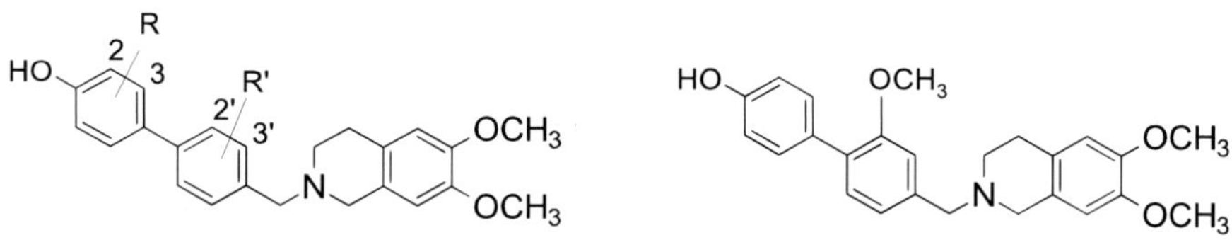

R or R' = OCH_3, F, NO_2, NH_2 3'-OCH_3 MC70 derivative

E) Decoration of MC70 in 2,3- or 2',3' and the corresponding 3'-OCH3 derivative.

Figure 8. MC70 and its derivatives: general structures and the most potent P-gp modulators within the series.

P-GP RADIOTRACERS

As widely discussed, P-gp has an important role not only in physiological conditions, as first line of defence in different compartments of our body, but mainly in several types of pathologies as in cancers and in neurodegeneration; thus, the availability of specific and highly active tools towards the pump is an important issue and several efforts have been made to develop radiotracers to image and detect the *active* or *inactive* state of the protein.

PET radiotracers to image P-gp, either as [^{11}C]- or [^{18}F]-radiolabelled, have been developed considering that the type of radioisotope ([^{11}C] or [^{18}F]) have an impact on the utility because of the different half life ($t_{1/2}$), that is about 20 minutes for [^{11}C] and about 2 hours for [^{18}F] -tracers. [^{11}C]-tracers are mostly used as experimental tools whereas [^{18}F]-tracers have a clinical perspective. Consequently, several promising [^{11}C]-tracers have been identified as starting point for the development of the corresponding [^{18}F]-tracers.

P-gp radiotracers are classified on the basis of their P-gp interacting mechanism as substrates and inhibitors, even if, as reported in the biological chapter, this classification is still controversial. A P-gp substrate may lead to detect the activity of P-gp while a P-gp inhibitor may give important information about the expression of the protein. These findings may be helpful to early detect the onset of some pathological conditions due to a down- or over-expression of the protein or to its dysfunction (i.e., cancer or Alzheimer's disease).

P-gp Substrates

Among the P-gp substrates, "off label" drugs such as verapamil [162, 163], metoclopramide [164, 165], desmethylloperamide [166, 167] are the most reported, together with MC225, a MC18 analogue [158, 168-170] that is a promising radiotracer now in clinical trials in humans [171].

As widely mentioned above, verapamil is a Ca^{++} L-type channel blocker employed for hypertension treatment. The enantiomers (*S*)-verapamil and (*R*)-verapamil display different pharmacokinetic profile and different potency in blocking Ca^{++} channel. (*S*)-Verapamil, the most active channel blocker, is metabolized more quickly than (*R*)-verapamil that is less potent in blocking the Ca^{++} channel. Since (*R*)-verapamil, (*S*)-verapamil and their racemic mixture display the same binding properties towards P-gp, (*R*)-verapamil was chosen as PET radiotracer because of its more convenient metabolism and activity as Ca^{++} channel blocker compared to the other enantiomer. [^{11}C]-(*R*)-Verapamil (Figure 9) has been studied in animal models and in humans, alone and in co-administration with a P-gp modulating agent (cyclosporine) or with a P-gp inhibitor, such as tariquidar, to evaluate its activity as P-gp radiotracer. The results were ambiguous and species-correlated [172]. Additionally, the metabolism due to cytochrome P450 could produce radiolabelled metabolites that bind P-gp either as substrates or inhibitors, leading to another pitfall together with the low half-life of [^{11}C]-tracer [173].

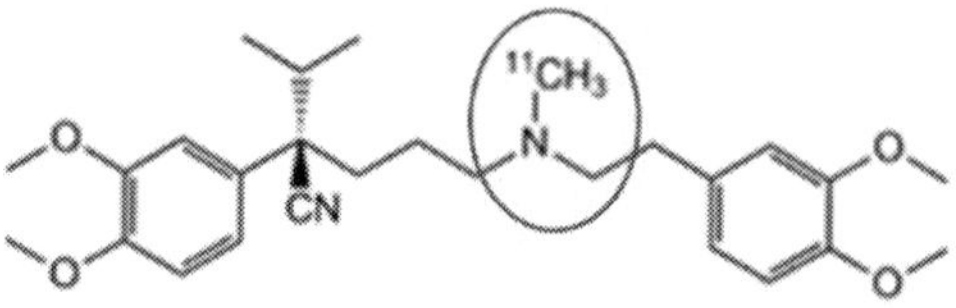

Figure 9. [^{11}C]-(*R*)-Verapamil PET tracer.

Metoclopramide is a mixed dopaminergic/serotonergic drug (D_2/5-HT_3 receptor, respectively) with antiemetic properties. [^{11}C]-Metoclopramide (Figure 10) has been studied in humans alone and in the presence of a P-gp inhibitor [174], displaying a good ability to detect P-gp only in specific areas of the CNS. This possibly beneficial behaviour is accompanied by the short [^{11}C]-tracer half-life and a very fast metabolism [164].

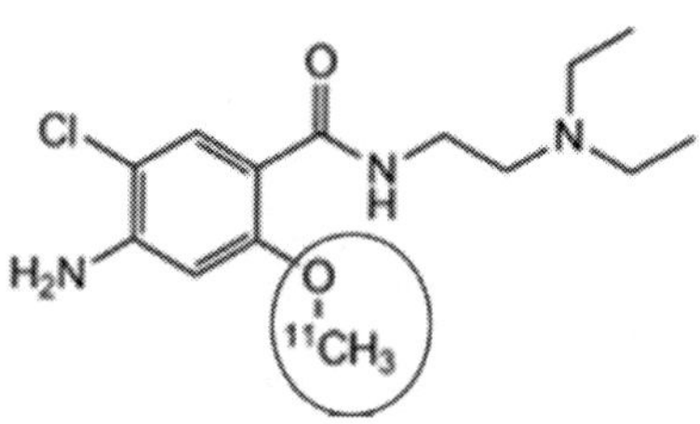

Figure 10. [^{11}C]-Metoclopramide PET tracer.

Loperamide is an agonist towards μ receptor (opioid receptor family), displaying antidiarreal properties. Loperamide is actively metabolized to the corresponding *N*-desmethyl derivative and both loperamide and the corresponding desmethyl metabolite were *in vivo* found as P-gp substrates.

[^{11}C]-dLop (Figure 11) presents several controversial aspects: it behaves as a P-gp substrate or a P-gp inhibitor depending on the dose and seems to accumulate into acidic organelles and lysosomes, not allowing an easy elimination [175-177]. Moreover, as for metoclopramide and verapamil, also [^{11}C]-dLop is a [^{11}C]-tracer with low baseline uptake.

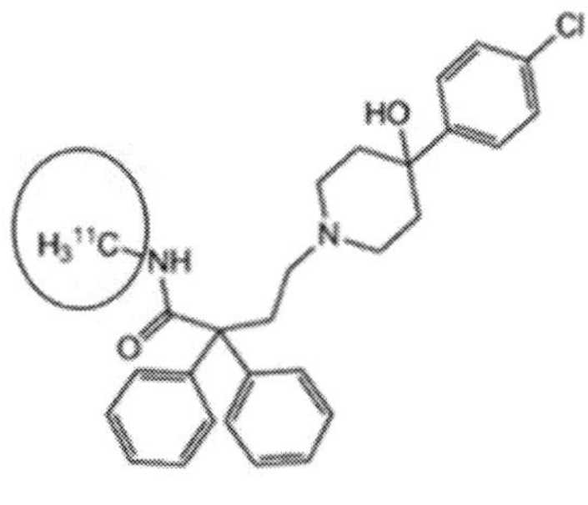

Figure 11. [^{11}C]-dLoperamide PET tracer.

All the presented P-gp substrates share several aspects as they are all: (*i*) [^{11}C]-tracers; (*ii*) off label drugs; (*iii*) derivatives with low metabolic stability.

Recently, a new ligand bearing a 6,7-dimethoxytetrahydroisoquinoline moiety (see the Medicinal Chemistry paragraph), named MC225, has been developed as [^{18}F]-radiotracer, through several lead optimization studies [40, 161]. [^{18}F]-MC225 (Figure 12) is a promising P-gp substrate that presents several advantages compared to the [^{11}C]-tracers previously reported.

Preliminary results were encouraging since [^{18}F]-MC225 had an uptake higher than the [^{11}C]-tracer in rat and showed a good metabolic stability. Additional studies with [^{18}F]-MC225 are ongoing, and among them the clinical trial entitled:" "First in human study of [^{18}F]-MC225" [171] aimed to demonstrate the altered function of P-gp at the BBB in AD patients.

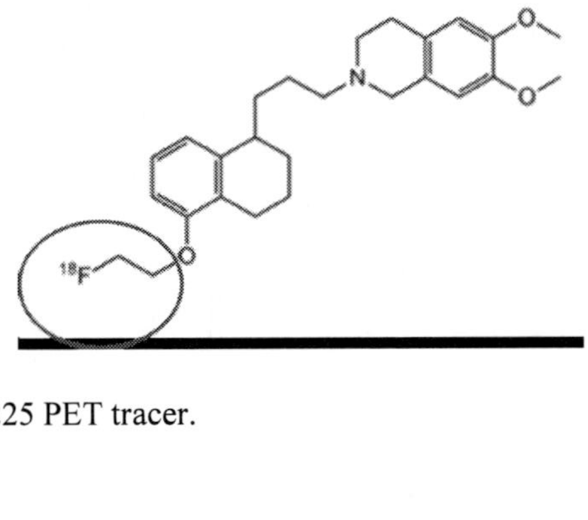

Figure 12. [^{18}F]-MC225 PET tracer.

P-gp Inhibitors

Elacridar and tariquidar are the P-gp inhibitors commonly used as PET radiotracers to evaluate the expression of P-gp. [^{11}C] and [^{18}F] -tracers have been developed for both the ligands [178-182].

The PET tracer [^{11}C]-elacridar (Figure 13) has been studied in healthy human subjects and the results of this study displayed several drawbacks since the radiotracer has a dual activity as BCRP substrate and P-gp substrate/inhibitor in a dose dependent manner [179]. For this reason, it is not useful to study P-gp expression at BBB level. Also the [^{18}F]-fluorethylelacridar (Figure 13), planned to overcome the limits of the [^{11}C]-tracer and with a clinical perspective, led to the same results observed with [^{11}C]-elacridar in an *in vivo* study performed in P-gp/BCRP knockout mice and in P-gp/BCRP wild-type mice [180].

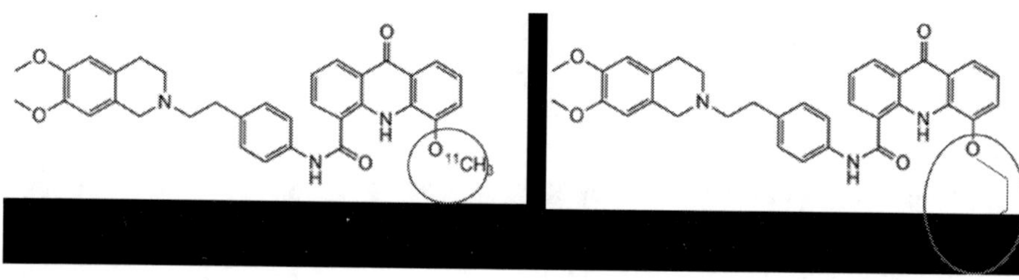

Figure 13. [^{11}C]-Elacridar (left) and [^{18}F]-Fluoroethylelacridar (right) PET tracers.

The same disappointing results were obtained with tariquidar and its fluoroethyl derivative [178, 179, 181]. Since [^{11}C] and [^{18}F] -radiolabelled elacridar and tariquidar were the most promising P-gp tracers acting as inhibitors (Figure 14), the imaging of P-gp expression with PET radiotracer is still open. Several attempts are ongoing to identify radiotracers acting as specific P-gp inhibitors to study *in vivo* P-gp expression [182].

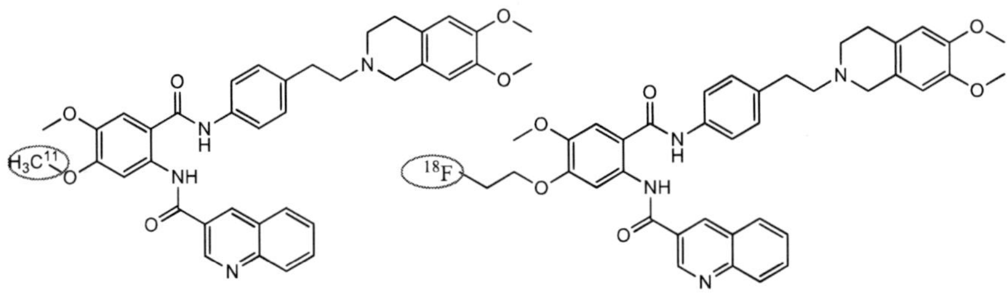

Figure 14. [^{11}C]-Tariquidar (left) and [^{18}F]-Fluoroethytariquidar (right) PET tracers.

CONCLUSION

Development of selective P-gp inhibitors is crucial in defeating MDR together with studies toward the inhibition of other MDR transporters such as BCRP and MRP1. The goal of obtaining selective drugs to inhibit P-gp or to modify or design anticancer drugs devoid of P-gp activity is still challenging because of the accommodating nature of the binding site(s). However, several progresses have been made during the decades, with subnanomolar ligands obtained and computational studies helping to elucidate the modes of interaction with the flexible binding site(s). All of these pieces of information from SAR studies together with the application of modern high-resolution techniques such as the recently obtained near-atomic resolution cryo-em of P-gp with zosuquidar or taxol bound can provide more solid bases for molecular modeling studies and dynamic simulations, in contrast to what has been going on so far.

As for the therapeutic strategies in oncology, together with the common and "old" approach to co-administrate a P-gp ligand (substrate or inhibitor) in order to rehabilitate the antitumour therapy, new perspectives are now possible thanks to the ability of some P-gp agents to exert collateral sensitivity, offering to the anticancer therapy a new escape to the pharmacokinetic limitation of the combined administration. Moreover, in the neurodegeneration field, the use of a P-gp inducer/stimulator agent may open a new scenario, taking into account the possibility to overcome the side-effects that can occur through the activation of the pump also in other regions of our body, by the planning of a site-directed delivery systems.

Conflict of Interest

The authors declare that there are no conflicts of interest.

References

[1] Leopoldo, M.; Nardulli, P.; Contino, M.; Leonetti, F.; Luurtsema, G.; Colabufo, N. A. An update patent review on P-glycoprotein inhibitor (2011-2018). *Expert Opin. Ther. Pat.* 2019, *29*, 455-461.

[2] Amawi, H.; Sim, H. M.; Tiwari, A. K.; Ambudkar, S. V.; Shukla, S. ABC Transporter-Mediated Multidrug-Resistant Cancer. *Adv. Exp. Med. Biol.* 2019, *1141*, 549-580.

[3] Yano, K.; Tomono, T.; Ogihara, T. Advances in studies of P-glycoprotein and its expression Regulators. *Bio. Pharm. Bull.* 2018, *41*, 11-19.

[4] Futamata, R.; Ogasawara, F.; Ichikawa, T.; Kodan, A.; Kimura, Y.; Kioka, N.; Ueda, K. In vivo FRET analyses reveal a role of ATP hydrolysis-associated conformational changes in human P-glycoprotein. *J. Biol. Chem.* 2020, *295*, 5002-5011.

[5] Dastvan, R.; Mishra, S.; Peskova, Y. B.; Nakamoto, R. K.; Mchaourab, H. S. Mechanism of allosteric modulation of P-glycoprotein by transport substrates and inhibitors. *Science*, 2019, *364*, 689-692.

[6] Thiel-Demby, V. E.; Humphreys, J. E.; St John Williams L. A.; Ellens, H. M.; Shah, N.; Ayrton, A. D.; Polli, J. W. Biopharmaceutics classification system: validation and learnings of an in vitro permeability assay. *Mol. Pharm.* 2009, *6*, 11-18.

[7] Bahadduri, P. M.; Polli, J. E.; Swaan, P. W.; Ekins, S. Targeting drug transporters - combining in silico and in vitro approaches to predict in vivo. *Methods Mol. Biol.* 2010, *637*, 65-103.

[8] Cantore, M.; Leopoldo, M.; Berardi, F.; Perrone, R.; Colabufo, N. A. Design and Synthesis of New Selective P-gp Substrates and Inhibitors. *Curr. Pharm. Des.* 2016, *22*, 5774-5778.

[9] Chai, A. B.; Leung, G. K. F.; Callaghan, R.; Gelissen, I. C. P-glycoprotein: a role in the export of amyloid-β in Alzheimer's disease? *FEBS J.* 2020, *287*, 612-625.

[10] Harilal, S.; Jose, J.; Parambi, D. G. T.; Kumar, R.; Mathew, G. E.; Uddin, M. S.; Kim, H.; Mathew, B. Advancements in nanotherapeutics for Alzheimer's disease: current perspectives. *J. Pharm. Pharmacol.* 2019, *71*, 1370-1383.

[11] Pan, Y.; Nicolazzo, J. A. mpact of aging, Alzheimer's disease and Parkinson's disease on the blood-brain barrier transport of therapeutics. *Adv. Drug Deliv. Rev.* 2018, *135*, 62-74.

[12] Sui, Y. T.; Bullock, K. M.; Erickson, M. A.; Zhang, J.; Banks, W. A. Alpha synuclein is transported into and out of the brain by the blood-brain barrier. *Peptides* 2014, *62*, 197-202.

[13] Mora Lagares, L.; Minovski, N.; Novič, M. Multiclass Classifier for P-Glycoprotein Substrates, Inhibitors, and Non-Active Compounds. *Molecules*, 2019, *24*, 1-22.

[14] Colabufo, N. A.; Berardi, F.; Cantore, M.; Contino, M.; Inglese, C.; Niso, M.; Perrone, R. Perspectives of P-glycoprotein modulating agents in oncology and neurodegenerative diseases: pharmaceutical, biological, and diagnostic potentials. *J. Med. Chem.* 2010, *53*, 1883-1897.

[15] Colabufo, N. A.; Berardi, F.; Perrone, M. G.; Capparelli, E.; Cantore, M.; Inglese, C.; Perrone, R. Substrates, inhibitors and activators of P-glycoprotein: candidates for radiolabeling and imaging perspectives. *Curr. Top. Med. Chem.* 2010, *10*, 1703-1714.

[16] Cantore, M.; Leopoldo, M.; Berardi, F.; Perrone, R.; Colabufo, N. A. Design and synthesis of new selective P-gp substrates and inhibitors. *Curr. Pharm. Des.* 2016, *22*, 5774-5778.

[17] Syvänen, S.; Eriksson, J. Advances in PET imaging of P-glycoprotein function at the blood-brain barrier. *ACS Chem. Neurosci.* 2013, *4*, 225-237.

[18] Kannan, P.; John, C.; Zoghbi, S. S.; Halldin, C.; Gottesman, M. M.; Innis, R. B.; Hall, M. D. Imaging the Function of P-Glycoprotein With Radiotracers: Pharmacokinetics and in vivo applications. *Clin. Pharmacol. Ther.* 2009, *86*, 368-377.

[19] Rahmim, A.; Lodge, M. A.; Karakatsanis, N. A.; Panin, V. Y.; Zhou, Y.; McMillan, A.; Cho, S.; Zaidi, H.; Casey, M. E.; Wahl, R. L. Dynamic whole-body PET imaging: principles, potentials and applications. *Eur. J. Nucl. Med. Mol. Imaging* 2019, *46*, 501-518.

[20] Wang, G-X.; Wang, D-W.; Liu, Y.; Ma, Y-H. Intractable epilepsy and the P-glycoprotein hypothesis. *Int. J. Neurosci.* 2016, *126*, 385-92.

[21] van Vliet, E. A.; Redeker, S.; Aronica, E.; Edelbroek, P. M.; Gorter, J. A. Expression of multidrug transporters MRP1, MRP2, and BCRP shortly after status epilepticus, during the latent period, and in chronic epileptic rats. *Epilepsia* 2005, *46*, 1569-1580.

[22] Hartz, A. M. S.; Pekcec, A.; Soldner, E. L. B.; Zhong, Y.; Schlichtiger, J.; Bauer, B. P-gp protein expression and transport activity in rodent seizure models and human epilepsy. *Mol. Pharm.* 2017, *14*, 999-1011.

[23] Haimeur, A.; Conseil, G.; Deeley, R. G.; Cole, S. P. C. The MRP-related and BCRP/ABCG2 multidrug resistance proteins: biology, substrate specificity and regulation. *Curr. Drug Metab.* 2004, *5*, 21-53.

[24] Ni, Z.; Bikadi, Z.; Rosenberg, M. F.; Mao, Q. Structure and function of the human breast cancer resistance protein (BCRP/ABCG2). *Curr. Drug Metab.* 2010, *11*, 603-317.

[25] Milane, A.; Fernandez, C.; Dupuis, L.; Buyse, M.; Loeffler, J. P.; Farinotti, R.; Meininger, V.; Bensimon. G. P-glycoprotein expression and function are increased in an animal model of amyotrophic lateral sclerosis. *Neurosci. Lett.* 2010, *472*, 166-170.

[26] Bernstein, H-G.; Hildebrandt, J.; Dobrowolny, H.; Steiner, J.; Bogerts, B.; Pahnke, J. Morphometric analysis of the cerebral

expression of ATP-binding cassette transporter protein ABCB1 in chronic schizophrenia: Circumscribed deficits in the habenula. *Schizophr. Res.* 2016, *177*, 52-58.

[27] Vogelgesang, S.; Glatzel, M.; Walker, L. C.; Kroemer, H. K.; Aguzzi, A.; Warzok, R. W. Cerebrovascular P-glycoprotein expression is decreased in Creutzfeldt–Jakob disease. *Acta Neuropathol.* 2006, *111*, 436-443.

[28] Matzneller, P.; Kussmann, M.; Eberl, S.; Maier-Salamon, A.; Jäger, W.; Bauer, M.; Langer, O.; Zeitlinger, M.; Poeppl, W. Pharmacokinetics of the P-gp inhibitor tariquidar in rats after intravenous, oral, and intraperitoneal administration. *Eur. J. Drug Metab. Pharmacokinet.* 2018, *43*, 599-606.

[29] Vraka, C.; Dumanic, M.; Racz, T.; Pichler, F.; Philippe, C.; Balber, T.; Klebermass, E. M.; Wagner, K. H.; Hacker, M.; Wadsak, W.; Mitterhauser, M. A new method measuring the interaction of radiotracers with the human P-glycoprotein (P-gp) transporter. *Nucl. Med. Biol.* 2018, *60*, 29-36.

[30] Martin, C.; Berridge, G.; Mistry, P.; Higgins, C.; Charlton, P.; Callaghan, R. Drug binding sites on P-glycoprotein are altered by ATP binding prior to nucleotide hydrolysis. *Biochemistry* 2000, *39*, 11901-11906.

[31] Aller, S. G.; Yu, J.; Ward, A.; Weng, Y.; Chittaboina, S.; Zhuo, R.; Harrell, P. M.; Trinh, Y. T.; Zhang, Q.; Urbatsch, I. L.; Chang, G. Structure of P-glycoprotein reveals a molecular basis for poly-specific drug binding. *Science* 2009, *323*, 1718-1722.

[32] Colabufo, N. A.; Berardi, F.; Cantore, M.; Contino, M.; Inglese, C.; Niso, M.; Perrone, R. Perspectives of P-glycoprotein modulating agents in oncology and neurodegenerative diseases: pharmaceutical, biological and diagnostic potentials. *J. Med. Chem.* 2010, *53*, 1883-1897.

[33] Colabufo, N. A.; Berardi, F.; Cantore, M.; Perrone, M. G.; Contino, M.; Inglese, C.; Niso, M.; Perrone, R. Multi-Drug-Resistance-reverting agents: 2-aryloxazole and 2-arylthiazole derivatives as potent BCRP or MRP1 inhibitors. *Chem Med Chem* 2009, *4*, 188-195.

[34] Colabufo, N. A.; Contino, M.; Cantore, M.; Capparelli, E.; Perrone, M. G.; Cassano, G.; Gasparre, G.; Leopoldo, M.; Berardi, F.; Perrone, R. Naphthalenyl derivatives for hitting P-gp/MRP1/BCRP transporters. *Bioorg. Med. Chem.* 2013, *21*, 1322-1330.

[35] Contino, M.; Zinzi, L.; Perrone, M. G.; Leopoldo, M.; Berardi, F.; Perrone, R.; Colabufo, N. A. Potent and selective tariquidar bioisosters as potential PET radiotracers for imaging P-gp. *Bioorg. Med. Chem. Lett.* 2013, *23*, 1369-1373.

[36] Contino, M.; Zinzi, L.; Cantore, M.; Perrone, M. G.; Leopoldo, M.; Berardi, F.; Perrone, R.; Colabufo N A. Activity-Lipophilicity relationship studies on P-gp ligands designed as simplified Tariquidar bulky fragments. *Bioorg. Med. Chem. Lett.* 2013, *23*, 3728-3731.

[37] Teodori E, Contino M, Riganti C, Bartolucci G, Braconi L, Manetti D, Romanelli MN, Trezza A, Athanasios A, Spiga O, Perrone MG, Giampietro R, Gazzano E, Salerno M, Colabufo NA, Dei S. Design, synthesis and biological evaluation of stereo- and regioisomers of amino aryl esters as multidrug resistance (MDR) reversers. *Eur. J. Med. Chem.* 2019, *182*, 111655.

[38] Capparelli, E.; Zinzi, L.; Cantore, M.; Contino, M.; Perrone, M. G.; Luurtsema, G.; Berardi, F.; Perrone, R.; Colabufo, N. A. SAR studies on tetrahydroisoquinoline derivatives: the role of flexibility and bioisosterism to raise potency and selectivity on P-gp protein. *J. Med. Chem.* 2014, *57*, 9983-9994.

[39] Teodori, E.; Dei, S.; Floriddia, E, Perrone MG, Manetti D, Romanelli MN, Contino M, Colabufo NA. Arylamino Esters As P-Glycoprotein Modulators: SAR Studies to Establish Requirements for Potency and Selectivity. *Chem Med Chem* 2015, *10*, 1339-13432.

[40] Capparelli, A.; Contino, M.; Perrone, M. G.; Berardi, F.; Perrone, R.; Leopoldo, M.; Colabufo, N. A. Functionalized coumarine fragment to obtain fluorescent and selective P-Glycoprotein ligands. *Arch. Pharm. Chem. Life Sci.* 2016, *348*, 1-7.

[41] Guglielmo, S.; Lazzarato, L.; Contino, M.; Perrone, M. G.; Chegaev, K.; Carrieri A.; Fruttero, R.; Colabufo, N. A.; Gasco, A. Structure-Activity Relationship Studies on Tetrahydroisoquinoline Derivatives:

[4′-(6,7-Dimethoxy-3,4-dihydro-1*H*-isoquinolin-2-ylmethyl)biphenyl-4-ol] (MC70) Conjugated through Flexible Alkyl Chains with Furazan Moieties Gives Rise to Potent and Selective Ligands of P-glycoprotein. *J. Med. Chem.* 2016, *59*, 6729-6738.

[42] Guglielmo, S.; Contino, M.; Lazzarato, L.; Perrone, M. G.; Blangetti, M.; Fruttero, R.; Colabufo, N. A. A Potent and selective P-gp modulator for altering Multidrug Resistance due to pump overexpression. *Chem Med Chem* 2016, *11*, 374–376.

[43] Teodori, E.; Dei, S.; Bartolucci, G.; Perrone, M. G.; Manetti, D.; Romanelli, M. N.; Contino, M.; Colabufo, N. A. Structure-Activity Relationship Studies on 6,7-Dimethoxy-2-phenethyl-1,2,3,4-tetrahydroisoquinoline Derivatives as Multidrug Resistance (MDR) reversers. *Chem Med Chem* 2017, *12*, 1369-1379.

[44] Riganti, C.; Contino, M.; Guglielmo, S.; Perrone, M. G.; Salaroglio, I. C.; Milosevic, V.; Giampietro, R.; Leonetti, F.; Rolando, B.; Lazzarato, L.; Colabufo, N. A.; Fruttero, R. Design, Biological Evaluation, and Molecular Modeling of Tetrahydroisoquinoline Derivatives: Discovery of A Potent P-Glycoprotein Ligand Overcoming Multidrug Resistance in Cancer Stem Cells. *J. Med. Chem.* 2019, *62*, 974-986.

[45] Braconi, L.; Bartolucci, G.; Contino, M.; Chiaramonte, N.; Giampietro, R.; Manetti, D.; Perrone, M. G.; Romanelli, M. N.; Colabufo, N. A.; Riganti, C.; Dei, S.; Teodori, E. 6,7-Dimethoxy-2-phenethyl-1,2,3,4-tetrahydroisoquinoline amides and corresponding ester isosteres as Multidrug Resistance (MDR) reversers. *Journal Of Enzyme Inhibition And Medicinal Chemistry* 2020, *35*, 974–992.

[46] Krishna, R.; Mayer, L. D. Multidrug resistance (MDR) in cancer. Mechanisms, reversal using modulators of MDR and the role of MDR modulators in influencing the pharmacokinetics of anticancer drugs. *Eur. J. Pharm. Sci.* 2000, *11*, 265-283.

[47] Salaroglio, I. C.; Abate, C.; Rolando, B.; Battaglia, L.; Gazzano, E.; Colombino, E.; Costamagna, C.; Annovazzi, L.; Mellai, M.; Berardi, F.; Capucchio, M. T.; Schiffer, D.; Riganti, C. Validation of thiosemicarbazone compounds as P-glycoprotein inhibitors in human

primary brain-blood barrier and glioblastoma stem cells. *Mol. Pharmaceutics* 2019, *16*, 3361-3373.

[48] Amiri-Kordestani, L.; Basseville, A.; Kurdziel, K.; Fojo, A. T.; Bates, S. E. Targeting MDR in breast and lung cancer: discriminating its potential importance from the failure of drug resistance reversal studies. *Drug. Resist. Updates* 2012, *15*, 50-61.

[49] Hall, M. D.; Handley, M. D.; Gottesman, M. M. Is resistance useless? Multidrug resistance and collateral sensitivity. *Trends Pharmacol Sci* 2009, *30*, 546-556.

[50] Szybalski, W.; Bryson, V. Genetic studies on microbial cross resistance to toxic agents: I. Cross resistance of Escherichia coli to fifteen antibiotics. *J. Bacteriol.* 1952, *64*, 489-499.

[51] Pluchino, K. M.; Hall, M. D.; Goldsborough, A. S.; Callaghan, R. Gottesman M. M. Collateral sensitivity as a strategy against cancer multidrug resistance. *Drug Resistance Updates* 2012, *15*, 98-105.

[52] Szakàcs, G.; Paterson, J. K.; Ludwig, J. A.; Booth-Genthe, C.; Gottesman, M. M. Targeting multidrug resistance in cancer. *Nat. Rev. Cancer* 2006, *5*, 219-234.

[53] Szakàcs, G.; Hall, M. D.; Gottesman, M. M.; Boumendjel, A.; Kachadourian, R.; Day, B. J.; Baubichon-Cortay, H.; Di Pietro A. Targeting the Achilles Heel of Multidrug-Resistant Cancer by Exploiting the Fitness Cost of Resistance. *Chem. Rev.* 2014, *114*, 5753-5774.

[54] Silva, R.; Vilas-Boas, V.; Carmo, H.; Jorge Dinis-Oliveira, R.; Carvalho, F.; de Lourdes Bastos, M.; Remião, F. Modulation of P-glycoprotein efflux pump: induction and activation as a therapeutic strategy. *Pharmacology & Therapeutics* 2015, *149*, 1-123.

[55] Sterz, K.; Mollmann, L.; Jacobs, A.; Baumert, D.; Wiese, M. Activators of P-glycoprotein: Structure-activity relationships and investigation of their mode of action. *ChemMedChem* 2009, *4*, 1897-1911.

[56] Vilas-Boas, V.; Silva, R.; Palmeira, A.; Sousa, E.; Ferreira, L. M.; Branco, P. S.; Carvalho, F.; Bastos Mde, L.; Remião F. Development of novel rifampicin-derived P-glycoprotein activators/inducers.

Synthesis, in silico analysis and application in the RBE4 cell model, using paraquat as substrate. *PLoS One* 2013, *8*, e74425.

[57] Silva, R.; Carmo, H.; Dinis-Oliveira, R.; Cordeiro-da-Silva, A.; Lima, S. C.; Carvalho, F.; Bastos Mde L.; Remião F. In vitro study of P-glycoprotein induction as an antidotal pathway to prevent cytotoxicity in Caco-2 cells. *Arch. Toxicol.* 2011, *85*, 315-326.

[58] Silva, R.; Vilas-Boas, V.; Carmo, H.; Dinis-Oliveira, R. J.; Carvalho, F.; Bastos, M. L.; Remião, F. P-glycoprotein induction by hypericin protects Caco-2 cells against paraquat toxicity. *Toxicology Letters* 2011, *205*, S93-S94.

[59] Dinis-Oliveira, R. J.; Duarte, J. A.; Remiao, F.; Sanchez-Navarro, A.; Bastos, M. L.; Carvalho, F. Single high dose dexamethasone treatment decreases the pathological score and increases the survival rate of paraquat-intoxicated rats. *Toxicology* 2006, *227*, 73-85.

[60] Dinis-Oliveira, R. J.; Remiao, F.; Duarte, J. A.; Ferreira, R.; Sanchez Navarro, A.; Bastos, M. L.; Carvalho, F. P-glycoprotein induction: an antidotal pathway for paraquat-induced lung toxicity. *Free Radic. Biol. Med.* 2006, *41*, 1213-1224.

[61] Dinis-Oliveira, R. J.; Duarte, J. A.; Sanchez-Navarro, A.; Remiao, F.; Bastos, M. L.; Carvalho, F. Paraquat poisonings: mechanisms of lung toxicity, clinical features, and treatment. *Crit. Rev. Toxicol.* 2008, *38*, 13-71.

[62] Zerin, T.; Kim, Y. S;, Hong, S. Y.; Song, H. Y. Protective effect ofmethylprednisolone on paraquat-induced A549 cell cytotoxicity via induction of efflux transporter, P-glycoprotein expression. *Toxicol. Lett.* 2012, *208*, 101-107.

[63] Silva, R.; Carmo, H.; Vilas-Boas, V.; Pinho, P. G.; Dinis-Oliveira, R. J.; Carvalho, Silva, I.; Correia-de-Sá, P.; Bastos, Mde L.; Remião, F. Doxorubicin decreases paraquat accumulation and toxicity in Caco-2 cells. *Toxicol. Lett.* 2013, *217*, 34-41.

[64] Arias, A.; Rigalli, J. P.; Villanueva, S. S.; Ruiz, M. L.; Luquita, M. G.; Perdomo, V. G., Vore, M.; Catania, V. A.; Mottino, AD. Regulation of expression and activity of multidrug resistance proteins MRP2 and MDR1 by estrogenic compounds in Caco-2 cells. Role in

prevention of xenobioticinduced cytotoxicity. *Toxicology* 2014, *320*, 46-55.

[65] Abuznait, A. H.; Kaddoumi, A. Role of ABC transporters in the pathogenesis of Alzheimer's disease. *ACS Chem. Neurosci.* 2012, *3*, 820-831.

[66] Pan, Y.; Nicolazzo, J. A. Impact of aging, Alzheimer's disease and Parkinson's disease on the blood-brain barrier transport of therapeutics. *Advanced Drug Delivery Reviews* 2018, *135*, 62-74.

[67] van Assema, D. M.; Lubberink, M.; Bauer, M.; van der Flier, W. M.; Schuit, R. C.; Windhorst, A. D.; Comans, E. F.; Hoetjes, N. J.; Tolboom, N.; Langer, O.; Muller, M.; Scheltens, P.; Lammertsma, A. A.; van Berckel, B. N. Blood-brain barrier P-glycoprotein function in Alzheimer's disease. *Brain* 2012, *135*, 181-189.

[68] Deo, A. K.; Borson, S.; Link, J. M.; Domino, K.; Eary, J. F.; Ke, B.; Richards, T. L.; Mankoff, D. A.; Minoshima, S.; O'Sullivan, F.; Eyal, S.; Hsiao, P.; Maravilla, K.; Unadkat, J. D. Activity of P-glycoprotein, a beta-amyloid transporter at the bloodbrain barrier, is compromised in patients with mild Alzheimer disease, *J. Nucl. Med.* 2014, 55, 1106-1111.

[69] Kortekaas, R.; Leenders, K. L.; van Oostrom, J. C.; Vaalburg, W.; Bart, J.; Willemsen, A. T.; Hendrikse, N. H. Blood-brain barrier dysfunction in parkinsonian midbrain in vivo. *Ann. Neurol.* 2005, *57*, 176-179.

[70] Bartels, A. L.; van Berckel, B. N. M.; Lubberink, M.; Luurtsema, G.; Lammertsma, A. A.; Leenders, K. L. Blood–brain barrier P-glycoprotein function is not impaired in early Parkinson's disease. *Parkinsonism Relat. Disord.* 2008, 14, 505-508.

[71] Colabufo, N. A.; Contino, M.; Cantore, M.; Berardi, F.; Perrone, R.; Tonazzi, A.; Console, L.; Panaro, M.; Savolainen, H.; Luurtsema, G. An innovative small molecule for promoting neuroreparative strategies. *RSC Adv.* 2018, *8*, 5451-5458.

[72] Alam, A.; Küng, R.; Kowal, J.; McLeod, R. A.; Tremp, N.; Broude, E. V; Roninson, I. B.; Stahlberg, H.; Locher, K. P. Structure of a

zosuquidar and UIC2-bound human-mouse chimeric ABCB1. *Proc. Natl. Acad. Sci. U S A.* 2018, *115*, 1973-1982.

[73] Alam, A.; Kowal, J.; Broude, E.; Roninson, I.; Locher, K. P. Structural insight into substrate and inhibitor discrimination by human P-glycoprotein. *Science*, 2019, *363*, 753-756.

[74] Loo, T. W.; Bartlett, M. C.; Clarke, D. M. Drug binding in human P-glycoprotein causes conformational changes in both nucleotide-binding domains. *J. Biol. Chem.* 2003, *278*, 1575-1578.

[75] Mollazadeh, S.; Sahebkar, A.; Hadizadeh, F.; Behravan, J.; Arabzadeh, S. Structural and functional aspects of P-glycoprotein and its inhibitors. *Life Sciences*, 2018, *214*, 118-123.

[76] Pluchino, K. M.; Hall, M. D.; Moen, J. K.; Chufan, E. E.; Fetsch, P. A.; Shukla, S.; Gill, D. R.; Hyde, S. C.; Xia, D.; Ambudkar, S. V.; Gottesman, M. M. Human-Mouse chimeras with normal expression and function reveal that major domain swapping is tolerated by P-Glycoprotein (ABCB1). *Biochemistry* 2016, *55*, 10101023.

[77] Wang, R.; Kuo, C.; Lien, L.; Lien, E. Structure–activity relationship: analyses of p-glycoprotein substrates and inhibitors. *J. Clin. Pharm. Ther.* 2003, 203-228.

[78] Waghray, D.; Zhang, Q. Inhibit or Evade Multidrug Resistance P-glycoprotein in Cancer Treatment. *J. Med. Chem.* 2018, 5108-5121.

[79] Palmeira, A; Sousa, E.; Vasconcelos, M. H.; Pinto, M. M. Three decades of P-gp inhibitors: skimming through several generations and scaffolds. *Curr. Med. Chem.* 2012, *19*, 1946-2025

[80] Hollt, V.; Kouba, M; Dietel, M.; Vogt,G. Stereoisomers of calcium antagonists which differ markedly in their potencies as calcium blockers are equally effective in modulating drug transport by P-glycoprotein. *Biochem. Pharmacol.* 1992, *43*, 2601-2608.

[81] List, A. F.; Kopecky, K. J.; Willman, C. L.; Head, D. R.; Persons, D. L.; Slovak, M. L.; Dorr, R.; Karanes, C.; Hynes, H. E.; Doroshow, J. H.; Shurafa, M.; Appelbaum, F. R. Benefit of cyclosporine modulation of drug resistance in patients with poor-risk acute myeloid leukemia: a Southwest Oncology Group study. *Blood* 2001, *98*, 32123220.

[82] Solary, E.; Velay, I.; Chauffert, B.; Caillot, D.; Bidan, J. M.; Dumas, M.; Casasnovas, O.; Guy, H. Quinine circumvents the doxorubicin resistance of a multidrug resistant human leukemic cell-line, K562/DXR. *Nouv. Rev. Fr. Hematol.* 1990, *32*, 361–363.

[83] Hu, X. F.; Nadalin, G.; De Luise, M.; Martin, T. J.; Wakeling, A.; Huggins, R.; Zalcberg, J. R. Circumvention of doxorubicin resistance in multi-drug resistant human leukaemia and lung cancer cells by the pure antiestrogen ICI 164384. *Eur. J. Cancer* 1991, *27*, 773-777.

[84] Stupp, R.; Bauer, J.; Pagani, O.; Gerard, B.; Cerny, T.; Sessa, C.; Bastian, G.; Sarkany, M.; Schlapfer, J.; Giroux, B.; Leyvraz, S. Ventricular arrhythmia and torsade de pointe: dose limiting toxicities of the MDR-modulator S9788 in a phase I trial. *Ann. Oncol.* 1998, *9*, 1233-1242.

[85] Wandel, C.; Kim, R. B.; Kajiji, S.; Guengerich, P.; Wilkinson, G. R.; Wood, A. J. P-glycoprotein and cytochrome P-450 3A inhibition: dissociation of inhibitory potencies. *Cancer Res.* 1999, *59*, 3944-3948.

[86] Berger, D.; Citarella, R.; Dutia, M.; Greenberger, L.; Hallett, W.; Paul, R.; Powell, D. Novel multidrug resistance reversal agents. *J. Med. Chem.* 1999, *42*, 2145-2461.

[87] Bisi, A.; Gobbi, S.; Rampa, A.; Belluti, F.; Piazzi, L.; Valenti, P.; Gyemant, N.; Molnar, J. New potent P-glycoprotein inhibitors carrying a polycyclic scaffold. *J. Med. Chem.* 2006, *49*, 3049-3051.

[88] Schmidt, M.; Ungvari, J.; Glode, J.; Dobner, B.; Langner, A. New 1,3-dioxolane and 1,3-dioxane derivatives as effective modulators to overcome multidrug resistance. *Bioorg. Med. Chem.* 2007, *15*, 2283-2297.

[89] Lee, B. D.; Li, Z.; French, K. J.; Zhuang, Y.; Xia, Z.; Smith, C. D. Synthesis and evaluation of dihydropyrroloquinolines that selectively antagonize P-glycoprotein. *J. Med. Chem.* 2004, *47*, 1413-1422.

[90] D'Elia, P.; De Matteis, F.; Dragoni, S.; Shah, A.; Sgaragli, G.; Valoti, M. DP7, a novel dihydropyridine multidrug resistance reverter, shows only weak inhibitory activity on human CYP 3A enzyme(s). *Eur. J. Pharmacol.* 2009, *614*, 7-13.

[91] Slate, D. L.; Bruno, N. A.; Casey, S. M.; Zutshi, N.; Garvin, L. J.; Wu, H.; Pfister, J. R. RS-33295–198: a novel, potent modulator of P-glycoprotein-mediated multidrug resistance. *Anticancer Res.* 1995, *15*, 811-814.

[92] Hyafil, F.; Vergely, C.; Du Vignaud, P.; Grand-Perret T. In vitro and in vivo reversal of multidrug resistance by GF120918, an acridone carboxamide derivative. *Cancer Res.* 1993, *53*, 4595-4602.

[93] Martin, C.; Berridge, G.; Mistry, P.; Higgins, C.; Charlton, P.; Callaghan, R. The molecular interaction of the high affinity reversal agent XR9576 with P-glycoprotein. *Br. J. Pharmacol.* 1999, *128*, 403-411.

[94] Shaffer, B. C.; Gillet, J. P.; Patel, C.; Baer, M. R.; Bates, S. E.; Gottesman, M. M. Drug resistance: still a daunting challenge to the successful treatment of AML. *Drug Resist. Update* 2012, *15*, 62-69.

[95] Dean, M.; Fojo, T.; Bates, S. Tumour stem cells and drug resistance. *Nat. Rev. Cancer* 2005, *5*, 275-284.

[96] Seelig, A. A general pattern for substrate recognition by P-glycoprotein. *Eur J Biochem.* 1998, *251*, 252-261.

[97] Seelig, A.; Landwojtowicz, E. Structure–activity relationship of P-glycoprotein substrates and modifiers. *Eur .J. Pharm. Sci.* 2000, *12*, 31-40.

[98] Bain, L. J.; McLachlan, J. B.; LeBlanc, G. A. Structure-activity relationships for xenobiotic transport substrates and inhibitory ligands of P-glycoprotein. *Environ. Health Perspect.* 1997, *105*, 812-818.

[99] Hou, T.; Xu, X. Recent development and application of virtual screening in drug discovery: an overview. *Curr. Pharm. Des.* 2004, 10, 1011-1033.

[100] Ekins, S.; Kim, R. B.; Leake, B. F.; Dantzig, A. H.; Schuetz, E. G.; Lan, L. B.; Yasuda K.; Shepard R. L.; Winter, M. A.; Schuetz, J. D.; Wikel, J. H.; Wrighton, S. A. Application of three-dimensional quantitative structure-activity relationships of Pglycoprotein inhibitors and substrates. *Mol. Pharmacol.* 2002, *61*, 974-981.

[101] Ekins, S.; Ecker, G. F.; Chiba, P.; Swaan, P. W. Future directions for drug transporter modelling. *Xenobiotica* 2007, *37*, 1152-1170.

[102] Chen, L.; Li, Y.; Yu, H.; Zhang, L.; Hou, T. Computational models for predicting substrates or inhibitors of P-glycoprotein. *Drug. Discov. Today* 2012, *17*, 343-351

[103] Penzotti, J. E.; Lamb, M. L.; Evensen, E.; Grootenhuis, P. D. J. A computational ensemble pharmacophore model for identifying substrates of P-glycoprotein. *J. Med. Chem.* 2002, 45, 1737-1740.

[104] Cianchetta, G.; Singleton, R. W.; Zhang, M.; Wildgoose, M.; Giesing, D.; Fravolini, A.; Cruciani, G.; Vaz, R. J. A pharmacophore hypothesis for P-glycoprotein substrate recognition using GRIND-based 3D-QSAR. *J. Med. Chem.* 2005, *48*, 2927-2935.

[105] Crivori, P.; Reinach, B.; Pezzetta, D.; Poggesi, I. Computational models for identifying potential P-glycoprotein substrates and inhibitors. *Mol. Pharm.* 2006, *3*, 33-44.

[106] Huang, J.; Ma, G.; Muhammad, I.; Cheng, Y. Identifying P-glycoprotein substrates using a support vector machine optimized by a particle swarm. *J. Chem. Inf. Model* 2007, *47*, 1638-1647.

[107] Poongavanam, V.; Haider, N.; Ecker, G. F. Fingerprint-based in silico models for the prediction of P-glycoprotein substrates and inhibitors. *Bioorg. Med. Chem.* 2012, *20*, 5388-5395.

[108] Prajapati, R.; Singh, U.; Patil, A.; Khomane, K. S.; Bagul, P.; Bansal, A. K. Sangamwar A. T. In silico model for P-glycoprotein substrate prediction: insights from molecular dynamics and in vitro studies. *J. Comput. Aided Mol. Des.* 2013, *27*, 347-363.

[109] Shahraki, O.; Zargari, F.; Edraki, N.; Khoshneviszadeh, M.; Firuzi, O.; Miri, R. Molecular dynamics simulation and molecular docking studies of 1, 4- Dihydropyridines as P-glycoprotein's allosteric inhibitors. *J. Biomol. Struct. Dyn.* 2017, 1-14.

[110] Pajeva, I. K.; Globisch, C.; Wiese, M. Combined pharmacophore modeling, docking, and 3D QSAR studies of ABCB1 and ABCC1 transporter inhibitors. *ChemMedChem* 2009, *4*, 1883–1896.

[111] Abate, C.; Pati, M. L.; Contino, M.; Colabufo, N. A.; Perrone, R.; Niso, M.; Berardi, F. From mixed sigma-2 receptor/P-glycoprotein targeting agents to selective P-glycoprotein modulators: small

structural changes address the mechanism of interaction at the efflux pump. *Eur. J. Med. Chem.* 2015, *89*, 606-615.

[112] Emmert, D.; Campos, C. R.; Ward, D.; Lu, P.; Namanja, H. A.; Bohn, K.; Miller, D. S.; Sharom, F. J.; Chmielewski, J.; Hrycyna, C. A. Reversible dimers of the atypical antipsychotic quetiapine inhibit pglycoprotein-mediated efflux in vitro with increased binding affinity and in situ at the blood-brain barrier. *ACS Chem. Neurosci.* 2014, *5*, 305–317.

[113] Bohn, K.; Lange, A.; Chmielewski, J.; Hrycyna, C. A. Dual Modulation of Human P-Glycoprotein and ABCG2 with Prodrug Dimers of the Atypical Antipsychotic Agent Paliperidone in a Model of the Blood-Brain Barrier. *Mol. Pharmacol.* 2017, *14*, 1107-1119.

[114] Colabufo, N. A.; Berardi, F.; Contino, M.; Inglese, C.; Perrone, R. Flavonoids as MDR Modulating Agents: SAR Studies. In Multidrug Resistance: Biological and Pharmaceutical Advance in the Antitumour Treatment; Colabufo, N. A., Ed.; Research Signpost: Kerala, India, 2008; pp 171-201.

[115] Duncan. R. Polymer therapeutics as nanomedicines: new perspectives. *Curr. Opin. Biotechnol.* 2011, *22*, 492–501.

[116] Ferrari, M. Cancer nanotechnology: opportunities and challenges. *Nat. Rev. Cancer*, 2005, *5*, 161–171.

[117] Peer, D.; Karp, J. M.; Hong, S.; Farokhzad, O. C.; Margalit, R.; Langer, R. Nanocarriers as an emerging platform for cancer therapy. *Nat. Nanotechnol.* 2007, *2*, 751–760.

[118] Huang, Y.; Cole, S. P.; Cai, T.; Cai, Y. U. Applications of nanoparticle drug delivery systems for the reversal of multidrug resistance in cancer. *Oncol. Lett.* 2016, *12*, 11–15.

[119] Shi, J.; Kantoff, P. W.; Wooster, R.; Farokhzad, O. C. Cancer nanomedicine: progress, challenges and opportunities. *Nat. Rev. Cancer*, 2017, *17*, 20–37.

[120] Saneja, A.; Dubey, R. D.; Alam, N.; Khare, V.; Gupta, P. N. Co-formulation of P-glycoprotein substrate and inhibitor in nanocarriers: an emerging strategy for cancer chemotherapy. *Curr. Cancer Drug Targets*, 2014,*14*, 419-433.

[121] Xia, D.; He, Y.; Li, Q.; Hu, C.; Huang, W.; Zhang, Y.; Wan, F.; Wang, C.; Gan, Y. Transport mechanism of lipid covered saquinavir pure drug nanoparticles in intestinal epithelium. *J. Control Release*, 2018, *269*, 159-170.

[122] Ma, X.; Zhao, Z.; Wang, H.; Liu, Y.; Xu, Y.; Zhang, J.; Chen, B.; Li, L.; Zhao, Y. P-Glycoprotein Antibody Decorated Porous Hydrogel Particles for Capture and Release of Drug-Resistant Tumor Cells. *Adv. Healthc. Mater*, 2019, *8*, e1900136.

[123] Barker, T. J.; Duncan, K. K.; Otrubova, K.; Boger, D. L. Potent Vinblastine C20' Ureas Displaying Additionally Improved Activity Against a Vinblastine-Resistant Cancer Cell Line. *ACS Med. Chem. Lett.* 2013, *4*, 985–988.

[124] Sears, J. E.; Boger, D. L. Total synthesis of vinblastine, related natural products, and key analogues and development of inspired methodology suitable for the systematic study of their structure-function properties. *Acc. Chem. Res.* 2015, *48*, 653–662.

[125] Voss, M. E.; Ralph, J. M.; Xie, D.; Manning, D. D.; Chen, X.; Frank, A. J.; Leyhane, A .J.; Liu, L.; Stevens, J. M.; Budde, C.; Surman, M. D.; Friedrich, T.; Peace, D.; Scott, I. L.; Wolf, M.; Johnson, R. Synthesis and SAR of vinca alkaloid analogues. *Bioorg. Med. Chem. Lett.* 2009, *19*, 1245–1249.

[126] Etievant, C.; Barret, J. M.; Kruczynski, A.; Perrin, D.; Hill, B. T. Vinflunine (20',20'-difluoro-3',4'- dihydrovinorelbine), a novel Vinca alkaloid, which participates in P-glycoprotein (Pgp)-mediated multidrug resistance in vivo and in vitro. *Inves. New Drugs,* 1998, *16*, 3–17.

[127] Gerullis, H.; Wawroschek, F.; Kohne, C. H.; Ecke, T. H. Vinflunine in the treatment of advanced urothelial cancer: clinical evidence and experience. *Ther. Adv. Urol.* 2017, *9*, 28–35.

[128] Wartmann, M.; Altmann, K. H. The biology and medicinal chemistry of epothilones. *Curr. Med. Chem: Anticancer Agents*, 2002, *2*, 123–148.

[129] Rak Tkaczuk K. H. Ixabepilone as monotherapy or in combination with capecitabine for the treatment of advanced breast cancer. *Breast Cancer (Auckl)*, 2011, *5*, 1–14.

[130] Lee, F. Y.; Borzilleri, R.; Fairchild, C. R.; Kamath, A.; Smykla, R.; Kramer, R.; Vite, G. Preclinical discovery of ixabepilone, a highly active antineoplastic agent. *Cancer Chemother. Pharmacol.* 2008, *63*, 157– 166.

[131] Lee, F. Y.; Borzilleri, R.; Fairchild, C. R.; Kim, S. H.; Long, B. H.; Reventos-Suarez, C.; Vite, G. D.; Rose, W. C.; Kramer, R. A. BMS-247550: a novel epothilone analog with a mode of action similar to paclitaxel but possessing superior antitumor efficacy. *Clin. Cancer Res.* 2001, *7*, 1429–1437.

[132] Abidi, A. Cabazitaxel: A novel taxane for metastatic castration-resistant prostate cancer-current implications and future prospects. *J. Pharmacol. Pharmacother.* 2013, *4*, 230–237.

[133] Bouchet, B. P.; Galmarini, C. M. Cabazitaxel, a new taxane with favorable properties. *Drugs Today (Barc.)*, 2010, *46*, 735–742.

[134] Vredenburg, M. R.; Ojima, I.; Veith, J.; Pera, P.; Kee, K.; Cabral, F.; Sharma, A.; Kanter, P.; Greco, W. R.; Bernacki, R. J. Effects of orally active taxanes on P-glycoprotein modulation and colon and breast carcinoma drug resistance. *J. Natl. Cancer Inst.* 2001, *93*, 1234–1245.

[135] Duran, G. E.; Wang, Y. C.; Francisco, E. B.; Rose, J. C.; Martinez, F. J.; Coller, J.; Brassard, D.; Vrignaud, P.; Sikic, B. I. Mechanisms of resistance to cabazitaxel. *Mol. Cancer Ther.* 2015, *14*, 193–201.

[136] Ojima, I.; Lichtenthal, B.; Lee, S.; Wang, C.; Wang, X. Taxane anticancer agents: a patent perspective. *Expert Opin. Ther. Pat.* 2016, *26*, 1–20.

[137] ClinicalTrials.gov Identifier: NCT01989884.

[138] Palmeira, A.; Vasconcelos, M. H.; Paiva, A.; Fernandes, M. X.; Pinto, M.; Sousa, E. Dual inhibitors of P-glycoprotein and tumor cell growth: (re)discovering thioxanthones. *Biochem. Pharmacol.* 2012, 57–68.

[139] Pati, M. L.; Niso, M.; Spitzer, D.; Berardi, F.; Contino, M.; Riganti, C.; Hawkins, WG; Abate, C. Multifunctional thiosemicarbazones and

deconstructed analogues as a strategy to study the involvement of metal chelation, sigma-2 (σ2) receptor and P-gp protein in the cytotoxic action: *in vitro* and *in vivo* activity in pancreatic tumors. *Eur. J. Med. Chem.* 2018, *144*, 359–371.

[140] Pati, M. L.; Niso, M.; Ferorelli, S.; Abate, C.; Berardi, F. Novel metal chelators thiosemicarbazones with activity at the 2 receptors and P-glycoprotein: an innovative strategy for resistant tumor treatment. *RSC Adv.* 2015, *5*, 103131.

[141] Niso, M.; Abate, C.; Contino, M.; Ferorelli, S.; Azzariti, A.; Perrone, R.; Colabufo, N. A.; Berardi, F. Sigma-2 receptor agonists as possible antitumor agents in resistant tumors: hints for collateral sensitivity. *ChemMedChem.* 2013, *8*, 2026-2035.

[142] Chegaev, K.; Fraix, A.; Gazzano, E.; Abd-Ellatef, G. E.; Blangetti, M.; Rolando, B.; Conoci, S.; Riganti, C.; Fruttero, R.; Gasco, A.; Sortino, S. Light-Regulated NO Release as a Novel Strategy To Overcome Doxorubicin Multidrug Resistance. *ACS Med. Chem. Lett.* 2017, *8*, 361-365.

[143] Riganti, C.; Rolando, B.; Kopecka, J.; Campia, I.; Chegaev, K.; Lazzarato, L.; Federico, A.; Fruttero, R.; Ghigo, D. Mitochondrial-targeting nitrooxy-doxorubicin: a new approach to overcome drug resistance. *Mol. Pharm.* 2013, *10*, 161-174.

[144] Teodori, E.; Braconi, L.; Bua, S.; Lapucci, A.; Bartolucci, G.; Manetti, D.; Romanelli, M. N.; Dei, S.; Supuran, C. T.; Coronnello, M. Dual P-Glycoprotein and CA XII Inhibitors: A New Strategy to Reverse the P-gp Mediated Multidrug Resistance (MDR) in Cancer Cells. *Molecules*, 2020, *25*, 1748.

[145] Sim, H. M.; Loh, K. Y.; Yeo, W. K.; Lee, C. Y.; Go, M. L. Aurones as modulators of ABCG2 and ABCB1: synthesis and structure-activity relationships. *ChemMedChem.* 2011, *6*, 713–724.

[146] Gu, X.; Ren, Z.; Peng, H.; Peng, S.; and Zhang, Y. Bifendate-chalcone hybrids: A new class of potential dual inhibitors of P-glycoprotein and breast cancer resistance protein. *Biochem. Biophys. Res. Commun.* 2014, *455*, 318–322.

[147] Li, X. Q., Wang, L., Lei, Y., Hu, T., Zhang, F. L., Cho, C. H., et al. (2015). Reversal of P-gp and BCRP-mediated MDR by tariquidar derivatives. *Eur. J. Med. Chem.* 101, 560–572.

[148] Dinić, J.; Podolski-Renić, A.; Jeremić, M.; Pešić, M. Potential of natural-based anticancer compounds for P-Glycoprotein inhibition. *Curr. Pharm. Des.* 2018, *24*, 4334-4354.

[149] Karthikeyan, S.; Hoti, S. Development of fourth generation ABC inhibitors from natural products: a novel approach to overcome cancer multidrug resistance. *Anticancer Agents Med. Chem.* 2015, *15*, 605–615.

[150] Silbermann, K.; Shah, C. P.; Sahu, N. U.; Juvale, K.; Stefan, S. M.; Kharkar, P. S.; Wiese, M. Novel chalcone and flavone derivatives as selective and dual inhibitors of the transport proteins ABCB1 and ABCG2. *Eur. J. Med. Chem.* 2019, *164*, 193-213.

[151] Iriti, M.; Kubina, R.; Cochis, A.; Sorrentino, R.; Varoni, E. M.; Kabała-Dzik, A., et al. Rutin, a quercetin glycoside, restores chemosensitivity in human breast cancer cells. *Phytother. Res.* 2017 *31*, 1529–1538.

[152] Yuan, J.; Wong, I. L. K.; Jiang, T.; Wang, S. W.; Liu, T.; Wen, B. J.; et al. Synthesis of methylated quercetin derivatives and their reversal activities on P-gp- and BCRP-mediated multidrug resistance tumour cells. *Eur. J. Med. Chem.* 2012, *54*, 413–422.

[153] Bisi, A.; Cappadone, C.; Rampa, A.; Farruggia, G.; Sargenti, A.; Belluti, F.; et al. Coumarin derivatives as potential antitumor agents: growth inhibition, apoptosis induction and multidrug resistance reverting activity. *Eur. J. Med. Chem.* 2017, *127*, 577–585.

[154] Combes, S.; Barbier, P.; Douillard, S.; McLeer-Florin, A.; Bourgarel-Rey, V.; Pierson, J. T.; et al. Synthesis and biological evaluation of 4-arylcoumarin analogues of combretastatins. Part 2. *J. Med. Chem.* 2011, *54*, 3153– 3162.

[155] Dei, S.; Romanelli, M. N.; Manetti, D.; Chiaramonte, N.; Coronnello, M.; Salerno, M.; Teodori, E. Design and synthesis of aminoester heterodimers containing flavone or chromone moieties as modulators

of P-glycoprotein-based multidrug resistance (MDR). *Bioorg. Med. Chem.* 2018, *26*, 50-64.

[156] Sachs, J.; Döhl, K.; Weber, A.; Bonus, M.; Ehlers, F.; Fleischer, E.; Klinger, A.; Gohlke, H.; Pietruszka, J.; Schmitt, L.; Teusch, N. Novel 3,4-Dihydroisocoumarins inhibit human P-gp and BCRP in multidrug resistant tumors and demonstrate substrate inhibition of yeast Pdr5. *Front. Pharmacol.* 2019, *10*, 400.

[157] Colabufo, N. A,; Berardi, F.; Cantore, M.; Perrone, M. G.; Contino, M.; Inglese, C.; Niso, M.; Perrone, R.; Azzariti, A.; Simone, G. M.; Paradiso, A. 4-Biphenyl and 2-naphthyl substituted 6,7-dimethoxytetrahydroisoquinoline derivatives as potent P-gp modulators. *Bioorg. Med. Chem.* 2008, *16*, 3732-3743.

[158] Colabufo, N. A.; Berardi, F.; Cantore, M.; Perrone, M. G.; Contino, M.; Inglese, C.; Niso, M.; Perrone, R.; Azzariti, A.; Simone, G. M.; Porcelli, L.; Paradiso, A. Small P-gp modulating molecules: SAR studies on tetrahydroisoquinoline derivatives. *Bioorg. Med. Chem.* 2008, *16*, 362-373.

[159] Fruttero, R.; Crosetti, M.; Chegaev, K.; Guglielmo, S.; Gasco, A.; Berardi, F.; Niso, M.; Perrone, R.; Panaro, M. A.; Colabufo, N. A. Phenylsulfonylfuroxans as modulators of multidrug-resistance-associated protein-1 and P-glycoprotein. *J. Med. Chem.* 2010, *53*, 5467-5475.

[160] Szewczyk, P.; Tao, H.; McGrath, A. P.; Villaluz, M.; Rees, S. D.; Lee, S. C.; Doshi, R.; Urbatsch, I. L.; Zhang, Q.; Chang, G. Snapshots of ligand entry, malleable binding and induced helical movement in Pglycoprotein. *Acta Crystallogr., Sect. D: Biol. Crystallogr.* 2015, *71*, 732– 741.

[161] Contino, M.; Guglielmo, S.; Perrone, M. G.; Giampietro, R.; Rolando, B.; Carrieri, A.; Zaccaria, D.; Chegaev, K.; Borio, V.; Riganti, C.; Zabielska-Koczywąs, K.; Colabufo, N. A.; Fruttero, R. New tetrahydroisoquinoline-based P-glycoprotein modulators: decoration of the biphenyl core gives selective ligands. *Medchemcomm.* 2018, *9*, 862-869.

[162] Luurtsema, G.; Molthoff, C. F. M.; Schuit, R. C.; Windhorst, A. D.; Lammertsma, A. A.; Franssen, E. J. F. Evaluation of (*R*)-[^{11}C]verapamil as PET-tracer of P-glycoprotein function in the blood-brain barrier: kinetics and metabolism in the rat. *Nucl. Med. Biol.* 2005, *32*, 87-93.

[163] Luurtsema, G.; Molthoff, C. F.; Windhorst, A. D.; Smit, J. W.; Keizer, H.; Boellaard, R.; Lammertsma, A. A.; Franssen, E. J. (*R*)- and (*S*)-[^{11}C]verapamil as PET-tracers for measuring P-glycoprotein function: *in vitro* and *in vivo* evaluation. *Nucl. Med. Biol.* 2003, *30*, 747-51

[164] Pottier, G.; Marie, S.; Goutal, S.; Auvity, S.; Peyronneau, M. A.; Stute, S.; Boisgard, R.; Dollé, F.; Buvat, I.; Caillé, F.; Tournier, N. Imaging the impact of the P-Glycoprotein (ABCB1) function on the brain kinetics of metoclopramide. *J. Nucl. Med.* 2016, *57*, 309-314.

[165] Zoufal, V.; Mairinger, S.; Brackhan, M.; Krohn, M.; Filip, T.; Sauberer, M.; Stanek, J.; Wanek, T.; Tournier, N.; Bauer, M.; Pahnke, J.; Langer, O. Imaging P-glycoprotein Induction at the Blood-Brain Barrier of a beta-amyloidosis mouse model with ^{11}C-Metoclopramide PET. *J. Nucl. Med.* 2019, 10.2967/jnumed.119.237198.

[166] Zoghbi, S. S.; Liow, J. S.; Yasuno, F.; Hong, J.; Tuan, E.; Lazarova, N.; Gladding, R. L.; Pike, V. W.; Innis, R. B. ^{11}C-loperamide and its N-desmethyl radiometabolite are avid substrates for brain permeability-glycoprotein efflux *J. Nucl. Med.* 2008, *49*, 649-56.

[167] Lazarova, N.; Zoghbi, S. S.; Hong, J.; Seneca, N.; Tuan, E.; Gladding RL, Liow JS, Taku A, Innis RB, Pike VW. Synthesis and evaluation of [*N*-methyl-^{11}C]-*N*-desmethyl-loperamide as a new and improved PET radiotracer for imaging P-gp function. *J. Med. Chem.* 2008, *51*, 6034-6043.

[168] Savolainen H., Windhorst A. D., Elsinga P. H., Cantore M., Colabufo N. A., Willemsen A. T., Luurtsema G. Evaluation of [18F]MC225 as a PET radiotracer for measuring P-glycoprotein function at the blood-brain barrier in rats: Kinetics, metabolism, and selectivity. *J. Cereb. Blood Flow Metab.* 2017, *37*, 1286-1298.

[169] Fusi F., Durante M., Gorelli B., Perrone M. G., Colabufo N. A., Saponara S. MC225, a Novel Probe for P-glycoprotein PET Imaging

at the Blood-brain Barrier: In Vitro Cardiovascular Safety Evaluation. *J. Cardiovasc. Pharmacol.* 2017, *70*, 405-410.

[170] García-Varela, L.; Vállez García, D.; Rodríguez-Pérez, M.; van Waarde, A.; Sijbesma, J. W. A.; Schildt, A.; Kwizera, C.; Aguiar, P.; Sobrino, T.; Dierckx, R. A. J. O.; Elsinga, P. H.; Luurtsema, G. Test-retest repeatability of [^{18}F]MC225-PET in rodents: a tracer for imaging of P-gp function. *ACS Chem. Neurosci.* 2020, *11*, 648-658.

[171] https://rctportal.niph.go.jp/en/detail?trial_id=jRCTs031190136.

[172] Schou M., Varnäs K., Lundquist S., Nakao R., Amini N., Takano A., Finnema S. J., Halldin C, Farde L. Large Variation in Brain Exposure of Reference CNS Drugs: a PET Study in Nonhuman Primates. *Int. J. Neuropsychopharmacol.* 2015, *18*, 1-11.

[173] Bauer M, Karch R., Zeitlinger M., Philippe C, Römermann K., Stanek J., Maier-Salamon A., Wadsak W., Jäger W., Hacker M., Müller M., Langer O. Approaching complete inhibition of P-glycoprotein at the human blood-brain barrier: an (*R*)-[^{11}C]verapamil PET study. *J. Cereb. Blood Flow Metab.* 2015, *35*, 743-746.

[174] Tournier, N.; Bauer, M.; Pichler, V.; Nics, L.; Klebermass, E. M.; Bamminger, K.; Matzneller, P.; Weber, M.; Karch, R.; Caillé, F.; Auvity, S.; Marie, S.; Jäger, W.; Wadsak, W.; Hacker, M.;, Zeitlinger, M.; Langer. ^{11}C-Metoclopramide assessed with PET imaging in humans. *J. Nucl. Med.* 2019, *60*, 985-991.

[175] Damont, A.; Goutal, S.; Auvity, S.; Valette, H.;, Kuhnast, B.; Saba, W.; Tournier, N. Imaging the impact of cyclosporin A and dipyridamole on P-glycoprotein (ABCB1) function at the blood-brain barrier: A [^{11}C]-*N*-desmethyl-loperamide PET study in nonhuman primates. *Eur. J. Pharm. Sci.* 2016, *91*, 98-104.

[176] Kaufmann, A. M.; Krise, J. P. Lysosomal Sequestration of Amine-Containing Drugs: Analysis and Therapeutic Implications. *J. Pharm. Sci.* 2007, *96*, 729-746.

[177] Macintyre, A. C.; Cutler, D. J. The potential role of lysosomes in tissue distribution of weak. *Biopharm. Drug Dispos.* 1988, *9*, 513-26.

[178] Bauer, M.; Karch, R.; Zeitlinger, M.; Stanek, J.; Philippe, C.; Wadsak, W.; Mitterhauser, M.; Jäger, W.; Haslacher, H.; Müller, M.; Langer,

O. Interaction of ^{11}C-tariquidar and ^{11}C-elacridar with P-glycoprotein and breast cancer resistance protein at the human blood-brain barrier. *J. Nucl. Med.* 2013, *54*, 1181-1187.
[179] Bankstahl, J. P.; Bankstahl, M.; Römermann, K.; Wanek, T.; Stanek, J.; Windhorst, A. D.; Fedrowitz, M.; Erker, T.; Müller, M.; Löscher, W.; Langer, O.; Kuntner, C. Tariquidar and elacridar are dose-dependently transported by P-glycoprotein and Bcrp at the blood-brain barrier: a small-animal positron emission tomography and in vitro study. *Drug Metab. Dispos.* 2013, *41*, 754-762.
[180] Dörner, B.; Kuntner, C.; Bankstahl, J. P.; Wanek, T.; Bankstahl, M.; Stanek, J.; Müllauer, J.; Bauer, F.; Mairinger, S.; Löscher, W.; Miller, D. W.; Chiba, P.; Müller, M.; Erker, T.; Langer, O. Radiosynthesis and in vivo evaluation of 1-[^{18}F]fluoroelacridar as a positron emission tomography tracer for P-glycoprotein and breast cancer resistance protein. *Bioorg. Med. Chem.* 2011, *19*, 2190-2198.
[181] Bauer, F.; Kuntner, C.; Bankstahl, J. P.; Wanek, T.; Bankstahl, M.; Stanek, J.; Mairinger, S.; Dörner, B.; Löscher, W.; Müller, M.; Erker, T.; Langer, O. Synthesis and in vivo evaluation of [^{11}C]tariquidar, a positron emission tomography radiotracer based on a third-generation P-glycoprotein inhibitor. *Bioorg. Med. Chem.* 2010, *18*, 5489-5497.
[182] Kawamura, K.; Yamasaki, T.; Konno, F.; Yui, J.; Hatori, A.; Yanamoto, K.; Wakizaka, H.; Ogawa, M.; Yoshida, Y.; Nengaki, N.; Fukumura, T.; Zhang, M. R. Synthesis and in vivo evaluation of ^{18}F-fluoroethyl GF120918 and XR9576 as positron emission tomography probes for assessing the function of drug efflux transporters. *Bioorg. Med. Chem.* 2011, *19*, 861-870.

In: An Introduction to P-Glycoprotein
Editors: M. Wahajuddin et al.
ISBN: 978-1-53619-488-3

Chapter 6

P-GLYCOPROTEIN: A NEW INSIGHT IN THE FIELD OF NEUROGENESIS WITH A DIFFERENT PERSPECTIVE

Virendra Tiwari[1,2], Akanksha Mishra[1,3], Sonu Singh[1,4] and Shubha Shukla[1,2,*]

[1]Neuroscience and Ageing Biology Division, CSIR-Central Drug Research Institute, (U.P.), India
[2]Academy of Scientific and Innovative Research (AcSIR), Ghaziabad, India
[3]Department of Cell Biology and Anatomy, New York Medical College, Valhalla, NY, US
[4]Department of Neuroscience, School of Medicine, University of Connecticut (Uconn) Health Center, Farmington, CT, US

ABSTRACT

P-glycoprotein (P-gp) is one of the most studied ATP-binding cassette transporters (ABC). The modulation of this efflux transporter at blood

* Corresponding Author's: Email: shubha_shukla@cdri.res.in.

brain barrier prevents entry of many xenobiotics, endogenous and exogenous compounds in brain. Alteration in P-gp protein is known to be involved in various neurodegenerative disorders and other central nervous system diseases. Some recent studied have also reported expression of P-gp (ABCB1/MDR1) in neuronal stem cells/ progenitor cells by cell sorting technique. These previous studies suggest that P-gp (ABCB1/MDR1) gene also contribute towards the pathology of stem cells. Therefore, in present chapter, the interconnection/regulation between P-gp protein and neurogenesis has been discussed, highlighting the background and mechanism of P-gp and neurogenesis regulation.

Keywords: P-gp, neurogenesis, NSCs, ABC transporter, dentate gyrus

INTRODUCTION

ATP binding cassette transporters (ABC) are one of the largest and most studied family of proteins. The known 48 human ABC transporters are further subdivided into seven families from ABC A to G depending upon the contribution of these transporters in various molecular and cellular processes like drug resistance, transportation of small and large peptides and other molecules. The ABC transporters are efflux transporters that export drugs out of the cells. These ABC transporters participate in diverse cellular processes, including drug resistance and metabolism, transport of lipids, organic anions and iron metabolism. There is a specific tissue distribution pattern for each and every transporter. Along with liver, kidney, small intestine, they are also present on some important blood tissue barriers such as blood brain barrier, fetal-maternal barrier and blood eye barrier, thereby protecting the sensitive tissues from any harmful substance and consequently maintaining cellular homeostasis. The major difference between various ABC transporter subfamilies is the arrangement of N-terminal extension of transmembrane domain. Among all known ABC transporters, ABCB1/P-gp (P-glycoprotein) is the most studied type and recognized as multidrug resistance 1 (MDR1) transporter. It is named as MDR due to its involvement in the molecular mechanism of multidrug resistance of many drugs.

Although the transporter is present at the membrane of most tissues and blood-tissue barriers, as discussed earlier, but, recently its presence is also observed in hematopoietic and neuronal stem cells with high genetic expression. Neural stem cells (NSCs) have capacity to self-renew and differentiate into neurons, astrocytes and oligodendrocytes to generate intermediate and mature neurons. NSCs are recently reported to differentiate into other hematopoietic cells also, which is an advantage to researchers for development of other human stem cells. Furthermore, apart from other neurotransmitter transporter presence at the blood brain barrier and progenitor/ neuronal cells, presence of P-gp has also been observed in NSCs. During embryonic period, NSCs proliferate, migrate and differentiate to form mature neurons. These findings triggered a new dimension of studies pertaining to postnatal neurogenesis that became important, especially when only three neurogenic niches are known in brain: subventricular zone (SVZ), sub-granular zone (SGZ) of hippocampus and striatum. In the present chapter, neuronal stem cells, neurogenesis, P-gp and interlinking between them has been briefly discussed.

Neurogenesis and Its Regulation

Over the last three decades, several studies have reported that mammals do possess the capacity of generation of new neurons throughout their life time. These findings were reinvestigation of the discovery done around five decades earlier. Neurogenesis is a natural phenomenon through which generation of new neurons takes place and was first described by Altman and Das in 1965 (Altman and Das 1965). The SGZ of the hippocampal DG is one of the important neuronal stem cells (NSCs) containing niches, that are pluripotent in nature and have regenerative capacity. Hippocampal neurogenesis can be affected by several environmental and chemical factors (Kuhn, Dickinson-Anson et al., 1996, Kempermann, Kuhn et al., 1997, Eriksson, Perfilieva et al., 1998, Gould, Beylin et al., 1999). Other studies have confirmed the role of stressors including both physical and psychosocial stress, resulting in decreased hippocampal neurogenesis in mammals (Gould, McEwen et al., 1997, Gould, Tanapat et al., 1998). Similarly decreased cell proliferation was also observed in acute and chronic stress conditions (Fuchs, Flugge et al., 1997).

The disease pattern of neuronal and synaptic loss at early stage of neurodegenerative disorders such as Parkinson's disease (PD), Alzheimer's disease (AD), and Huntington's disease (HD) is responsible for the associated symptoms like depression, anxiety, cognitive decline, olfactory dysfunction and functional depression of hippocampus (Simuni and Sethi 2008, Stout, Paulsen et al., 2011, Hinnell, Hurt et al., 2012). Therefore, increased susceptility of these neurogenenic niches could be the underlying cause of progresssion of neurodegenerative disorders (Braak, Del Tredici et al., 2003, Carlesimo, Piras et al., 2012). It has been observed that apart from neuronal degeneration, changes are also seen in the neuronal vicinity, where the major key player are glial cells. All in all, the newly generated neurons in a diseased brain or regeneration of new neurons, work in co-ordination with other neighboring cells.

As discussed earlier, adult hippocampal neurogenesis is a process that consist of generation of new functional neurons from neural stem cells (NSCs) through the advancement of neural progenitor and neuroblast cells and subsequent incorporation of these newly formed neurons into existing neuronal circuitry. Various factors trigger the quiescent radial glial like cells (RGLs) and expedite their proliferation. These active RGLs are pluripotent in nature and mediate generation of neural progenitors (NPs) that differentiate into neuroblasts and finally leads to formation of either mature neurons or glial cells. All these steps such as proliferation, differentiation, migration and final integration into neuronal circuitry are governed by a number of locally and distally present factors.

Factors Regulating Neurogenesis

It is still debatable whether which cell population in SGZ is a true NSCs. Several studies have revealed different regulator of neurogenesis in brain. These key regulators may be internal and external in nature. The internal factor encompasses neurotrophic regulator (e.g.: BDNF), inflammatory mediators, transcriptional factors, neurotransmitters and hormones (Lee,

Duan et al., 2002, Tonchev and Yamashima 2007, Kohman and Rhodes 2013, Triviño-Paredes, Patten et al., 2016). The external regulators include exercise, antioxidants (flavonoids) and NSCs implantation (Maltman, Hardy et al., 2011, Murphy, Dias et al., 2014, Triviño-Paredes, Patten et al., 2016). Here we will discuss briefly about theses regulators and their effect on neurogenesis.

Neurotransmitters are the chemical messenger that plays a crucial role in synaptic transmission. The 5-HT (5-hydroxy tryptophan; serotonin) is a monoamine neurotransmitter synthesized mainly in raphe nuclei and lower mid brain of the medulla oblongata (Gaspar, Cases et al., 2003). Serotonergic neurons are present throughout the brain as well as in hippocampus (Sahay and Hen 2007). Long term treatment of SSRIs has been shown to remarkably enhance adult neurogenesis (Malberg, Eisch et al., 2000, Wang, David et al., 2008). Dopamine (DA) is mainly secreted from SNpc (Substantia nigra pars compacta) and VTA (ventral tegmental area) (Gasbarri, Sulli et al., 1997, Baker, Baker et al., 2004). Accumulating evidences have shown reduced level of proliferation of NPCs in both neurogenic niches of hippocampus followed by destruction of dopaminergic (DAergic) neurons in SNpc and VTA, or after decrease in dopamine level by neurotoxin such as 1-methyl-4-phenyl-1,2,3,6-tetrahydropyridine (MPTP) or 6-hydroxydopamine (6-OHDA) injection (Gasbarri, Sulli et al., 1997, Höglinger, Rizk et al., 2004).

GABA is the one of the major inhibitory neurotransmitters present abundantly in the adult brain, it acts via two subtypes namely GABA-A and GABA-B (Giachino, Barz et al., 2014). GABAergic signals are crucial for modulation of spatially and temporally regulated network activities underlying hippocampus-dependent memory (Paulsen and Moser 1998). In vitro studies have reported that GABA-A subtype of receptor is well expressed in NPCs (Paulsen and Moser 1998, Ge, Pradhan et al., 2007).

Another important neurotransmitter is Acetylcholine (Ach), majorly found in medial septum, nucleus basalis of Meynert, vertical limbs of diagonal band of Broca and substantia innominate, which further elongates to the different brain regions including hippocampus, thalamus, olfactory bulb and cortical regions (Paul, Jeon et al., 2015). Inhibition of forebrain cholinergic signal, mediated by selective neurotoxic, 192 IgG-saporin, has been shown to reduce hippocampal neurogenesis significantly, while subsequent administration of cholinergic agonist (physostigmine) restored the diminished hippocampal neurogenesis in adult and aged rodents (Harrist, Beech et al., 2004, Mohapel, Leanza et al., 2005, Itou, Nochi et al., 2011). Taking all in consideration, these studies elucidate that neurotransmitter system plays vital role in adult hippocampus neurogenesis.

Brain derived neurotrophic factor (BDNF) modulate neuronal development in the hippocampus and participate in maturation of GABAergic inhibitory networks in the cortex (Gillespie, Crair et al., 2000, Hong, McCord et al., 2008, Waterhouse and Xu 2009). Higher mammals brain studies have revealed increased level of BDNF in hippocampus region (Mori, Shimizu et al., 2004). Furthermore, deletion of BDNF diminshes adult neurogenesis in adult DG, which was again recovered after exogenous administration of BDNF (Scharfman, Goodman et al., 2005, Taliaz, Stall et al., 2010).

Exercise enhance blood flow that subsequently increase trophic factors in the neurogenic niches. Studies have shown that running leverages adult hippocampal neurogenesis by enhancing cell proliferation, differentiation and survival of new born neurons in DG region. Furthermore, studies have revealed that exercise enhance BDNF and FGF-2 both peripherally as well as centrally (Gomez-Pinilla, Dao et al., 1997, Russo-Neustadt, Beard et al., 1999). Another pathological condition is stress, a panic situation that is associated with altered homeostasis of an organism and subsequent physiological and behavioral responses. It is evident by different studies that exposure of mild to chronic stress at different life stages may lead to impaired hippocampal neurogenesis by subsequent reduction in cell proliferation, survival and neuronal differentiation in the DG region (Heine, Zareno et al., 2005, Mirescu and Gould 2006).

P-glycoprotein

P-gp (ABCB1/MDR1), one of the most studied ABC transporter, is a glycosylated membrane-associated efflux transporter. It is of 170kDa molecular weight and composed of 1280 amino acids. It is a single polypeptide consisting of two equal halves, each comprising six transmembrane helix and one nucleotide binding domain connected by a cytoplasmic linker. The transmembrane domain of P-gp enclose a very large cavity that has the capacity to lodge two substrates in concert. Thus, the transporter could bind to multiple drugs due to the large and flexible cavity (6000Å) present at the membrane of transporter using induced fit type of model (Figure 1).

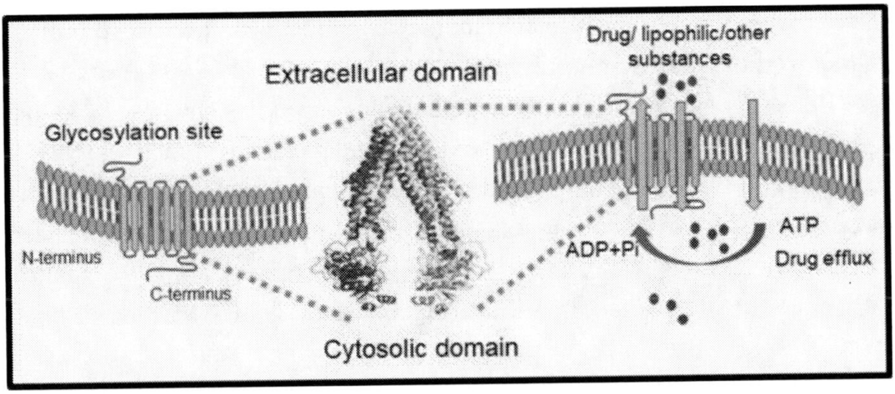

Figure 1. P-gp a multidrug transporter.

Involvement of P-Glycoprotein in Neurodegeneration

Progressive loss of neurons has been reported by several studies in sporadic and genetic form of neurodegenerative disorders. Apart from impaired adult neurogenesis i.e., the loss of existing neurons, the loss of self-renewal capacity is also been found to be compromised in neurodegeneration (Luo and O'Leary 2005, Winner and Winkler 2015). Previous research findings suggest that cerebral P-gp function declines with the progression of neurodegeneration in diseases including Parkinson's, Alzheimer's, Amyotrophic lateral sclerosis, Huntington's, Creutzfeldt-Jakob Disease and epilepsy (Vogelgesang, Cascorbi et al., 2002, Bartels, Willemsen et al., 2008). Furthermore, dysfunctioning of p-gp transporter may lead to neuronal degeneration mediated either by deposition of toxin, intracellularly as well extracellularly or by decreased clearance of toxins from neuronal cells. Accumulating evidences indicate that during early neurodegeneration phase P-gp expression enhances to combat inflammatory condition and the disease progression by activating BBB efflux of toxin materials from neuronal cells (McRae, Brouwer et al., 2003, Fernandez, Buyse et al., 2004). Another study suggest that Aβ protein modulates conformation of P-gp protein, similar observation was found by Cirrito and colleagues indicating decreased elimination of Aβ protein in P-gp knockout mice (Cirrito, Deane et al., 2005). Furthermore, drugs enhancing P-gp activity were found to be effective in increasing the clearance of Aβ protein and slowed the disease progression (Loeb, Molloy et al., 2004). Similar to AD, P-gp play a pivotal role in PD pathogenesis. Studies have revealed that P-gp enhance efflux of various toxicant and pesticides such as MPP^+, paraquat and DDT. Rat lung toxicity was decreased by P-gp activation by dexamethasone, while subsequent P-gp inhibition by verapamil enhanced the toxicity (Bain and LeBlanc 1996, Langston, Forno et al., 1999, Martel, Calhau et al., 2001, Shabbir, DiStasio et al., 2005, Dinis-Oliveira, Remiao et al., 2006). Similarly a postmortem study has revealed increased polymorphism of C3435T TT in MDR1 gene which was associated with decreased level of P-gp (Hoffmeyer, Burk et al., 2000). Similar to above diseases P-gp might play some role in disease pathogenesis in Huntington disease (HD), Creutzfeldt-Jakob Disease (CJD) and amyotrophic lateral sclerosis (ALS) (Vogelgesang, Glatzel et al., 2006). Although these diseases are less explored, however, CJD that is characterized by abnormal accumulation of isoform of prion protein (PrP), was found to be associated with decreased activity of P-gp suggesting the role of P-gp in neurodegenerative diseases.

Link Between P-Glycoprotein and Neurogenesis

P-gp is widely expressed at the membrane of most excretory organs such as liver, kidney and intestine and also other tissue blood barriers, but recently it has been observed that the transporter is functionally present in human neuronal/progenitor stem cells. The study was done under in vitro experimental conditions in progenitor cells, suggesting the involvement of P-gp which could play a vital role as functional biomarker in maintaining the human neuronal stem/progenitor cells in an undifferentiated state (Figure 2). Further, not only in vitro conditions, under in vivo conditions also the P-gp was found to be highly expressed. Yamamoto and colleagues had investigated the expression of P-gp in human fetal neural stem/progenitor cells during early development stage (Yamamoto, Shofuda et al., 2009). They found that P-gp is extensively expressed on the surface of cells under in vivo experimental conditions. Further thay have also revealed that expression of P-gp is direclty linked to the content of nestin in cytoplasm and also the level of CD133 gene present at cellular surface. During analysis in neurosphere cultures that are capable of expressing P-gp gene, it was observed that 53% of human neuronal stem/progenitor cells expresses P-gp gene on their surface. Moreover, in the same treated culture, the other markers were also examined such as nestin and CD133. The double staining of P-gp and CD133 on neuronal stem cells showed 68.6% cells positive for CD133 gene while 73.1% cells were found to be positively stained with P-gp. Also, 95.4% of stained cells were positive for nestin expression, whereas 50.8% of nestin positive cells expressed P-gp protein.

In the same experiment, the researchers also prformed FACS analysis for corelating the proliferative efficacy of cells through quantifying nestin as a marker during high and low expression of P-gp protein. They found that cells with low expression of P-gp also manifested less staining of nestin, in contrary, the cells with higher expression of P-gp revealed higher staining for nestin gene. Through this finding, it could be suggested that high percentage of P-gp in neuronal stem cells is somehow related to the proliferative efficacy of cells. Further, the microarray technique also proclaimed the differences in various gene expressions like CD24, during different cellular conditions such as neuronal stem cells with low and high expression of P-gp gene. Although, this analysis need further study for confirmation of results and finding out the exact molecular phenomenon behind the same.

The expression of P-gp was first evidenced by Chaudhary et al., (Chaudhary and Roninson 1991) in which they have demonstrated the localization of transporter in haematipoeitic stem cells positive for CD34 gene, through the use of rhodamine 1234, a fluorescent dye. Hoechst-33342 (another fluoresent dye) staining in the stem cells isolated from different tissues, is also used for determining the presence of P-gp transporter at the cellular membrane. Further, in a study, in ABCB1 (P-gp) deficient mice, revealed high expression of P-gp in stem cells, hence the efflux of xenobiotics could not be their only contribution, but they might be also participating in cell proliferation (Israeli, Ziaei et al., 2005).

Furthermore, during cell differentiation, it was observed that transporter (P-gp) expression was downregulated during cell differentiation process in human neuronal stem or progenitor cells alongwith downregulation of nestin and upregulation of GFAP (glial fibrillary acidic protein) (Islam, Kanemura et al., 2005). These studies support direct link between P-gp transporters and neurogenesis or cell proliferation and differentiation. In an another recent research, it was reported that deactivation of P-gp transporter does not influence astrogliosis and endogenous neurogenesis, but to affirm the same, more experiments are needed (Manrique-Castano, Sardari et al., 2019). Hence, the expression of transporters might or might not influence the neurogenesis cascade phenomenon. Schumacher and colleagues have determined brain related phenotypical alterations in P-gp deficient mice. They concluded that P-gp deficient mice show impeded differentiation of neuronal progenitors as the genetic or protein expression of doublecortin and calretinin was ameliorated in the cells, hence loss of P-gp transporter results into modulation of whole brain homeostasis and renegerative potency (Schumacher, Krohn et al., 2012).

Conclusion and Future Prospects

Although limited research has been carried out regarding the concept of P-glycoprotein, neural stem cells and neurogenesis, however, few investigators support the hypothesis that alteration of P-glycoprotein transporter modulate neurogenesis cascade process and there are reports denying this fact. Hence, there might be a possibility of both the mechanism, thusP-glycoprotein could be an interesting and ideal target for development of neuronal regenerative efficacious drugs and there may be a possibility of other side too. Therefore, more studies need to be conducted for confirmation of involvement of transporters in neurogenesis and neural stem cell proliferation and differentiation.

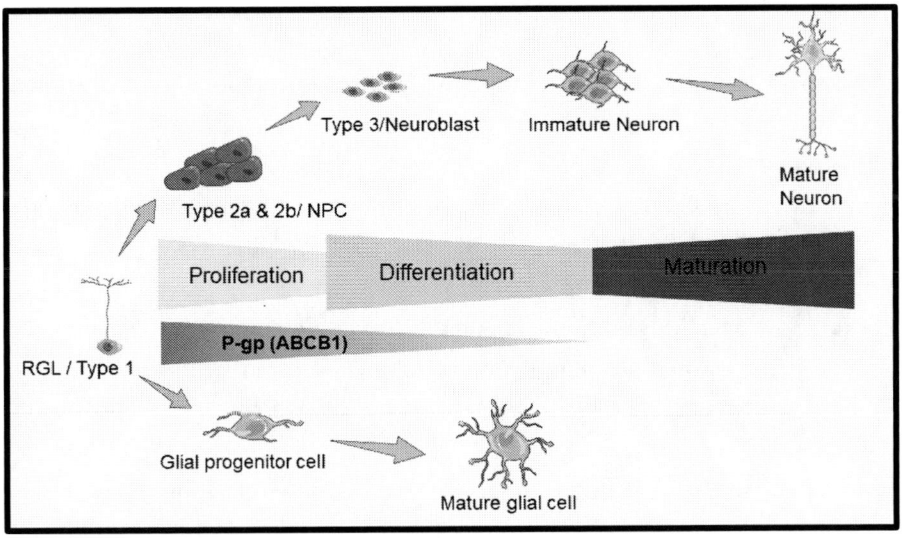

Figure 2. Orchestration of neurogenesis and possible role of P-gp transportor. RGL, Radial Glial like cells; NPC, Neural progenitor cells; ABCB1, ATP-binding cassette (ABC) transporter protein B1.

Acknowledgments

The authors are thankful to Director, CSIR-CDRI for continuous encouragement and support. Virendra Tiwari and Akanksha Mishra acknowledges CSIR, India, for providing the research fellowship. Sonu Singh is supported by a research fellowship from Indian Council of Medical Research (ICMR), New Delhi- India.

CONFLICT OF INTEREST

The authors declare that there are no conflicts of interest.

REFERENCES

Altman, J. and G. D. Das (1965). "Autoradiographic and histological evidence of postnatal hippocampal neurogenesis in rats." *J. Comp. Neurol.* 124(3): 319-335.

Bain, L. J. and G. A. LeBlanc (1996). "Interaction of structurally diverse pesticides with the human MDR1 gene product P-glycoprotein." *Toxicol. Appl. Pharmacol.* 141(1): 288-298.

Baker, S. A., K. A. Baker and T. Hagg (2004). "Dopaminergic nigrostriatal projections regulate neural precursor proliferation in the adult mouse subventricular zone." *European Journal of Neuroscience* 20(2): 575-579.

Bartels, A. L., A. T. Willemsen, R. Kortekaas, B. M. de Jong, R. de Vries, O. de Klerk, J. C. van Oostrom, A. Portman and K. L. Leenders (2008). "Decreased blood-brain barrier P-glycoprotein function in the progression of Parkinson's disease, PSP and MSA." *J. Neural. Transm. (Vienna)* 115(7): 1001-1009.

Braak, H., K. Del Tredici, U. Rüb, R. A. De Vos, E. N. J. Steur and E. Braak (2003). "Staging of brain pathology related to sporadic Parkinson's disease." *Neurobiology of aging* 24(2): 197-211.

Carlesimo, G., F. Piras, F. Assogna, F. Pontieri, C. Caltagirone and G. Spalletta (2012). "Hippocampal abnormalities and memory deficits in Parkinson disease: a multimodal imaging study." *Neurology* 78(24): 1939-1945.

Chaudhary, P. M. and I. B. Roninson (1991). "Expression and activity of P-glycoprotein, a multidrug efflux pump, in human hematopoietic stem cells." *Cell* 66(1): 85-94.

Cirrito, J. R., R. Deane, A. M. Fagan, M. L. Spinner, M. Parsadanian, M. B. Finn, H. Jiang, J. L. Prior, A. Sagare, K. R. Bales, S. M. Paul, B. V. Zlokovic, D. Piwnica-Worms and D. M. Holtzman (2005). "P-glycoprotein deficiency at the blood-brain barrier increases amyloid-beta deposition in an Alzheimer disease mouse model." *J. Clin. Invest.* 115(11): 3285-3290.

Dinis-Oliveira, R. J., F. Remiao, J. A. Duarte, R. Ferreira, A. Sanchez Navarro, M. L. Bastos and F. Carvalho (2006). "P-glycoprotein induction: an antidotal pathway for paraquat-induced lung toxicity." *Free Radic. Biol. Med.* 41(8): 1213-1224.

Eriksson, P. S., E. Perfilieva, T. Björk-Eriksson, A.-M. Alborn, C. Nordborg, D. A. Peterson and F. H. Gage (1998). "Neurogenesis in the adult human hippocampus." *Nature medicine* 4(11): 1313-1317.

Fernandez, C., M. Buyse, M. German-Fattal and F. Gimenez (2004). "Influence of the pro-inflammatory cytokines on P-glycoprotein expression and functionality." *J. Pharm. Pharm. Sci.* 7(3): 359-371.

Fuchs, E., G. Flugge, B. McEwen, P. Tanapat and E. Gould (1997). Chronic subordination stress inhibits neurogenesis and decreases the volume of the granule cell layer. *Soc. Neurosci. Abstr.*

Gasbarri, A., A. Sulli and M. G. Packard (1997). "The dopaminergic mesencephalic projections to the hippocampal formation in the rat." *Progress in Neuro-Psychopharmacology and Biological Psychiatry* 21(1): 1-22.

Gaspar, P., O. Cases and L. Maroteaux (2003). "The developmental role of serotonin: news from mouse molecular genetics." *Nature Reviews Neuroscience* 4(12): 1002-1012.

Ge, S., D. A. Pradhan, G.-l. Ming and H. Song (2007). "GABA sets the tempo for activity-dependent adult neurogenesis." *Trends in neurosciences* 30(1): 1-8.

Giachino, C., M. Barz, J. S. Tchorz, M. Tome, M. Gassmann, J. Bischofberger, B. Bettler and V. Taylor (2014). "GABA suppresses neurogenesis in the adult hippocampus through GABAB receptors." *Development* 141(1): 83-90.

Gillespie, D. C., M. C. Crair and M. P. Stryker (2000). "Neurotrophin-4/5 alters responses and blocks the effect of monocular deprivation in cat visual cortex during the critical period." *J. Neurosci.* 20(24): 9174-9186.

Gomez-Pinilla, F., L. Dao and V. So (1997). "Physical exercise induces FGF-2 and its mRNA in the hippocampus." *Brain Res.* 764(1-2): 1-8.

Gould, E., A. Beylin, P. Tanapat, A. Reeves and T. J. Shors (1999). "Learning enhances adult neurogenesis in the hippocampal formation." *Nature neuroscience* 2(3): 260-265.

Gould, E., B. S. McEwen, P. Tanapat, L. A. Galea and E. Fuchs (1997). "Neurogenesis in the dentate gyrus of the adult tree shrew is regulated by psychosocial stress and NMDA receptor activation." *Journal of Neuroscience* 17(7): 2492-2498.

Gould, E., P. Tanapat, B. S. McEwen, G. Flügge and E. Fuchs (1998). "Proliferation of granule cell precursors in the dentate gyrus of adult monkeys is diminished by stress." *Proceedings of the National Academy of Sciences* 95(6): 3168-3171.

Harrist, A., R. D. Beech, S. L. King, A. Zanardi, M. A. Cleary, B. J. Caldarone, A. Eisch, M. Zoli and M. R. Picciotto (2004). "Alteration of hippocampal cell proliferation in mice lacking the beta 2 subunit of the neuronal nicotinic acetylcholine receptor." *Synapse* 54(4): 200-206.

Heine, V. M., J. Zareno, S. Maslam, M. Joels and P. J. Lucassen (2005). "Chronic stress in the adult dentate gyrus reduces cell proliferation near the vasculature and VEGF and Flk-1 protein expression." *Eur. J. Neurosci.* 21(5): 1304-1314.

Hinnell, C., C. S. Hurt, S. Landau, R. G. Brown, M. Samuel and P. P. S. Group (2012). "Nonmotor versus motor symptoms: how much do they matter to health status in Parkinson's disease?" *Movement Disorders* 27(2): 236-241.

Hoffmeyer, S., O. Burk, O. von Richter, H. P. Arnold, J. Brockmoller, A. Johne, I. Cascorbi, T. Gerloff, I. Roots, M. Eichelbaum and U. Brinkmann (2000). "Functional polymorphisms of the human multidrug-resistance gene: multiple sequence variations and correlation of one allele with P-glycoprotein expression and activity in vivo." *Proc. Natl. Acad. Sci. U S A* 97(7): 3473-3478.

Höglinger, G. U., P. Rizk, M. P. Muriel, C. Duyckaerts, W. H. Oertel, I. Caille and E. C. Hirsch (2004). "Dopamine depletion impairs precursor cell proliferation in Parkinson disease." *Nature neuroscience* 7(7): 726-735.

Hong, E. J., A. E. McCord and M. E. Greenberg (2008). "A biological function for the neuronal activity-dependent component of Bdnf transcription in the development of cortical inhibition." *Neuron* 60(4): 610-624.

Islam, M. O., Y. Kanemura, J. Tajria, H. Mori, S. Kobayashi, T. Shofuda, J. Miyake, M. Hara, M. Yamasaki and H. Okano (2005). "Characterization of ABC transporter ABCB1 expressed in human neural stem/progenitor cells." *FEBS letters* 579(17): 3473-3480.

Israeli, D., S. Ziaei, P. Gonin and L. Garcia (2005). "A proposal for the physiological significance of mdr1 and Bcrp1/Abcg2 gene expression in normal tissue regeneration and after cancer therapy." *Journal of theoretical biology* 232(1): 41-45.

Itou, Y., R. Nochi, H. Kuribayashi, Y. Saito and T. Hisatsune (2011). "Cholinergic activation of hippocampal neural stem cells in aged dentate gyrus." *Hippocampus* 21(4): 446-459.

Kempermann, G., H. G. Kuhn and F. H. Gage (1997). "More hippocampal neurons in adult mice living in an enriched environment." *Nature* 386(6624): 493-495.

Kohman, R. A. and J. S. Rhodes (2013). "Neurogenesis, inflammation and behavior." *Brain, behavior, and immunity* 27: 22-32.

Kuhn, H. G., H. Dickinson-Anson and F. H. Gage (1996). "Neurogenesis in the dentate gyrus of the adult rat: age-related decrease of neuronal progenitor proliferation." *Journal of Neuroscience* 16(6): 2027-2033.

Langston, J. W., L. S. Forno, J. Tetrud, A. G. Reeves, J. A. Kaplan and D. Karluk (1999). "Evidence of active nerve cell degeneration in the substantia nigra of humans years after 1-methyl-4-phenyl-1,2,3,6-tetrahydropyridine exposure." *Ann. Neurol.* 46(4): 598-605.

Lee, J., W. Duan and M. P. Mattson (2002). "Evidence that brain-derived neurotrophic factor is required for basal neurogenesis and mediates, in part, the enhancement of neurogenesis by dietary restriction in the hippocampus of adult mice." *Journal of neurochemistry* 82(6): 1367-1375.

Loeb, M. B., D. W. Molloy, M. Smieja, T. Standish, C. H. Goldsmith, J. Mahony, S. Smith, M. Borrie, E. Decoteau, W. Davidson, A. McDougall, J. Gnarpe, O. M. O'D and M. Chernesky (2004). "A randomized, controlled trial of doxycycline and rifampin for patients with Alzheimer's disease." *J. Am. Geriatr. Soc.* 52(3): 381-387.

Luo, L. and D. D. O'Leary (2005). "Axon retraction and degeneration in development and disease." *Annu. Rev. Neurosci.* 28: 127-156.

Malberg, J. E., A. J. Eisch, E. J. Nestler and R. S. Duman (2000). "Chronic antidepressant treatment increases neurogenesis in adult rat hippocampus." *Journal of Neuroscience* 20(24): 9104-9110.

Maltman, D. J., S. A. Hardy and S. A. Przyborski (2011). "Role of mesenchymal stem cells in neurogenesis and nervous system repair." *Neurochemistry international* 59(3): 347-356.

Manrique-Castano, D., M. Sardari, T. Silva de Carvalho, T. R. Doeppner, A. Popa-Wagner, C. Kleinschnitz, A. Chan and D. M. Hermann (2019). "Deactivation of ATP-binding cassette transporters ABCB1 and ABCC1 does not influence post-ischemic neurological deficits, secondary neurodegeneration and neurogenesis, but induces subtle microglial morphological changes." *Frontiers in cellular neuroscience* 13: 412.

Martel, F., C. Calhau, P. Soares-da-Silva and I. Azevedo (2001). "Transport of [3H]MPP+ in an immortalized rat brain microvessel endothelial cell line (RBE 4)." *Naunyn Schmiedebergs Arch. Pharmacol.* 363(1): 1-10.

McRae, M. P., K. L. Brouwer and A. D. Kashuba (2003). "Cytokine regulation of P-glycoprotein." *Drug Metab. Rev.* 35(1): 19-33.

Mirescu, C. and E. Gould (2006). "Stress and adult neurogenesis." *Hippocampus* 16(3): 233-238.

Mohapel, P., G. Leanza, M. Kokaia and O. Lindvall (2005). "Forebrain acetylcholine regulates adult hippocampal neurogenesis and learning." *Neurobiology of aging* 26(6): 939-946.

Mori, T., K. Shimizu and M. Hayashi (2004). "Differential expression patterns of TrkB ligands in the macaque monkey brain." *Neuroreport* 15(16): 2507-2511.

Murphy, T., G. P. Dias and S. Thuret (2014). "Effects of diet on brain plasticity in animal and human studies: mind the gap." *Neural plasticity* 2014.

Paul, S., W. K. Jeon, J. L. Bizon and J.-S. Han (2015). "Interaction of basal forebrain cholinergic neurons with the glucocorticoid system in stress regulation and cognitive impairment." *Frontiers in aging neuroscience* 7: 43.

Paulsen, O. and E. Moser (1998). "A model of hippocampal memory encoding and retrieval: GABAergic control of synaptic plasticity." *Trends in neurosciences* 21(7): 273-278.

Russo-Neustadt, A., R. C. Beard and C. W. Cotman (1999). "Exercise, antidepressant medications, and enhanced brain derived neurotrophic factor expression." *Neuropsychopharmacology* 21(5): 679-682.

Sahay, A. and R. Hen (2007). "Adult hippocampal neurogenesis in depression." *Nature neuroscience* 10(9): 1110-1115.

Scharfman, H., J. Goodman, A. Macleod, S. Phani, C. Antonelli and S. Croll (2005). "Increased neurogenesis and the ectopic granule cells after intrahippocampal BDNF infusion in adult rats." *Exp. Neurol.* 192(2): 348-356.

Schumacher, T., M. Krohn, J. Hofrichter, C. Lange, J. Stenzel, J. Steffen, T. Dunkelmann, K. Paarmann, C. Fröhlich and A. Uecker (2012). "ABC transporters B1, C1 and G2 differentially regulate neuroregeneration in mice." *PloS one* 7(4): e35613.

Shabbir, A., S. DiStasio, J. Zhao, C. P. Cardozo, M. S. Wolff and A. J. Caplan (2005). "Differential effects of the organochlorine pesticide DDT and its metabolite p,p'-DDE on p-glycoprotein activity and expression." *Toxicol. Appl. Pharmacol.* 203(2): 91-98.

Simuni, T. and K. Sethi (2008). "Nonmotor manifestations of Parkinson's disease." *Annals of Neurology: Official Journal of the American Neurological Association and the Child Neurology Society* 64(S2): S65-S80.

Stout, J. C., J. S. Paulsen, S. Queller, A. C. Solomon, K. B. Whitlock, J. C. Campbell, N. Carlozzi, K. Duff, L. J. Beglinger and D. R. Langbehn (2011). "Neurocognitive signs in prodromal Huntington disease." *Neuropsychology* 25(1): 1.

Taliaz, D., N. Stall, D. E. Dar and A. Zangen (2010). "Knockdown of brain-derived neurotrophic factor in specific brain sites precipitates behaviors associated with depression and reduces neurogenesis." *Mol. Psychiatry* 15(1): 80-92.

Tonchev, A. B. and T. Yamashima (2007). ""Transcribing" postischemic neurogenesis: a tale revealing hopes of adult brain repair." *Journal of Molecular Medicine* 85(6): 539-542.

Triviño-Paredes, J., A. R. Patten, J. Gil-Mohapel and B. R. Christie (2016). "The effects of hormones and physical exercise on hippocampal structural plasticity." *Frontiers in neuroendocrinology* 41: 23-43.

Vogelgesang, S., I. Cascorbi, E. Schroeder, J. Pahnke, H. K. Kroemer, W. Siegmund, C. Kunert-Keil, L. C. Walker and R. W. Warzok (2002). "Deposition of Alzheimer's beta-amyloid is inversely correlated with P-glycoprotein expression in the brains of elderly non-demented humans." *Pharmacogenetics* 12(7): 535-541.

Vogelgesang, S., M. Glatzel, L. C. Walker, H. K. Kroemer, A. Aguzzi and R. W. Warzok (2006). "Cerebrovascular P-glycoprotein expression is decreased in Creutzfeldt-Jakob disease." *Acta Neuropathol.* 111(5): 436-443.

Wang, J.-W., D. J. David, J. E. Monckton, F. Battaglia and R. Hen (2008). "Chronic fluoxetine stimulates maturation and synaptic plasticity of adult-born hippocampal granule cells." *Journal of Neuroscience* 28(6): 1374-1384.

Waterhouse, E. G. and B. Xu (2009). "New insights into the role of brain-derived neurotrophic factor in synaptic plasticity." *Mol. Cell Neurosci.* 42(2): 81-89.

Winner, B. and J. Winkler (2015). "Adult neurogenesis in neurodegenerative diseases." *Cold Spring Harbor perspectives in biology* 7(4): a021287.

Yamamoto, A., T. Shofuda, M. O. Islam, Y. Nakamura, M. Yamasaki, H. Okano and Y. Kanemura (2009). "ABCB1 is predominantly expressed in human fetal neural stem/progenitor cells at an early development stage." *Journal of neuroscience research* 87(12): 2615-2623.

In: An Introduction to P-Glycoprotein ISBN: 978-1-53619-488-3
Editors: M. Wahajuddin et al.

Chapter 7

FORMULATION STRATEGIES TO BYPASS P-GLYCOPROTEIN MEDIATED DRUG EFFLUX

Viral Shah[1] and Manish Nivsarkar[2]
[1]Department of Pharmaceutics, B. V. Patel,
Pharmaceutical Education and Research Centre,
Ahmedabad, Gujarat, India
[2]Department of Pharmacology and Toxicology, B. V. Patel,
Pharmaceutical Education and Research Centre,
Ahmedabad, Gujarat, India

ABSTRACT

P-glycoprotein (P-gp), a member of ATP binding cassette (ABC) is a transmembrane permeability glycoprotein. P-gp is widely distributed throughout the body and functions as a carrier mediated primary active efflux transporter, which can extrude a broad range of structurally diverse compounds out of the cells. P-gp, therefore can potentially reduce the absorption, oral bioavailability and retention time of a number of therapeutic substances. As P-gp jeopardizes the success of drug delivery, strategies are being developed to overcome P-gp mediated drug efflux, in order to improve the delivery and thereby bioavailability of therapeutic agents. In general, P-gp can be inhibited by three mechanisms: (i) blocking drug binding site either allosterically, competitively or non-competitively (ii) interrupting ATP hydrolysis; (iii) altering integrity of cell membrane lipids.

Several generations of P-gp inhibitors have been developed to impede this multi-specific efflux protein but unfortunately, these inhibitors lack selectivity. To overcome this limitation, researchers are exploring nanocarrier based drug delivery systems with P-gp modulating activity to bypass P-gp mediated efflux. Another promising approach that can offer the advantage of bypassing P-gp mediated drug efflux is co-formulating P-gp inhibitors and substrate therapeutic agents in a unit formulation meant for delivery.

The present chapter is a brief overview of P-gp mediated drug transport mechanism that hinders the success of various therapies, with emphasis on formulation strategies that would overcome the P-gp mediated hurdles in the field of drug delivery and targeting.

INTRODUCTION

The therapeutic effectiveness of drug substances for numerous disease states such as infectious diseases, cancer, central nervous system (CNS) disorders (epilepsy, depression, and schizophrenia) is limited by poor therapeutic outcomes or drug resistance. Poor Therapeutic outcomes of drug substances are mainly related to the factors that affect the pharmacokinetics and pharmacodynamics profiles of drug substances. Oral bioavailability of drug substance is affected by both drug properties and the physiology of the gastrointestinal tract (GIT) [1, 2, 28]. Oral bioavailability is a cumulative outcome of fraction of drug absorbed, fraction undergoing hepatic elimination and fraction escaping gut-wall elimination. Physiological, physiochemical, and biopharmaceutical factors mainly affect drug bioavailability [3, 4, 5, 29]. Passive diffusion of drug substance into systemic circulation or target diseased organ is dependent on its physiochemical characteristics such as lipophilicity, molecular weight, and hydrophobic bonding [3]. However, active efflux of the drug is another important mechanism underlying in reduced bioavailability of active drug molecules post oral dosing [4]. The active transport pathway is mediated by transporters that are further categorized into influx and efflux transporters. The bioavailability of drug substance through various routes is determined by the compounds physiochemical properties and their relative affinity for these (influx/efflux) transport proteins. Several transporters belonging to the Adenosine triphosphate (ATP) binding cassette (ABC) superfamily and solute carrier (SC) super families, are expressed by entrecotes present on the apical and basolateral surface of membranes. These transporter proteins are responsible for influx and efflux of endogenous substances across the membrane. Efflux transporters mechanistically limit the levels of substrates into the respective tissue by reducing substrate uptake [6-10].

Various multispecific transport proteins, playing a dynamic role in limiting the bioavailability of orally administered drug substance have been identified in several organs. Some of these proteins belong to ATP-binding cassette (ABC) superfamily of transporters with P-glycoprotein (P-gp), multidrug resistance associated protein (MRP), and breast cancer resistance protein (BCRP) as representative examples [4, 6]. P-glycoprotein (P-gp), the permeability glycoprotein or plasma glycoprotein is an active, efflux, membrane bound transport protein pump discovered in 1976. P-gp is a member of ATP binding cassette (ABC) super family, multidrug resistance (MDR)/transporter associated with antigen processing (TAP), sub-family B, and member 1, abbreviated as ABCB1. [11-17]. It is also called as MDR1 and PGY1 and is recently designated as CD243. P-gp is widely distributed throughout the body and functions as a carrier mediated primary active efflux transporter, which can extrude a broad range of structurally diverse compounds out of the cells. A vast majority of bioactive agents do not readily permeate to the target diseased organ due to the existence of P-glycoprotein efflux transporter. Therefore, one of the determining factor for oral bioavailability and intestinal efflux of drugs is P-gp efflux transporter [18, 19, 3]. P-gp was found to be present on the surface of biliary canalicular hepatocytes, luminal surface of columnar epithelial cells of the lower gastrointestinal tract (GIT) including liver, pancreas, small and large intestines, jejunum and colon, apical surface of proximal convoluted tubular cells of kidney, capillary endothelial cells of blood-brain barrier (BBB), apical membrane of the placental fetal-membrane barrier function and in various other tissues like lungs, heart, adrenals, prostrate, skin, spleen and skeletal muscle. [20-28] P-gp efflux mechanism involves the protein binding to the ATP and requires energy derived by the hydrolysis of ATP to ADP in the presence of adenosine-triphosphatase enzyme (ATPase). Studies into several disorders have shown that the P-glycoprotein efflux transporter plays a vital role in the progression of disease by reducing therapeutic outcomes of drug substances. Various research findings are being made focusing on overcoming the P-glycoprotein drug efflux transporter by its inhibition or bypassing mechanisms [30-37].

P-gp Efflux Transporter Structure and Mechanism of Action

P-gp is presently the most widely studied member amongst the ABC transporter family, as it has shown the ability to transport an extensive list of substrates with a great degree of structural diversity [38, 39, 44]. P-gp is a 1280-long amino acid glycoprotein, type of energy-dependent ATPase transmembrane drug efflux transporter. Chemically it is a single chain structure with two equal length homologous portions. Each portion is separated by a flexible polypeptide linker portion and consist of 6 transmembrane domains and two ATP binding regions [45-48].

The efflux action of the protein follows a carrier mediated primary active transport mechanism. In this process, energy released from the ATP hydrolysis gives the driving force for extrusion process. The efflux transfers only one molecule at a time and takes place unidirectionally (out of the cells into the extracellular space) and. Thus, P-gp is a uniporter carrier protein. The mechanism of efflux by the P-gp transporter can be explained by several models. Pore, flippase and the hydrophobic vacuum cleaner models, are predominantly used to explain the mechanism of P-gp efflux (Figure 1 and 2). The pore model is described by interaction of P-gp with drugs within the boundaries of the cytosol, followed by cell efflux via protein channels. The flippase model explains drug efflux as "flipping" of drug molecules from inner leaflet to outer leaflet of the cell against a concentration gradient based diffusion process [49]. The vacuum cleaner model hypothesizes that P-gp binds directly to the substrate molecules that are located on the plasma membrane and pumps them out of the cell by recognizing the substrates as foreign bodies [49].

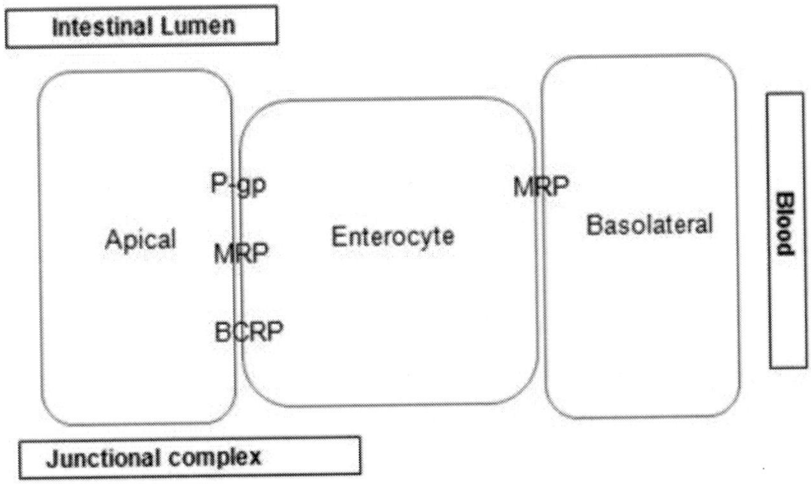

Figure 1. Drug efflux by P-glycoprotein in the intestine.

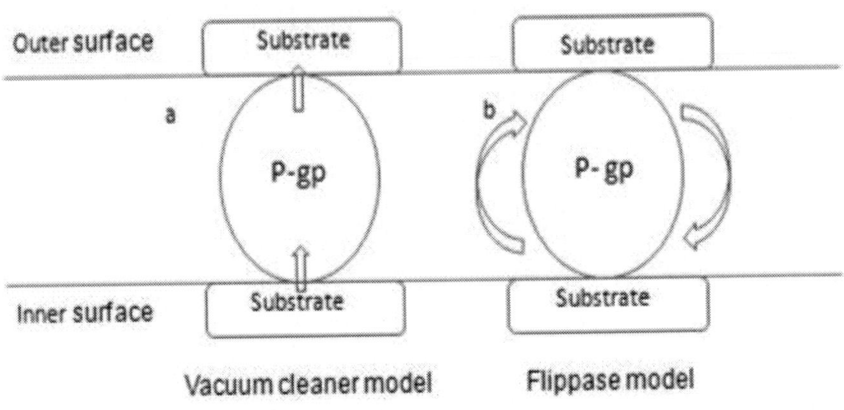

Figure 2. (a) Vacuum cleaner and (b) Flippase model of P- gp function.

P-gp Substrates and Inhibitors

P-gp exhibits capability to bind and transport a wide range of structurally and functionally dissimilar compounds. P-gp transporter has a diverse array of substrates which vary not only in size and structure but also in several chemical properties. Since the primary criterion subjecting a substrate to P-gp efflux is its interaction with the bilayer lipid membrane, a wide range of cationic, lipophilic and planar drugs become the protein substrates despite of their structural dissimilarity. P-gp can be inhibited by three mechanisms: (i) blocking drug binding site either allosterically, competitively or non-competitively (ii) interrupting ATP hydrolysis; (iii) altering integrity of cell membrane lipids [50-54]. P-gp inhibitors are classified into three generations: First generation inhibitors are pharmacological actives, which are in clinical use for other indications. Second generation inhibitors act as specific P-gp inhibitors and they do not exhibit any other pharmacological activity. The third generation inhibitors are similar to second generation inhibitors with a 10-fold higher affinity and potency to inhibit P-gp [55, 24]. To illustrate, First generation Chemosensitizers or reversal agents can inhibit the P-gp efflux pump and increase the absorption of drugs intracellularly [56, 57, 61]. Chemosensitizers act by competing at the P-gp substrate binding site. They also function by blockade of ATP hydrolysis; drugs such as verapamil, cyclosporine A, and antisteroidal agents such as tamoxifen are classified as first generation P-gp modulators [58-61]. However, high concentrations and pronounced side effects of these agents lead to the development of second generation chemosensitizers that exhibited similar limitations. Third generation chemosensitizers developed utilizing combinational chemistry and Structure Activity Relationships (SARs) approaches function as noncompetitive P-gp inhibitors. They result in alterations in protein conformation, thus modulating P-gp substrates [62]. Chemical constituents from natural origin, like epigallocatechin-3-gallate found in green tea is also reported for significant reduction in the expression and activity of P-gp, thereby subsequently improving the intestinal uptake and oral bioavailability of many drug substances [63, 64].

Table 1. List of P-gp inhibitors and substrates [57-65]

Inhibitor	**Substrates**
First generation: Verapamil, Doxorubicin, Clarithromycin, Sertralin, Omeprazole	Digoxin, Bromocriptine, Cimitidine
Second generation: Reversin, Valspoder,Gallopamil	
Third generation: Tariquidar, Biricodar, Annamycin, Mitotane	
Natural Origin: Green tea (epigallocatechin-3-gallate), grapes, citrus fruits, Kendarimide	

Range of *in vitro* P-gp assays has been developed so as to categorize compounds as P-gp substrates or inhibitors (Table 1). One of the assay method is the Transwell-based assays using polarized cell lines such as Madin-Darby Canine kidney (MDCK) cell line. This assay method provide a measure of the specific human P-gp-mediated efflux activity [57]. Another generally used P-gp *in vitro* assay is the P-gp ATPase assay for assessing drugs as P-gp substrates [58]. *In vitro* calcein AM P-gp inhibition assay can be utilized to detect compounds that inhibit the P-gp-mediated efflux, via employing a fluorescent P-gp substrate, calcein [58]. Another *in vitro* approach is the use of P-gp knockout mice that are genetically modified animals in which both genes that are homologous to the human MDR1 gene have been disrupted, resulting in a viable line of animal models. An assessment of the brain plasma area under the curve (AUC) ratio in knockout mice as compared to wild-type mice has become a standard experimental methodology to determine P-gp-mediated efflux [1, 59, 60].

Drug Delivery Strategies to Bypass P-Glycoprotein Mediated Drug Efflux

The development of drug delivery systems, involved in treatment of disorders requires a vital consideration of achievable therapeutic concentrations of drug substances in the required organ. Factors that impact the concentrations of drug substance in required organ include (i) the extent of intestinal absorption after oral administration, (ii) metabolic stability of the drug, and (iii) the active transport of drug via efflux pump transporters. To bypass the P-gp efflux pump, the formulation containing active drug molecule can be combined with a lipid, polymer or excipients which are capable of P-gp inhibition [50]. The following are the list of excipients which are potential P-gp inhibitors. Novel Drug Delivery Systems and Pharmaceutical Excipients Capable of bypassing P-gp efflux mechanism are discussed below:

Pharmaceutical Excipients Used In Drug Delivery Systems as P-gp Inhibitors

Natural Polymers

Natural gums, classified as polysaccharides consisting of multiple sugar groups bonded together have the ability of undergoing grafting and crosslinking reactions to form gels. Gums through such reactions may form hydrogels, xerogels, and nanoparticles which thereby can act as a potential P-gp efflux transporter inhibitor [64]. Chitosan, a cationic polysaccharide can be used as formulation component to form nanosystems, that may enhance the bioavailability of drug molecules by inhibiting P-gp efflux [65]. Anionic gums, such as xanthan and gellan gum, as well as alginates, can inhibit the action of the P-gp efflux pump at concentrations ranging from 0.05% and 0.5 mg/mL, respectively [66, 67].

Synthetic Polymers

Synthetic polymers such as polyethylene glycol 400, at a concentration range between between 1 and 20%, is reported to inhibit the P-gp drug efflux pump [68, 69]. Pluronic P85 and Vitamin E D-α-Tocopheryl polyethylene glycol 1000 succinate block copolymer have also been reported to inhibit P-gp efflux pump thereby enhancing substrate uptake [70]. Reports have been published for pluronic P85 as P-gp efflux pump protein inhibitor. It acts by inhibiting ATPase enzyme that is involved in the functioning of these proteins [71-74]. PEGylated sorbitans that are esterified with fatty acids are commonly known as polysorbates. The most extensively studied group of the Polysorbates is polyoxyethylene sorbitans monolaurates, known by the trade name Tween; these agents have been experimentally reported to be P-gp efflux pump inhibitors [66]. Poloxamers fall within the category of synthetic polymers are commonly known as Pluronics. Mixed micelles synthesized from a combination of poloxamer 407 and D-α-Tocopheryl polyethylene glycol 1000 succinate (TPGS 1000) have been reported to inhibit P-gp efflux transporters [76]. TPGS 1000 is a water soluble vitamin. It inhibits the P-gp pump by a combination of membrane fluidization, ATP depletion, and prevention of substrate binding mechanisms [76]. Thiomers, yet another group of synthetic polymers, containing a thiol moiety within their chemical structure are reported as potential P-gp efflux pump inhibitors with no systemic side effects. Thiomers enter the channels of the P-gp pump and thereafter form disulfide bonds with the cysteine subunits in P-gp; thereby there is an inhibition of P-gp efflux pump action hence the transport of drug molecules out of the cell is hindered [66].

Solvents and Surfactants

Both surfactants and solvents act as P-gp pump inhibitors by interaction with the polar heads of the lipid bilayers present in P-gp, thereby adjusting hydrogen bonding and ionic forces. They have the potential to insert themselves between the nonpolar tails of the lipid bilayer. These interactions cause the fluidization of the lipid membrane and thus P-gp inhibition. Nonionic surfactants such as Tween and Span are hydrophobic, less toxic and possess P-gp transporter inhibitory potential [77-79].

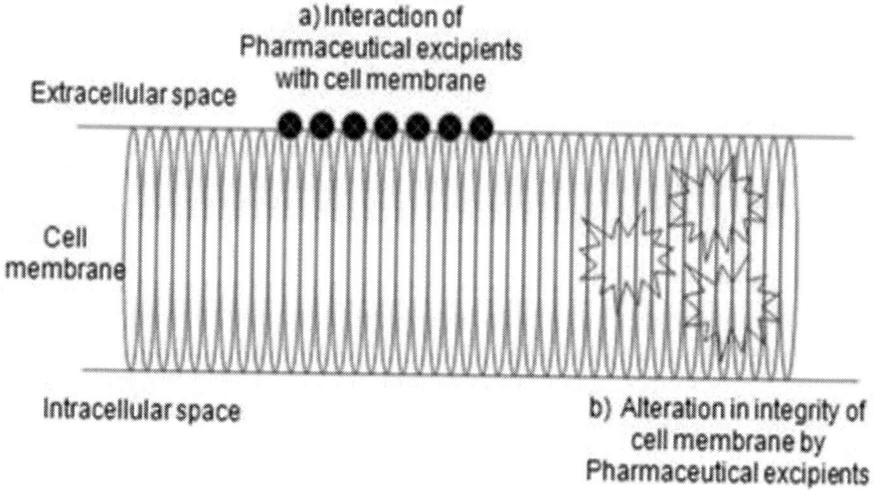

Figure 3. Cell membrane based mechanisms by which pharmaceutical excipients inhibit P-gp mediated efflux (a) by interacting with membrane (b) By altering the integrity of membrane.

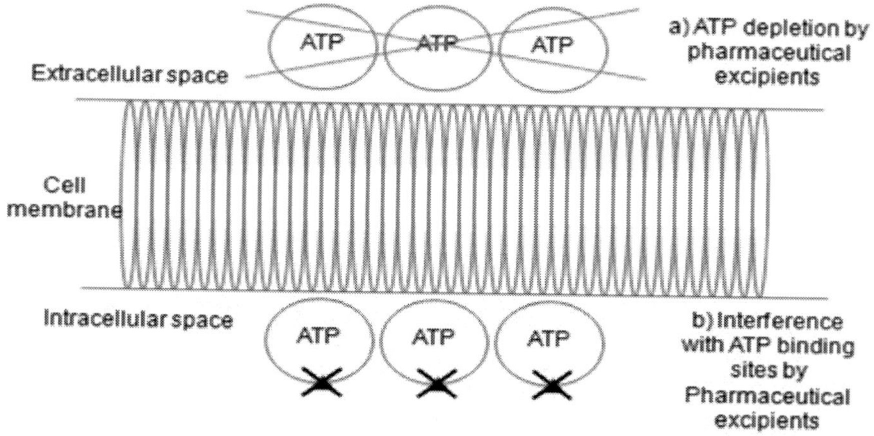

Figure 4. ATP based mechanisms by which pharmaceutical excipients inhibit P-gp mediated efflux (a) by ATP depletion (b) By interfering with ATP binding sites.

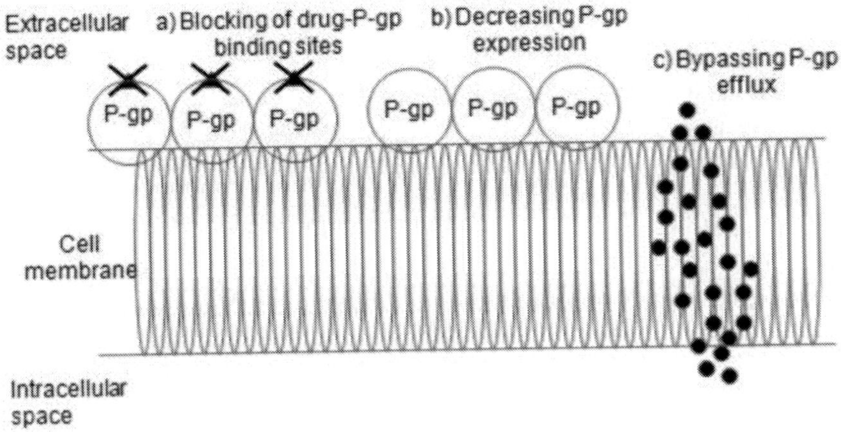

Figure 5. Mechanisms by which pharmaceutical excipients inhibit P-gp mediated efflux (a) by blocking drug-P-gp binding sites (b) By decreasing P-gp expression (c) by bypassing P-gp efflux.

Table 2. List of pharmaceutical excipients used as P-gp inhibitors []

	Excipients
Synthetic Origin	Tween 20/80, Polyethylene Glycol, Cremophor, Gelucire 44/14, Triton X, Polaxamers, Pluronics, Thiomers, Span, polyamidoamine (PAMAM), Myrj-52
Natural Origin	Anionic gums, Sodium alginate, chitosan, Falvicam, Ascophyllum

Formulations with P-gp Modulatory Applications

Self-Emulsifying Drug Delivery Systems

SMEDD's consisting of vitamin E (oil phase) and surfactants have been shown to enhance the solubility and bioavailability of paclitaxel (a P-gp substrate) owing to P-gp inhibitor activity [80, 81]. An advantage of using SMEDD's as a drug delivery system for P-gp inhibition is its capability to incorporate and solubilize high concentrations of P-gp inhibitors.

Double Coated Nanocapsules for Enhanced Intestinal Absorption and Bioavailability of a P-gp Substrate

An experimental study performed by Nassar and coworkers [2] proposes the use of double coated nanocapsules to improve the bioavailability of a P-gp substrate, Tacrolimus. The double coated nanocapsules prevented the molecular recognition of Tacrolimus by the P-gp efflux transporter. The conclusive results proved that the nanocapsule delivery system is a great platform for intestinal absorption of lipophilic drugs which are P-gp substrates [2].

Nanocarriers

Nanocarriers based colloidal systems include polymeric micelles, nanoparticles, lipid nanocapsules, and liposomes. Many of these systems have been designed and developed for indications in various CNS disorders to enhance brain uptake of the CNS targeted bioactives via P-gp transporter activity modulation. Nanoparticulate based formulations hold the potential of increasing the bioavailability of drug substances undergoing P-gp efflux [80-84]. These drug delivery systems due to their large surface area and good surface binding properties can be coated with specific P-gp inhibitory substances, such as polysorbate 80 that may possibly inhibit the P-gp efflux pump. Surfactant-Polymer based Nanoparticles are also reported to improve the therapeutic efficacy of an encapsulated drug by acting as P-gp inhibitors [85, 86]. Paclitaxel loaded lipid nanoparticles utilizing Brij 78 displayed IC50 values 9-fold greater than when formulated with taxol. The study established that lipid nanoparticles were able to inhibit P-gp due to the presence of Brig 78, which was utilized in the synthesis of the microemulsion precursor. Temporary and reversible reductions in ATP were observed with blank nanoparticles and free Brig 78. Therefore, the greater degree of P-gp substrate accumulation was elucidated by a synergistic combination of nanoparticle with Brig 78, where nanoparticles improve the uptake of the bioactive by partially bypassing the P-gp transporter and drug efflux is restricted via the release of Brig 78 from the nanoparticles [50, 62, 89]. In another research findings, Lipid nanocapsules loaded etoposide were synthesized due to their hypothesized reversal of multidrug resistance by the use of P-gp inhibitory surfactants during formulation. P-gp inhibitory activity of the etoposide loaded lipid nanocapsules was independent of size. The proposed mechanism was cell uptake followed by intracellular P-gp inhibition thus allowing for a higher intracellular drug concentration [90]. In a further research study the formulation of lipid nanocapsules was achieved by the use of tricaprylic acid, polyethylene glycol 660, and soybean lecithin, for the delivery of the therapeutic agent, paclitaxel, to caco-2 cells; results showed that the oral bioavailability of paclitaxel was greatly improved possibly due to the ability of lipid nanocapsules to inhibit the P-gp efflux activity; this mechanism is primarily due to the fact that the surface layer of nanocapsules being phospholipids thus resulting in P-gp inhibition via P-gp substrate site competition [91].

Polymeric Micelles

Micelles form from the spontaneous association of amphiphilic copolymers in aqueous phase, are characterized by a diameter no greater than 100 nm. The attractive force that leads to micellization is based on the interaction between the electrostatically neutral and hydrophobic portions of the copolymer. Self-assembly of the micelle only begins when the copolymer concentration reaches a threshold value generally referred to as the critical micelle concentration (CMC) [92, 93]. Mixed micelles of hydrophobic and hydrophilic pluronic L61 and F127 with encapsulated drug substance were reported to exhibit elevated cellular concentrations of drug due to P-gp inhibition displayed via modification of intracellular drug transport [88, 94].

Polyethylene Glycol-660 Hydroxystearate Nanocapsules

Nanocapsules encapsulated with etoposide (substrate) in combination with P-gp inhibiting surfactants, namely, PEG-HS (polyethylene glycol-660 hydroxystearate), were formulated and reported to exhibit increased bioavailability of etoposide [91, 94].

Immunoliposomes

The over expression of P-gp has been associated with the development of multidrug resistance in cancer cells. Methods employed in overcoming the multidrug resistance frequently involve the co administration of inhibitors of the P-gp transporter. Immunoliposome based drug delivery systems may be employed as alternatives to overcome multidrug resistance, since immunoliposomes penetrate target cells via receptor-mediated endocytosis, which in turn allows for the bypass of membrane related P-gp transporters. Targeting of immunoliposomes can be accomplished via the use of an antitransferrin receptor monoclonal antibody (OX26 mAb).

Table 3. List of formulations used as P-gp inhibitors []

Sr. No.	Formulation
1	Conventional Matrix Tablets
2	Miceller Systems
3	Hydrogel
4	Nanoparticulate system
5	Liposomes and Solid lipid Nanoparticles
6	Dendrimers
7	Lipid Nanocapsules
8	Self Emulsifying Drug Delivery System
9	Copolymer Conjugates
10	Films

The reported *in vitro* study depicted that immunoliposome based drug delivery systems can be utilized to bypass P-gp and therefore deliver bioactives to the cytosol of target cells [96]. Furthermore there is the novel approach of combining substrates and P-gp inhibitors within liposomal delivery systems; clinical trials were performed via the formulation of liposomes encapsulating PSC 8339, a recognized P-gp efflux inhibitor in combination with the drug molecule, doxorubicin; results observed depicted an increase in drug delivery potential with no alteration to the pharmacokinetic or pharmacodynamic character of the drug molecule [97, 98].

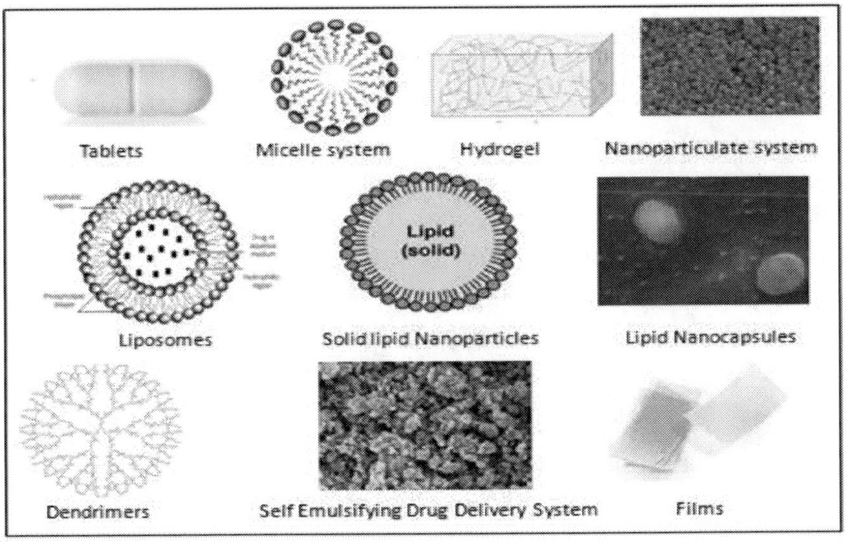

Figure 6. Formulation strategies used *to bypass* p-glycoprotein mediated drug efflux.

Dendrimers

Dendrimers are defined as synthetic macromolecules that have a well-defined structural configuration. They are made up of a centrally located core and branched units that stem from the core [68, 99]. The mechanism by which dendrimers inhibit P-gp is via endocytosis; the dendrimer passes into the cell interior; this inhibition process could be due to cell membrane alterations and ATPase inhibition; it has been reported that P-gp substrates that are encapsulated within dendrimers show an increased intracellular concentration [61]. Polyamidoamine (PAMAM) dendrimers belong to a new avenue of P-gp inhibition research; these dendrimers are known to improve the solubility of low solubility drugs [100].

Poly(D,L-lactide) Nanosuspensions

Nanosuspensions are dispersed systems comprising fine particles of drug molecules in the form of crystals. Nanosuspensions are known commonly to incorporate highly lipophilic compounds; these therapeutic agents are stabilized in solution via the use of surfactants. The large surface area afforded by the fine particles assists in enhancing bioavailability of drug substance [85, 101, 102]. Nanosuspensions formulated employing Pluronic F-68 (P-gp inhibitor) have been found to display better clinical outcomes in psychotic disorders via P-gp inhibition [103].

Exosomes

Extracellular vesicles (exosomes) are defined as cell derived membrane vesicles with a characteristic (phospho) lipid bilayer that allows for cell to cell communication. Exosomes are sized between 40 and 150 nm. Exosomes are produced by the formation of intraluminal vesicles in multivesicular bodies. Fusion of multivesicular bodies with the plasma membrane results in secretion of intraluminal vesicles which are in turn referred to as exosomes once released into the extracellular space. Due to their size and surface functionality, microvesicles and exosomes seem to be model candidates for drug delivery [104]. Exosome based formulations hold the potential of increasing the bioavailability of drug substances undergoing P-gp efflux. These drug delivery systems due to their large surface area and good surface binding properties can be coated with specific P-gp inhibitory substances that may possibly inhibit the P-gp efflux pump. [105].

References

[1] Löscher, Wolfgang, and Heidrun Potschka. 2005. Drug Resistance in Brain Diseases and the Role of Drug Efflux Transporters. *Nature Reviews. Neuroscience* 6, no. 8: 591–602. doi: 10.1038/nrn1728, PubMed: 16025095.

[2] Nassar, Taher, Alona Rom, Abraham Nyska, and Simon Benita. 2009. Novel Double Coated Nanocapsules for Intestinal Delivery and Enhanced Oral Bioavailability of Tacrolimus, a P-gp Substrate Drug. *Journal of Controlled Release* 133, no. 1: 77–84. doi: 10.1016/j.jconrel.2008.08.021, PubMed: 18822327.

[3] Takano, Mikihisa, Ryoko Yumoto, and Teruo Murakami. 2006. Expression and Function of Efflux Drug Transporters in the Intestine. *Pharmacology & Therapeutics* 109, no. 1–2: 137–61. doi: 10.1016/j.pharmthera.2005.06.005, PubMed: 16209890.

[4] Elsinga, Philip H., N. Harry Hendrikse, Joost Bart, Willem Vaalburg, and Aren van Waarde. 2004. PET Studies on *P*-Glycoprotein Function in the Blood–Brain Barrier: How It Affects Uptake and Binding of Drugs Within the CNS. *Current Pharmaceutical Design* 10, no. 13: 1493–503. doi: 10.2174/1381612043384736, PubMed: 15134571.

[5] Taylor, Eve M. 2002. The Impact of Efflux Transporters in the Brain on the Development of Drugs for CNS Disorders. *Clinical Pharmacokinetics* 41, no. 2: 81–92. doi: 10.2165/00003088-200241020-00001, PubMed: 11888329.

[6] De Van De Wetering, Koen, Alexander Burkon, Wouter Feddema, Alice Bot, Hugo de Jonge, Veronika Somoza, and Piet Borst. 2009. Intestinal Breast Cancer Resistance Protein (BCRP)/Bcrp1 and Multidrug Resistance protein 3 (MRP3)/Mrp3 Are Involved in the

Pharmacokinetics of Resveratrol. *Molecular Pharmacology* 75, no. 4: 876–85. doi: 10.1124/mol.108.052019, PubMed: 19114588.

[7] Demeule, Michel, Anthony Régina, Julie Jodoin, Alain Laplante, Claude Dagenais, France Berthelet, Albert Moghrabi, and Richard Béliveau. 2002. Drug Transport to the Brain: Key Roles for the Efflux Pump *P*-Glycoprotein in the Blood–Brain Barrier. *Vascular Pharmacology* 38, no. 6: 339–48. doi: 10.1016/s1537-1891(02)00201-x, PubMed: 12529928.

[8] Bartels, Anna L., Rudie Kortekaas, Joost Bart, Antoon T. M. Willemsen, Onno L. de Klerk, Jeroen J. de Vries, Joost C. H. van Oostrom, and Klaus L. Leenders. 2009. Blood–Brain Barrier *P*-Glycoprotein Function Decreases in Specific Brain Regions with Aging: a Possible Role in Progressive Neurodegeneration. *Neurobiology of Aging* 30, no. 11: 1818–24. doi: 10.1016/j.neurobiolaging.2008.02.002, PubMed: 18358568.

[9] Lin, Ying-Chi, Vicki L. Ellingrod, Jeffrey R. Bishop, and Del D. Miller. 2006. The Relationship Between *P*-Glycoprotein (PGP) Polymorphisms and Response to Olanzapine Treatment in Schizophrenia. *Therapeutic Drug Monitoring* 28, no. 5: 668–72. doi: 10.1097/01.ftd.0000246761.82377.a6, PubMed: 17038883.

[10] Stolp, H. B., and K. M. Dziegielewska. 2009. Review: Role of Developmental Inflammation and Blood–Brain Barrier Dysfunction in Neurodevelopmental and Neurodegenerative Diseases. *Neuropathology & Applied Neurobiology* 35, no. 2: 132–46. doi: 10.1111/j.1365-2990.2008.01005.x, PubMed: 19077110.

[11] Roberts, Derek J., and Kerry B. Goralski. 2008. A Critical Overview of the Influence of Inflammation and Infection on *P*-Glycoprotein Expression and Activity in the Brain. *Expert Opinion on Drug Metabolism & Toxicology* 4, no. 10: 1245–64. doi: 10.1517/17425255.4.10.1245, PubMed: 18798696.

[12] Van Os, Jim, Gunter Kenis, and Bart P F P. F. Rutten. 2010. The Environment and Schizophrenia. *Nature* 468, no. 7321: 203–12. doi: 10.1038/nature09563, PubMed: 21068828.

[13] Pharoah, F., J. J. Mari, J. Rathbone, and W. Wong. 2006. Family Intervention for Schizophrenia. *Cochrane Database of Systematic Reviews* 4: article ID CD000088. doi: 10.1002/14651858. CD000088.pub3.

[14] Nnadi, Charles U., and Anil K. Malhotra. 2007. Individualizing Antipsychotic Drug Therapy in Schizophrenia: the Promise of Pharmacogenetics. *Current Psychiatry Reports* 9, no. 4: 313–8. doi: 10.1007/s11920-007-0038-2, PubMed: 17880863.

[15] American Psychiatric Association, 1994. *Diagnostic and Statistical Manual of Mental Disorders*. 4th ed. Washington, DC: American Psychiatric Association.

[16] Kulhara, P., and S. Chakrabarti. 2001. Culture and Schizophrenia and Other Psychotic Disorders. *Psychiatric Clinics of North America* 24, no. 3: 449–64. doi: 10.1016/s0193-953x(05)70240-9, PubMed: 11593856.

[17] Khin, N. A., Yeh-Fong Chen, Yang Yang, Peiling Yang, and Thomas P. Laughren. 2012. Exploratory Analyses of Efficacy Data from Schizophrenia Trials in Support of New Drug Applications Submitted to the US Food and Drug Administration. *Journal of Clinical Psychiatry* 73, no. 6: 856–64. doi: 10.4088/JCP.11r07539, PubMed: 22687813.

[18] Kingdon, David G., Katie Ashcroft, Bharathi Bhandari, Stefan Gleeson, Nishchint Warikoo, Matthew Symons, Lisa Taylor, Eleanor Lucas, Ravi Mahendra, Soumya Ghosh, Anthony Mason, Raja Badrakalimuthu, Claire Hepworth, John Read, and Raj Mehta. 2010. Schizophrenia and Borderline Personality Disorder: Similarities and Differences in the Experience of Auditory Hallucinations, Paranoia, and Childhood Trauma. *Journal of Nervous & Mental Disease* 198, no. 6: 399–403. doi: 10.1097/NMD.0b013e3181e08c27, PubMed: 20531117.

[19] Falkai, P., and H. J. Möller. 2012. Neurobiology of Schizophrenia: from Outcome to Pathophysiological Insights. *European Archives of Psychiatry & Clinical Neuroscience* 262, no. 2: 93–4. doi: 10.1007/s00406-012-0294-y, PubMed: 22271345.

[20] Insel, Thomas R. 2010. Rethinking Schizophrenia. *Nature* 468, no. 7321: 187–93. doi: 10.1038/nature09552, PubMed: 21068826.

[21] Tandon, R., H. A. Nasrallah, and M. S. Keshavan. 2009. Schizophrenia. *Just the Facts' 4. Clinical Features and Conceptualization. Schizophrenia Research* 110, no. 1– 3: 1–23.

[22] Bebawy, Mary, and Manoranjenni Chetty. 2008. Differential Pharmacological Regulation of Drug Efflux and Pharmacoresistant Schizophrenia. *BioEssays: News & Reviews in Molecular, Cellular & Developmental Biology* 30, no. 2: 183–8. doi: 10.1002/bies.20706, PubMed: 18200566.

[23] Boulton, David W., C. Lindsay DeVane, Heidi L. Liston, and John S. Markowitz. 2002. In Vitro *P*-Glycoprotein Affinity for Atypical and Conventional Antipsychotics. *Life Sciences* 71, no. 2: 163–9. doi: 10.1016/s0024-3205(02)01680-6, PubMed: 12031686.

[24] Schmitt, U., A. Abou El-Ela, L. J. Guo, H. Glavinas, P. Krajcsi, J. M. Baron, C. Tillmann, C. Hiemke, P. Langguth, and S. Härtter. 2006. Cyclosporine A (CsA) Affects the Pharmacodynamics and Pharmacokinetics of the Atypical Antipsychotic Amisulpride Probably via Inhibition of *P*-Glycoprotein (P-gp). *Journal of Neural Transmission* 113, no. 7: 787–801. doi: 10.1007/s00702-005-0367-4, PubMed: 16252067.

[25] Pang, K. Sandy. 2003. Modeling of Intestinal Drug Absorption: Roles of Transporters and Metabolic Enzymes (for the Gillette Review Series). *Drug Metabolism & Disposition: the Biological Fate of Chemicals* 31, no. 12: 1507–19. doi: 10.1124/dmd.31.12.1507, PubMed: 14625347.

[26] Schlessinger, N., and K. M. Khuri. 2013. Giacomini, and A. Sali, "Molecular Modeling and Ligand Docking for Solute Carrier (SLC) Transporters". *Current Topics in Medicinal Chemistry* 13, no. 7: 843–56.

[27] Wagner, H., A. Spahn-Langguth, and A. Hanafy. 2001. Koggel, and P. Langguth, "Intestinal Drug Efflux: Formulation and Food Effects," *Advanced Drug Delivery Reviews* 50, no. 1 Suppl. 1: S13–S31.

[28] Kaur, Indu Pal, Rohit Bhandari, Swati Bhandari, and Vandita Kakkar. 2008. Potential of Solid Lipid Nanoparticles in Brain Targeting. *Journal of Controlled Release* 127, no. 2: 97–109. doi: 10.1016/j.jconrel.2007.12.018, PubMed: 18313785.

[29] Hawkins, Brian T., and Thomas P. Davis. 2005. The Blood–Brain Barrier/Neurovascular Unit in Health and Disease. *Pharmacological Reviews* 57, no. 2: 173–85. doi: 10.1124/pr.57.2.4, PubMed: 15914466.

[30] Löscher, Wolfgang, and Heidrun Potschka. 2005. Blood–Brain Barrier Active Efflux Transporters: ATP-Binding Cassette Gene Family. *Neurorx* 2, no. 1: 86–98. doi: 10.1602/neurorx.2.1.86, PubMed: 15717060.

[31] Löscher, Wolfgang, and Heidrun Potschka. 2005. Role of Drug Efflux Transporters in the Brain for Drug Disposition and Treatment of Brain Diseases. *Progress in Neurobiology* 76, no. 1: 22–76. doi: 10.1016/j.pneurobio.2005.04.006, PubMed: 16011870.

[32] Lee, G., S. Dallas, M. Hong, and R. Bendayan. 2001. Drug Transporters in the Central Nervous System: Brain Barriers and Brain Parenchyma Considerations. *Pharmacological Reviews* 53, no. 4: 569–96. PubMed: 11734619.

[33] Scherrmann, J. M. 2002. Drug Delivery to Brain via the Blood–Brain Barrier. *Vascular Pharmacology* 38, no. 6: 349–54. doi: 10.1016/s1537-1891(02)00202-1, PubMed: 12529929. View at Publisher · la Fougère, Christian, Guido Böning, Hero Bartmann, Björn Wängler, Sebastian Nowak, Theresa Just, Erika Wagner, Petra Winter, Axel Rominger, Stefan Förster, Franz-Josef Gildehaus, Pedro Rosa-Neto, Luciano Minuzzi, Peter Bartenstein, Heidrun Potschka, and Paul Cumming. 2010. Uptake and Binding of the Serotonin 5-HT1A Antagonist [18F]-MPPF in Brain of Rats: Effects of the Novel *P*-Glycoprotein Inhibitor Tariquidar. *NeuroImage* 49, no. 2: 1406–15. doi: 10.1016/j.neuroimage.2009.09.048, PubMed: 19796699.

[34] Aller, Stephen G., Jodie Yu, Andrew Ward, Yue Weng, Srinivas Chittaboina, Rupeng Zhuo, Patina M. Harrell, Yenphuong T. Trinh, Qinghai Zhang, Ina L. Urbatsch, and Geoffrey Chang. 2009. Structure

of *P*-Glycoprotein Reveals a Molecular Basis for Poly-Specific Drug Binding. *Science* 323, no. 5922: 1718–22. doi: 10.1126/science.1168750, PubMed: 19325113.

[35] Miller, David S., Björn Bauer, and Anika M S M. S. Hartz. 2008. Modulation of *P*-Glycoprotein at the Blood–Brain Barrier: Opportunities to Improve CNS Pharmacotherapy. *Pharmacological Reviews* 60, no. 2: 196–209. doi: 10.1124/pr.107.07109, PubMed: 18560012.

[36] Gabathuler, Reinhard. 2010. Approaches to Transport Therapeutic Drugs Across the Blood–Brain Barrier to Treat Brain Diseases. *Neurobiology of Disease* 37, no. 1: 48–57. doi: 10.1016/j.nbd.2009.07.028, PubMed: 19664710.

[37] Matsson, P. är, Jenny M. Pedersen, Ulf Norinder, Christel A S A. S. Bergström, and Per Artursson. 2009. Identification of Novel Specific and General Inhibitors of the Three Major Human ATP-Binding Cassette Transporters P-gp, BCRP and MRP2 Among Registered Drugs. *Pharmaceutical Research* 26, no. 8: 1816–31. doi: 10.1007/s11095-009-9896-0, PubMed: 19421845.

[38] Varma, Manthena V S V. S., Yasvanth Ashokraj, Chinmoy S. Dey, and Ramesh Panchagnula. 2003. *P*-Glycoprotein Inhibitors and Their Screening: a Perspective from Bioavailability Enhancement. *Pharmacological Research* 48, no. 4: 347–59. doi: 10.1016/s1043-6618(03)00158-0, PubMed: 12902205.

[39] Rosenberg, Mark F., Alhaji Bukar Kamis, Richard Callaghan, Christopher F. Higgins, and Robert C. Ford. 2003. Three-Dimensional Structures of the Mammalian Multidrug Resistance *P*-Glycoprotein Demonstrate Major Conformational Changes in the Transmembrane Domains upon Nucleotide Binding. *Journal of Biological Chemistry* 278, no. 10: 8294–9. doi: 10.1074/jbc.M211758200, PubMed: 12501241.

[40] Aouali, Nassera, Lahcen Eddabra, J. érôme Macadré, and Hamid Morjani. 2005. Immunosuppressors and Reversion of Multidrug-Resistance. *Critical Reviews in Oncology/Hematology* 56, no. 1: 61–70. doi: 10.1016/j.critrevonc.2004.12.010, PubMed: 15978826.

[41] Sharom, Frances Jane. 2014. Complex Interplay Between the *P*-Glycoprotein Multidrug Efflux Pump and the Membrane: Its Role in Modulating Protein Function. *Frontiers in Oncology* 4: 41: article ID Article. doi: 10.3389/fonc.2014.00041, PubMed: 24624364.

[42] Fardel, O., V. Lecureur, and A. Guillouzo. 1996. The *P*-Glycoprotein Multidrug Transporter. *General Pharmacology* 27, no. 8: 1283–91. doi: 10.1016/s0306-3623(96)00081-x, PubMed: 9304397.

[43] Constantinides, Panayiotis P., and Kishor M. Wasan. 2007. Lipid Formulation Strategies for Enhancing Intestinal Transport and Absorption of *P*-Glycoprotein (P-gp) Substrate Drugs: In Vitro/In Vivo Case Studies. *Journal of Pharmaceutical Sciences* 96, no. 2: 235–48. doi: 10.1002/jps.20780, PubMed: 17051593.

[44] Higgins, C. F., and M. M. Gottesman. 1992. Is the Multidrug Transporter a Flippase? *Trends in Biochemical Sciences* 17, no. 1: 18–21. doi: 10.1016/0968-0004(92)90419-a, PubMed: 1374941.

[45] Sauna, Z. E., M. M. Smith, M. Müller, K. M. Kerr, and S. V. Ambudkar. 2001. The Mechanism of Action of Multidrug-Resistance-Linked *P*-Glycoprotein. *Journal of Bioenergetics & Biomembranes* 33, no. 6: 481–91. doi: 10.1023/a:1012875105006, PubMed: 11804190.

[46] Wang, Jun-Sheng, Hao-Jie Zhu, Jennifer L. Donovan, Hong-Jie Yuan, John S. Markowitz, Mark E. Geesey, and C. Lindsay Devane. 2009. Aripiprazole Brain Concentration Is Altered in *P*-Glycoprotein Deficient Mice. *Schizophrenia Research* 110, no. 1–3: 90–4. doi: 10.1016/j.schres.2009.01.011, PubMed: 19239981.

[47] De Klerk, O. L., A. T. M. Willemsen, F. J. Bosker, A. L. Bartels, N. H. Hendrikse, J. A. den Boer, and R. A. Dierckx. 2010. Regional Increase in *P*-Glycoprotein Function in the Blood–Brain Barrier of Patients with Chronic Schizophrenia: a. *Psychiatry Research: Neuroimaging* 183, no. 2: 151–6. doi: 10.1016/j.pscychresns.2010.05.002.

[48] Wang, Jun-Sheng, Ying Ruan, Robin M. Taylor, Jennifer L. Donovan, John S. Markowitz, and C. Lindsay DeVane. 2004. The Brain Entry of Risperidone and 9-Hydroxyrisperidone Is Greatly

Limited by *P*-Glycoprotein. *International Journal of Neuropsychopharmacology* 7, no. 4: 415–9. doi: 10.1017/S1461145704004390, PubMed: 15683552.

[49] Nakagami, Taku, Norio Yasui-Furukori, Manabu Saito, Tomonori Tateishi, and Sunao Kaneo. 2005. Effect of Verapamil on Pharmacokinetics and Pharmacodynamics of Risperidone: In Vivo Evidence of Involvement of *P*-Glycoprotein in Risperidone Disposition. *Clinical Pharmacology & Therapeutics* 78, no. 1: 43–51. doi: 10.1016/j.clpt.2005.03.009, PubMed: 16003291.

[50] Kirschbaum, Katrin M., Stefanie Henken, Christoph Hiemke, and Ulrich Schmitt. 2008. Pharmacodynamic Consequences of P-glycoprotein-Dependent Pharmacokinetics of Risperidone and Haloperidol in Mice. *Behavioural Brain Research* 188, no. 2: 298–303. doi: 10.1016/j.bbr.2007.11.009, PubMed: 18164477.

[51] Feng, B., Jessica B. Mills, Ralph E. Davidson, Rouchelle J. Mireles, John S. Janiszewski, Matthew D. Troutman, and Sonia M. de Morais. 2008. In Vitro *P*-Glycoprotein Assays to Predict the In Vivo Interactions of *P*-Glycoprotein with Drugs in the Central Nervous System. *Drug Metabolism & Disposition: the Biological Fate of Chemicals* 36, no. 2: 268–75. doi: 10.1124/dmd.107.017434, PubMed: 17962372.

[52] Hitchcock, Stephen A. 2012. Structural Modifications That Alter the *P*-Glycoprotein Efflux Properties of Compounds. *Journal of Medicinal Chemistry* 55, no. 11: 4877–95. doi: 10.1021/jm201136z, PubMed: 22506484.

[53] Gohel, M., S. Modi, K. G. Vyas, and K. S. Rajesh. 2011. Delivery Approaches to Bypass *P*-Glycoprotein Efflux Pump. *Pharmaceutical Information* 9: 1.

[54] Nieto Montesinos, Rita, Arnaud Béduneau, Yann Pellequer, and Alf Lamprecht. 2012. Delivery of *P*-Glycoprotein Substrates Using Chemosensitizers and Nanotechnology for Selective and Efficient Therapeutic Outcomes. *Journal of Controlled Release* 161, no. 1: 50–61. doi: 10.1016/j.jconrel.2012.04.034, PubMed: 22562066.

[55] Choo, Edna F., Daniel Kurnik, Mordechai Muszkat, Tadashi Ohkubo, Sheila D. Shay, James N. Higginbotham, Hartmut Glaeser, Richard B. Kim, Alastair J. J. Wood, and Grant R. Wilkinson. 2006. Differential In Vivo Sensitivity to Inhibition of *P*-Glycoprotein Located in Lymphocytes, Testes, and the Blood–Brain Barrier. *Journal of Pharmacology & Experimental Therapeutics* 317, no. 3: 1012–8. doi: 10.1124/jpet.105.099648, PubMed: 16537797.

[56] Werle, Martin, and Andreas Bernkop-Schnürch. 2008. Thiolated Chitosans: Useful Excipients for Oral Drug Delivery. *Journal of Pharmacy & Pharmacology* 60, no. 3: 273–81. doi: 10.1211/jpp.60.3.3001, PubMed: 18284806.

[57] Hunter, R. L., J. McNicholl, and A. A. Lal. 1994. Mechanisms of Action of Nonionic Block Copolymer Adjuvants. *AIDS Research & Human Retroviruses* 10, no. 2 Suppl. 2: S95–8. PubMed: 7865341.

[58] Werle, Martin. 2008. Natural and Synthetic Polymers as Inhibitors of Drug Efflux Pumps. *Pharmaceutical Research* 25, no. 3: 500–11. doi: 10.1007/s11095-007-9347-8, PubMed: 17896100.

[59] Shen, Q., Yulian Lin, Takahiro Handa, Masamichi doi, Masami Sugie, Kana Wakayama, Naoki Okada, Takuya Fujita, and Akira Yamamoto. 2006. Modulation of Intestinal *P*-Glycoprotein Function by Polyethylene Glycols and Their Derivatives by In Vitro Transport and In Situ Absorption Studies. *International Journal of Pharmaceutics* 313, no. 1–2: 49–56. doi: 10.1016/j.ijpharm.2006.01.020, PubMed: 16500056.

[60] Hugger, Erin D., Kenneth L. Audus, and Ronald T. Borchardt. 2002. Effects of Poly(Ethylene Glycol) on Efflux Transporter Activity in Caco-2 Cell Monolayers. *Journal of Pharmaceutical Sciences* 91, no. 9: 1980–90. doi: 10.1002/jps.10175, PubMed: 12210045.

[61] Johnson, B. M., W. N. Charman, and C. J. H. Porter. 2002. An In Vitro Examination of the Impact of Polyethylene Glycol 400, Pluronic p85, and Vitamin E *d-a*-Tocopheryl Polyethylene Glycol 1000 Succinate on *p*-Glycoprotein Efflux and Enterocyte-Based Metabolism in Excised Rat Intestine. *AAPS PharmSci* 4, no. 4: 193–205. doi: 10.1208/ps040440.

[62] Batrakova, E. V., S. Li, S. V. Vinogradov, V. Y. Alakhov, D. W. Miller, and A. V. Kabanov. 2001. Mechanism of Pluronic Effect on *P*-Glycoprotein Efflux System in Blood Brain Barrier: Contributions of Energy Depletion and Membrane Fluidization. *Journal of Pharmacology & Experimental Therapeutics* 299, no. 2: 483–93. PubMed: 11602658.

[63] Dash, Ranjeet Prasad, Bhanuchander Ellendula, Milee Agarwal, and Manish Nivsarkar. 2015. Increased Intestinal *P*-Glycoprotein Expression and Activity with Progression of Diabetes and Its Modulation by Epigallocatechin-3-Gallate: Evidence from Pharmacokinetic Studies. *European Journal of Pharmacology* 767: 67–76. doi: 10.1016/j.ejphar.2015.10.009, PubMed: 26460146.

[64] Dash, R. P. and Nivsarkar, M. N. 2015. Intestinal *P*-Glycoprotein: Pharmacokinetic Implications and Approaches for Enhancement of Oral Bioavailability of Its Substrates. *Journal of Pharmaceutics & Therapeutics* 1, no. 1: 19–30. doi: 10.18314/jpt.v1i1.34.

[65] Batrakova, E. V., D. W. Miller, S. Li, V. Y. Alakhov, A. V. Kabanov, and W. F. Elmquist. 2001. Pluronic P85 Enhances the Delivery of Digoxin to the Brain: In Vitro and In Vivo Studies. *Journal of Pharmacology & Experimental Therapeutics* 296, no. 2: 551–7. PubMed: 11160643.

[66] Iqbal, J., and B. Hombach. 2010. Matuszczak, and A. Bernkop-Schnürch, "Design and In Vitro Evaluation of a Novel Polymeric *P*-Glycoprotein (P-gp) Inhibitor," *Journal of Controlled Release* 147, no. 1: 62–9.

[67] Batrakova, Elena V., Shu Li, Yili Li, Valery Yu Alakhov, and Alexander V. Kabanov. 2004. Effect of Pluronic P85 on ATPase Activity of Drug Efflux Transporters. *Pharmaceutical Research* 21, no. 12: 2226–33. doi: 10.1007/s11095-004-7675-5, PubMed: 15648254.

[68] Saxena, Vipin, and M. Delwar Hussain. 2012. Poloxamer 407/TPGS Mixed Micelles for Delivery of Gambogic Acid to Breast and Multidrug-Resistant Cancer. *International Journal of Nanomedicine* 7: 713–21. doi: 10.2147/IJN.S28745, PubMed: 22359450.

[69] Werle, Martin, and Martin Hoffer. 2006. Glutathione and Thiolated Chitosan Inhibit Multidrug Resistance *P*-Glycoprotein Activity in Excised Small Intestine. *Journal of Controlled Release* 111, no. 1–2: 41–6. doi: 10.1016/j.jconrel.2005.11.011, PubMed: 16377016.

[70] Bansal, Tripta, Naseem Akhtar, Manu Jaggi, Roop K. Khar, and Sushama Talegaonkar. 2009. Novel Formulation Approaches for Optimising Delivery of Anticancer Drugs Based on *P*-Glycoprotein Modulation. *Drug Discovery Today* 14, no. 21–22: 1067–74. doi: 10.1016/j.drudis.2009.07.010, PubMed: 19647803.

[71] Rege, Bhagwant D., Joseph P Y P. Y. Kao, and James E. Polli. 2002. Effects of Nonionic Surfactants on Membrane Transporters in Caco-2 Cell Monolayers. *European Journal of Pharmaceutical Sciences* 16, no. 4–5: 237–46. doi: 10.1016/s0928-0987(02)00055-6, PubMed: 12208453.

[72] Huo, Xiaokui, Q. Liu, Changyuan Wang, Qiang Meng, Huijun Sun, Jinyong Peng, Xiaochi Ma, and Kexin Liu. 2013. Enhancement Effect of P-gp Inhibitors on the Intestinal Absorption and Antiproliferative Activity of Bestatin. *European Journal of Pharmaceutical Sciences* 50, no. 3–4: 420–8. doi: 10.1016/j.ejps.2013.08.010, PubMed: 23981338.

[73] Li, Ming, Luqin Si, Hongping Pan, Abdullah K. Rabba, Fang Yan, Jun Qiu, and Gao Li. 2011. Excipients Enhance Intestinal Absorption of Ganciclovir by P-gp Inhibition: Assessed In Vitro by Everted Gut Sac and In Situ by Improved Intestinal Perfusion. *International Journal of Pharmaceutics* 403, no. 1–2: 37–45. doi: 10.1016/j.ijpharm.2010.10.017, PubMed: 20969937.

[74] Woo, Jong Soo, Chang Hyun Lee, Chang Koo Shim, and Sung-Joo Hwang. 2003. Enhanced Oral Bioavailability of Paclitaxel by Coadministration of the *p*-Glycoprotein Inhibitor KR30031. *Pharmaceutical Research* 20, no. 1: 24–30. doi: 10.1023/a:1022286422439, PubMed: 12608532.

[75] Wong, Ho Lun, Xiao Yu Wu, and Reina Bendayan. 2012. Nanotechnological Advances for the Delivery of CNS Therapeutics.

Advanced Drug Delivery Reviews 64, no. 7: 686–700. doi: 10.1016/j.addr.2011.10.007, PubMed: 22100125.

[76] Agarwal, N., G. Lariya, N. Saraogi, and H. Dubey. 2009. Agrawal, and G. P. Agrawal, "Nanoparticles as Novel Carrier for Brain Delivery: a Review," *Current Pharmaceutical Design* 15, no. 8: 917–25.

[77] Chavanpatil, Mahesh D., Ayman Khdair, Brigitte Gerard, Corbin Bachmeier, Donald W. Miller, Malathy P. V. Shekhar, and Jayanth Panyam. 2007. View at Publisher. Surfactant-Polymer Nanoparticles Overcome P-glycoprotein-Mediated Drug Efflux. *Molecular Pharmaceutics* 4, no. 5: 730–8. doi: 10.1021/mp070024d, PubMed: 17705442.

[78] Fortuna, G. 2011. Alves, and A. Falcao, "In Vitro and In Vivo Relevance of the *p*-Glycoprotein Probe Substrates in Drug Discovery and Development: Focus on Rhodamine 123, Digoxin and Talinolol," *Journal of Bioequivalence & Bioavailability* 01, no. 2.

[79] Mandal, Bivash, Himanshu Bhattacharjee, Nivesh Mittal, Hongkee Sah, Pavan Balabathula, Laura A. Thoma, and George C. Wood. 2013. Core-Shell-Type Lipid-Polymer Hybrid Nanoparticles as a Drug Delivery Platform. *Nanomedicine: Nanotechnology, Biology, & Medicine* 9, no. 4: 474–91. doi: 10.1016/j.nano.2012.11.010, PubMed: 23261500.

[80] Lamprecht, Alf, and Jean-Pierre Benoit. 2006. Etoposide Nanocarriers Suppress Glioma Cell Growth by Intracellular Drug Delivery and Simultaneous *P*-Glycoprotein Inhibition. *Journal of Controlled Release* 112, no. 2: 208–13. doi: 10.1016/j.jconrel.2006.02.014, PubMed: 16574265.

[81] Roger, E., F. Lagarce, E. Garcion, and J. P. Benoit. 2010. Reciprocal Competition Between Lipid Nanocapsules and P-gp for Paclitaxel Transport Across Caco-2 Cells. *European Journal of Pharmaceutical Sciences* 40, no. 5: 422–9. doi: 10.1016/j.ejps.2010.04.015, PubMed: 20438839.

[82] Gan, Chee Wee, and Si-Shen Feng. 2010. Transferrin-Conjugated Nanoparticles of Poly(Lactide)-*d*-α-Tocopheryl Polyethylene Glycol

Succinate Diblock Copolymer for Targeted Drug Delivery Across the Blood–Brain Barrier. *Biomaterials* 31, no. 30: 7748–57. doi: 10.1016/j.biomaterials.2010.06.053, PubMed: 20673685.

[83] Wang, Feihu, Dianrui Zhang, Qiang Zhang, Yuxuan Chen, Dandan Zheng, Leilei Hao, Cunxian Duan, Lejiao Jia, Guangpu Liu, and Yue Liu. 2011. Synergistic Effect of Folate-Mediated Targeting and Verapamil-Mediated P-gp Inhibition with Paclitaxel -Polymer Micelles to Overcome Multi-Drug Resistance. *Biomaterials* 32, no. 35: 9444–56. doi: 10.1016/j.biomaterials.2011.08.041, PubMed: 21903258.

[84] Danson, S., D. Ferry, V. Alakhov, J. Margison, D. Kerr, D. Jowle, M. Brampton, G. Halbert, and M. Ranson. 2004. Phase I Dose Escalation and Pharmacokinetic Study of Pluronic Polymer-Bound Doxorubicin (SP1049C) in Patients with Advanced Cancer. *British Journal of Cancer* 90, no. 11: 2085–91. doi: 10.1038/sj.bjc.6601856, PubMed: 15150584.

[85] Huwyler, J. örg, Andrin Cerletti, Gert Fricker, Alex N. Eberle, and J. ürgen Drewe. 2002. By-Passing of *P*-Glycoprotein Using Immunoliposomes. *Journal of Drug Targeting* 10, no. 1: 73–9. doi: 10.1080/10611860290007559, PubMed: 11996089.

[86] Krishna, R., N. McIntosh, K. W. Riggs, and L. D. Mayer. 1999. Doxorubicin Encapsulated in Sterically Stabilized Liposomes Exhibits Renal and Biliary Clearance Properties That Are Independent of Valspodar (PSC 833) Under Conditions That Significantly Inhibit Nonencapsulated Drug Excretion. *Clinical Cancer Research* 5, no. 10: 2939–47. PubMed: 10537363.

[87] Lee, K. D., K. Hong, and D. Papahadjopoulos. 1992. Recognition of Liposomes by Cells: *In Vitro* Binding and Endocytosis Mediated by Specific Lipid Headgroups and Surface Charge Density. *Biochimica & Biophysica Acta* 1103, no. 2: 185–97. doi: 10.1016/0005-2736(92)90086-2, PubMed: 1543703.

[88] Gillies, Elizabeth R., and Jean M J M. J. Fréchet. 2005. Dendrimers and Dendritic Polymers in Drug Delivery. *Drug Discovery Today* 10,

no. 1: 35–43. doi: 10.1016/S1359-6446(04)03276-3, PubMed: 15676297.

[89] Cui, Q., S. Xu, J. Shi Gu, and X. Che. 2009. PAMAM-Drug Complex for Delivering Anticancer Drug Across Blood–Brain Barrier *In-Vitro* and *In-Vivo*. *African Journal of Pharmacy & Pharmacology* 3, no. 5: 227–33.

[90] Svenson, Sonke. 2009. Dendrimers as Versatile Platform in Drug Delivery Applications. *European Journal of Pharmaceutics & Biopharmaceutics* 71, no. 3: 445–62. doi: 10.1016/j.ejpb.2008.09.023, PubMed: 18976707.

[91] Muthu, M. S., and S. Singh. 2009. Poly (D, L-Lactide) Nanosuspensions of Risperidone for Parenteral Delivery: Formulation and *In-Vitro* Evaluation. *Current Drug Delivery* 6, no. 1: 62–8. doi: 10.2174/156720109787048302, PubMed: 19418957.

[92] Van der Meel, Roy, Marcel H A M H. A. M. Fens, Pieter Vader, Wouter W. van Solinge, Omolola Eniola-Adefeso, and Raymond M. Schiffelers. 2014. Extracellular Vesicles as Drug Delivery Systems: Lessons from the Liposome Field. *Journal of Controlled Release* 195: 72–85. doi: 10.1016/j.jconrel.2014.07.049, PubMed: 25094032.

[93] Van Dommelen, Susan M., Pieter Vader, Samira Lakhal, S. A. A. Kooijmans, Wouter W. van Solinge, Matthew J. A. Wood, and Raymond M. Schiffelers. 2012. Microvesicles and Exosomes: Opportunities for Cell-Derived Membrane Vesicles in Drug Delivery. *Journal of Controlled Release* 161, no. 2: 635–44. doi: 10.1016/j.jconrel.2011.11.021, PubMed: 22138068.

[94] Haney, Matthew J., Natalia L. Klyachko, Yuling Zhao, Richa Gupta, Evgeniya G. Plotnikova, Zhijian He, Tejash Patel, Aleksandr Piroyan, Marina Sokolsky, Alexander V. Kabanov, and Elena V. Batrakova. 2015. Exosomes as Drug Delivery Vehicles for Parkinson's Disease Therapy. *Journal of Controlled Release* 207: 18–30. doi: 10.1016/j.jconrel.2015.03.033, PubMed: 25836593.

[95] Mahar Doan, Kelly M., Joan E. Humphreys, Lindsey O. Webster et al. 2002. Passive Permeability and P-glycoprotein-Mediated Efflux Differentiate Central Nervous System (CNS) and non-CNS Marketed

Drugs. *Journal of Pharmacology & Experimental Therapeutics* 303, no. 3: 1029–37. doi: 10.1124/jpet.102.039255, PubMed: 12438524.

[96] Wong, Ho Lun, Reina Bendayan, Andrew Mike Rauth, and Xiao Yu Wu. 2006. Simultaneous Delivery of Doxorubicin and GG918 (Elacridar) by New Polymer-Lipid Hybrid Nanoparticles (PLN) for Enhanced Treatment of Multidrug-Resistant Breast Cancer. *Journal of Controlled Release* 116, no. 3: 275–84. doi: 10.1016/j.jconrel. 2006.09.007, PubMed: 17097178.

[97] Kuo, Yung-Chih, and Hung-Hao Chen. 2006. Effect of Nanoparticulate Polybutylcyanoacrylate and Methylmethacrylate-Sulfopropylmethacrylate on the Permeability of Zidovudine and Lamivudine Across the In Vitro Blood–Brain Barrier. *International Journal of Pharmaceutics* 327, no. 1–2: 160–9. doi: 10.1016/j.ijpharm.2006.07.044, PubMed: 16939704.

[98] Yallapu, Murali Mohan, Meena Jaggi, and Subhash C. Chauhan. 2011. Design and Engineering of Nanogels for Cancer Treatment. *Drug Discovery Today* 16, no. 9–10: 457–63. doi: 10.1016/j.drudis. 2011.03.004, PubMed: 21414419.

[99] Nasongkla, Norased, Erik Bey, Jimin Ren, Hua Ai, Chalermchai Khemtong, Jagadeesh Setti Guthi, Shook-Fong Chin, A. Dean Sherry, David A. Boothman, and Jinming Gao. 2006. Multifunctional Polymeric Micelles as Cancer-Targeted, MRI-Ultrasensitive Drug Delivery Systems. *Nano Letters* 6, no. 11: 2427–30. doi: 10.1021/nl061412u, PubMed: 17090068.

[100] Mo, Ran, Xiang Jin, Nan Li et al. 2011. View at Publisher · S.-H. Kim and C.-C. Chu, “Synthesis and characterization of dextran-methacrylate hydrogels and structural study by SEM,” *Journal of Biomedical Materials Research,* vol. 49, no. 4, pp. 517–527, 2000. The Mechanism of Enhancement on Oral Absorption of Paclitaxel by *N*-Octyl-*O*-Sulfate Chitosan Micelles. *Biomaterials* 32, no. 20: 4609–20. doi: 10.1016/j.biomaterials.2011.03.005, PubMed: 21440934.

[101] Zhuang, X., X. Tian, Y. Zheng, N. Lan, L. Liu, R. Zhang, and Y. Liu. 2011. Formulation and Physicochemical Characterisation of a Novel Self-Microemulsifying Delivery System as Hydrotropic and

Solubilising Agent for Penfluridol. *Procedia Engineering. Proceedings of the 2nd SREE Conference on Chemical Engineering (CCE 2011)* 18: 59–65. doi: 10.1016/j.proeng.2011.11.010.

[102] Negi, Lalit Mohan, Mohammad Tariq, and Sushama Talegaonkar. 2013. Nano Scale Self-Emulsifying Oil Based Carrier System for Improved Oral Bioavailability of Camptothecin Derivative by *P*-Glycoprotein Modulation. *Colloids & Surfaces. B, Biointerfaces* 111: 346–53. doi: 10.1016/j.colsurfb.2013.06.001, PubMed: 23850745. ·.

[103] Estudante, Margarida, José G. Morais, Graça Soveral, and Leslie Z. Benet. 2013. Intestinal Drug Transporters: an Overview. *Advanced Drug Delivery Reviews* 65, no. 10: 1340–56. doi: 10.1016/ j.addr.2012.09.042, PubMed: 23041352.

[104] Neesse, Albrecht, Patrick Michl, Kristopher K. Frese, Christine Feig, Natalie Cook, Mike A. Jacobetz, Martijn P. Lolkema, Malte Buchholz, Kenneth P. Olive, Thomas M. Gress, and David A. Tuveson. 2011. Stromal Biology and Therapy in Pancreatic Cancer. *Gut* 60, no. 6: 861–8. doi: 10.1136/gut.2010.226092, PubMed: 20966025.

[105] Haj-Salem, I., S. Plante, A. S. Gounni, M. Rouabhia, and J. Chakir. 2018. Fibroblast-Derived Exosomes Promote Epithelial Cell Proliferation Through TGF-β2 Signaling Pathway in Severe Asthma. *Allergy* 1416: 55–87.

In: An Introduction to P-Glycoprotein
Editors: M. Wahajuddin et al.
ISBN: 978-1-53619-488-3

Chapter 8

MARINE SOURCES POTENTIATE TO INHIBIT P-GLYCOPROTEIN FOR THE MANAGEMENT OF CANCERS AND MULTIDRUG RESISTANCE

Varish Ahmad[1,*], Qazi Mohammad Sajid Jamal[2], Sohail Akhtar[3], Aftab Ahmad[1], Zaiba Naseem[4], Mohammed F. Abuzinadah[5] and Shahid Karim[6]

[1]Health Information Technology Department, Faculty of Applied Studies, King Abdulaziz University, Jeddah, Kingdom of Saudi Arabia
[2]Department of Health Informatics, College of Public Health and Health Informatics, Qassim University, Al Bukayriyah, Saudi Arabia
[3]Department of Biochemistry, Faculty of Science, King Abdulaziz University, Jeddah, Saudi Arabia
[4]Faculty of Pharmacy, Integral University, Lucknow, Uttar Pradesh, India
[5]Department of Medical Laboratory Technology, Faculty of Applied Medical Sciences, King Abdulaziz University, Jeddah, Kingdom of Saudi Arabia

* Corresponding Author's Email: ahmad.varish@gmail.com.

[6]Department of Pharmacology, Faculty of Medicine, King Abdulaziz University, Jeddah, Kingdom of Saudi Arabia

ABSTRACT

Marine-derived natural pharmaceutical active molecules are one of the significant sources of drug discovery and development. P-Glycoprotein (P-GP) inhibitors play an active role dominantly in cancer prevention and overcoming of multidrug resistance. Marine sources particularly, from marine microbes contributed a lot in the management of various diseases through different mechanisms and have been developed as a significant therapeutic molecule.

Many marine products were reported with potential P-GP inhibitory activity through the inhibition of the ATPase pump activity. P-GP can out flux a large number of different exogenous chemical molecules to the outside of the cellular environments. As a result of outflow, drug delivery to the target site become complex. Thus, inhibition of P-glycoprotein could be beneficial in the administration of a low amount of drug, increase permeability and drug transport to the desired site of infection with reduce toxicity.

Keywords: marine products, P-glycoproteins, inhibitors, cancer, drug resistance

1. INTRODUCTION

P-glycoprotein (P-gp), of the large ATP-binding cassette (ABC) family, is a transmembrane protein incorporated by ATP-binding cassette sub-family B member 1 (ABCB1). This protein is composed of 1,280 amino acids (170 kDa) arranged in two transmembrane domains, each comprising twelve highly potent hydrophobic α-helices and two intracellular nucleotide-binding regions with ATPase activity and involvement in cellular transport [1-2]. The drug-binding site (DBS) is found in the main protein component, and when ATP utilizes P-gp, the active organ is released by a flip-flop‖ to the luminal side. Its subsequent dephosphorylation leads to the reversal of the protein [3].

Not all P-gp functions are known; however, there is a growing understanding of the role of P-gp in many functions. In the blood-brain barrier and blood-placental barrier, for example, P-gp inhibits xenobiotic accumulation in the brain and uterus, respectively [3-4]. Moreover, P-gp typically binds xenobiotics taken along with urine components in the urine, bile, and intestinal lumen and transmits hormones. The appearance of P-gp in normal uterine cells in the abdomen also prevents drug absorption after oral administration, and P-gp in the brain inhibits the penetration of antiviral drugs. Finally, P-gp is therapeutically significant due to its key role in multi-drug resistance (MDR) in cancer as well as drug metabolism in several human diseases and pathogens, including the AIDS virus, epilepsy, and parasitic diseases [1-4].

Natural sources, including plants, animals, and microbes, undoubtedly produce a large number of therapeutic molecules. The molecular diversity of different therapeutics molecules originating from diverse sources must be explored. Nearly 70% of the Earth is covered by water and enriched with 80% of the biological diversity of life on the planet. The commonly used P-gp inhibitor has clinical limitations and insignificant specificity and potency with anticancer drugs; furthermore, computational studies have also not supported their safe and effective use in cancer [5]. A continuous search for a novel ecosystem that provides potential molecules for the management of drug-resistant and cancer-like dangerous diseases is crucial. The marine ecosystem is an excellent natural source, providing polyoxygenated diketopiperazines, sterols, alkaloids, terpenoids, polyketides, and peptides, which are widely reported for P-gp inhibitory activity [1-5].

MDR is one of the key reasons for the failure of cancer therapy in humans and is developed by different mechanisms, such as decreased drug transportation inside the cell, increased efflux, the activation of enzymes for toxin reduction, and a change in the molecular target of drugs. Molecules from the sea consist of scaffolds and unique features that have attracted scientists to use them as an excellent platform for the discovery and development of drugs [6]. The synthetic derivatives of marine molecules have also been documented as involving significant ABC transporter inhibitory activity as well as tumor cell growth. Marine molecules could, therefore, be of significant value in the rational drug design of derivatives with high potential and reduced pharmacokinetic interactions. P-gp is encoded by the human MDR-1 gene, which is located in chromosome 7. It contains 1,280 amino acids, arranged in two halves, each encompassing a transmembrane domain (TMD) which spans the membrane and an intracellular nucleotide-binding domain [5-7].

A recent study conducted by Sachs et al. (2019) identified that 3,4-dihydroisocoumarins can inhibit P-gp and breast cancer resistance proteins (BCRPs) after testing different human cancer cell lines [8]. In their study, 3,4-dihydroisocoumarins, previously unexplored as potential MDR-reversing agents, were tested as potential inhibitors of human and yeast ABC transporters. After observation, among the experimented natural products, three novel 3,4-dihydroisocoumarins were discussed as having inhibitory properties against two human transporters, P-gp and BCRP. The most effective inhibitor, the derivative, suggested an inhibitory property against the transporters of between 80 and 90% when compared to the positive controls at the main test concentration (50 μM). The study indicated that P-gp-expressing HCT-15 cells and BCRP-expressing MCF-7/MX cells were treated with a compound of chemotherapeutic drugs, doxorubicin and mitoxantrone, also known as transporter substrates for P-gp and BCRP. Subsequently, the combined dose treatment with 50 μM of derivative prepared chemotherapy-resistant cancer cells HCT-15 colon carcinoma cells for doxorubicin by reducing the IC_{50} value of doxorubicin-stimulated cytotoxicity by 3.7-fold and sensitized MCF-7/MX breast carcinoma cells to mitoxantrone by reducing the IC_{50} value of mitoxantrone-caused cytotoxicity by 5.6-fold. Furthermore, enantiomers (*R*)-substituted at 19 and (*S*)-19 inhibited transport function of P-gp and BCRP, though with a lower potency compared to the derivative. Sachs et al. also stated that several different analogous structure-activity relationships for transporter inhibition could be derived, and they execute in equivalence for P-gp and BCRP: their results proved that the hydroxy group at position 6 is compulsory for transporter inhibition and substitution by a methoxy group significantly trims down the activity. They also observed that a hydrophobic carbon chain at position 3 is vital for inhibition; this replacement seemed to need a specific chain length. Compounds without alkyl substituent derivatives, or with a methyl group 6-methoxymellein and angelicin B, as well as compounds with a hydrophilic chain derivatives (*R*) and (*S*)—notably reduced the inhibition of studied transporters. The study found that the effects were better defined by the inhibition of BCRP rather than that of P-gp [8].

A computational virtual screening study identified *frigocyclinone* from *Streptomyces griseus,* which is found in deep-sea environments, as a potent inhibitor against Kaposi's sarcoma. The authors suggested that the bioactive compounds were extracted and derived from marine organisms: a most interesting research study. Furthermore, approximately 30,000 natural compounds from different marine micro-organisms species are reported to have anti-bacterial, anti-inflammatory, and mainly anti-cancerous properties.

2. Mechanism of the Drug Resistance

The mechanism by which P-gp activates its pump function is not fully understood; however, there are several models to explain this process, two of which are widely accepted. The first model states that P-gp gives its effect to a flippase-type machine [9]. This approach is based on the assumption that drugs on the surface and the inside of the membrane should adhere to the outer and inner layers of the membrane. Based on this equilibrium method, P-gp exchanges drugs from the inner membrane to the outer membrane. In contrast, the hydrophobic vacuum cleaner model, which is currently most widely accepted, suggests that P-gp removes hydrophobic molecules internally [9-10]. The high-resolution crystal structure of a mouse P-gp is not the same among the models, but instead, can be used to support any of them. The structure of the protein contains two sites within the P-gp cavity that connect to the inner layer of the membrane and can allow hydrophobic drugs to pass directly from the lipid bilayer to the cavity. In the absence of external components, P-gp involves an ATPase cognitive function [3, 11].The role of Pgp inhibitors to prevent the out flux of drug from cell is represented in Figure 1.

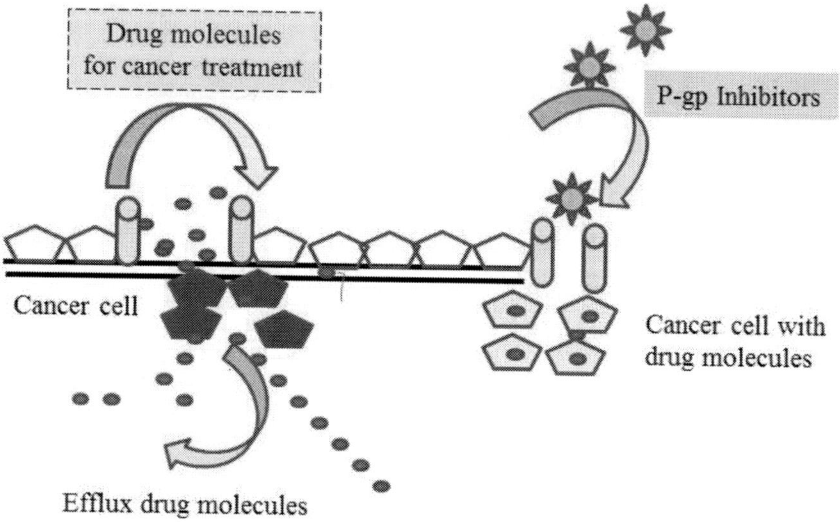

Figure 1. P-gp inhibitor preventing outflux of Drug from cancer cell.

In addition, substrates of P-gp can accurately measure this activity and consequently measure ATP hydrolysis. Ingredients that measure P-gp ATPase activity are formulated in three groups: (1) computers stimulate the basal activity of ATPase at low concentrations as well as restrict activity in highly concentrated areas (e.g., vinblastine, verapamil, and paclitaxel); (2) a meeting which increases ATPase activity in a dose-dependent manner (e.g., bisantrene, valinomycin, and tetraphenylphospho-nium); and (3) computers block both basic and integrated power of ATPase activity (e.g., cyclosporin A, rapamycin, and gramicidin D). Each of these types predicts that the inhibition of protein activity may impair the P-gp efflux function. However, this is not a general rule: some P-gp inhibitors rather increase the protein ATPase function. Furthermore, preliminary studies have suggested that P-gp inhibitors should bind to a nucleotide protein binding site (NBS) that inhibits ATPase activity [12-14]. Because of its role in drug function, P-gp has a high clinical relevance; it affects the absorption, distribution, and availability of drugs, and plays a key role in the fight against multi-drug resistance (MDR) in cancer.

3. Chemical Nature of Marine-Derived P-gp Inhibitors

The first generation, second generation, and third generation of P-gp have been well explored, and each class has its own distinct features and clinical applications. The first-generation P-gp inhibitors have been reported as nonselective to P-gp and substrates for other transporters, as well as enzymes; unpredictable pharmacokinetic interactions with other drugs have also been observed. The safe use by clinical trial and therapeutic investigation of first-generation P-gp inhibitors like quinidine, verapamil, and cyclosporine A has been conducted. To increase the efficacy and reduce the toxicity, each enantiomer of first-generation P-gp has been evaluated and grouped as second-generation P-gp inhibitors. Examples include the use of an enantiomeric form (R type) of verapamil as dexverapamil. The clinical trial of elacridar (GF 120918), biricodar, and valspodar (PSC-833) has been initiated, although it has limited use because substrates of cytochrome P450 3A revealed a problem not only with metabolism but also with the excretion of co-administered drugs [3-7].

A novel class of P-gp inhibitors has recently been introduced as ABC inhibitors: these consist mainly of plant, animal, and microbe-derived natural molecules of protein, surfactants, dual lipids ligands nature, or their mimics, such as peptidomimetics. Although the outdated resources of microbes and terrestrial plants will certainly produce new therapeutic molecules, it is also necessary to discover all other possible significant pools of molecular diversity. This approach will be beneficial in determining new environments for bioprospecting and it also offers the chance to search for extraordinary bioactive molecules and known mechanisms of drug resistance [15-18]. Marine-derived bioactive molecules are one of the most attractive goals in the discovery and development of global drugs. Indeed, they have unique structural, chemical features, novel scaffolds, and both increase efficacy and reduce toxicity, making them fit for drug development [19]. The synthetic compounds of marine-derived products have been well tested as ABC-P-gp transporter inhibitors. Thus, different classes including terpenoids, sterols, alkaloids, and peptides, as well as derivatives of marine-based molecules, have been reported to inhibit P-gp. Example include sipholane triterpenoids and derivatives, parguerenes and derivatives, ergosterol and derivatives, polyoxygenated steroids and derivatives, polyketides, bryostatin and derivatives, discodermolide, halichondrin B and derivatives, lamellarins and derivatives, ningalins and derivatives, welwitindolinones and derivatives, harmine and derivatives, indolocarbazoles and derivatives, ecteinascidin 743 (Trabectedin) and derivatives, diketopiperazine, fumitremorgins and derivatives, halimide and derivatives, hapalosin and derivatives, botryllamides and derivatives, kendarimide, patellamide and derivatives, irciniasulfonic acid derivatives, terreins, and shornephine A [3, 7, 20-21].

4. Microorganisms as Sources of P-Glycoproteins

Several marine organisms have been reported to produce compounds or analogs with P-gp inhibitory activity. Indeed, examples include the therapeutic use of vidarabine for herpes simplex virus and mediated superficial keratitis, cytarabine used in cancer treatment, ziconotide used for the treatment of severe chronic pain in patients with cancer or AIDS, and the use of Halaven and trabectedin in testing for metastatic breast cancer and soft tissue sarcoma. Furthermore, *Leptogorgia sarmentosa, Isis hippuris, echinoderms, Sarcophyton sp.,* sponges, and *Sinularia sp.* have also been reported to produce some polyoxygenated steroids that inhibit the overexpression of P-gp [22-25]. The marine sources of Pgp inhibitors represented in Figure 2.

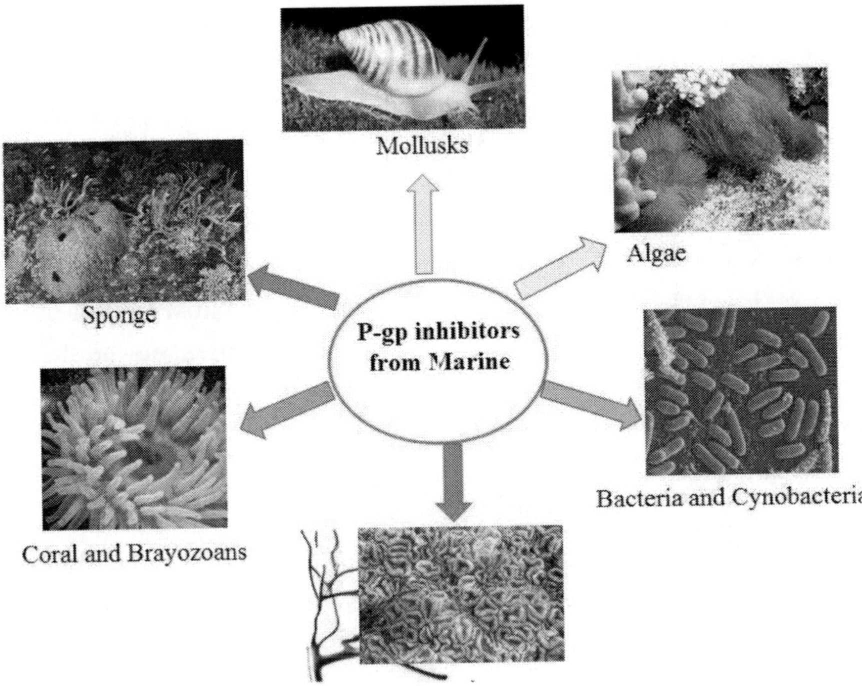

Figure 2. The potentential sources of marine for P-gp inhibitor.

4.1. P-gp Inhibitors from Sponge

Callyspongia siphonella, a red sea sponge, has been reported to produce sipholane triterpenoids such as sipholenol A, sipholenol L, sipholenone E, and siphonellinol, and these triterpenoids are suggested to have the potential to reverse the MDR along with antiproliferative and anti-migratory activities, as shown by in-vitro experimentation using breast cancer cells. The effects were due to the overexpression of P-gp and were more significant as the increased level of expression indicated. The *Spongia* species of marine sponge has been stated to produce a P-gp inhibitor, the polyhydroxy sterol acetate, ergosterol A. The sterol acetate reserved MDR to colchicine and vincristine in KB-C2 human carcinoma cells and KB-CV 60 respectively, by overexpression of MRP1 [25-26].

Bromoditerpenes Laurencia filiformis is an Australian red alga reported to produce bromoditerpenes and parguerenes. It also increases the activity of anticancer drugs such as vinblastine, taxol, actinomycin D, colchicine, and daunomycin in cell lines of MDR ovarian adenocarcinoma (NCI/ADR-RES). Another member of the alkaloid family, welwitindolinone C isothiocyanate derivative, exhibited weak activity, indicating that the methyl group is important for biological functions. Moreover, when the isonitrile group replaced the isothiocyanate group, the compound was ineffective, indicating that the isothiocyanate group is also important in the natural functions exhibited by these alkaloids. Found in the Australian red marine algae, *Laurencia filiformis*, were non-cytotoxic inhibitors of P-gp and MRP1 synthetic drugs [22, 26]. These two, small molecules reported a reversal of the absorption of P-gp vinblastine, doxorubicin, and paclitaxel MDR, without altering the P-gp levels. This suggests that 19 and 20 inhibit P-gp efflux through action mechanism or at least mechanically; this is very different from other inhibitors, such as verapamil and cyclosporin A, due to the interactions of 19 and 20 and inhibiting of extracellular antibody binding epitope to P-gp. A detailed analysis of the relationship between the structural functions of 19 and 20 suggests that it is possible to manipulate and optimize the pharmacophore value of these molecules to increase their function [27-28].

4.2. P-gp Inhibitors from Bryozoans

From a species of bryozoan, *Bugula neritina* has been isolated from a group of macrolide lactones called bryostatins. These compounds are powerful modulators of protein kinase C, and they are also anticancer and memory-enhancing agents [29-30]. Perhaps the most important member of this computerized family is bryostatin 1, a modulator of protein kinase C with a potency similar to tumor-enhancing phorbol ester, 12-O-Tetradecanoylphorbol-13-acetate (TPA) [31-32]. Compound 21 also has the potential to replace the P-gp-mediated MDR. In a trial using two rows of extracellular MDR1-induced MDR1 cells, the MDR Clone of the KB (KB-

C1) cells and the human epofuid cervix carcinoma (HeLa) were transmitted via an MDR1-V185 build (HeLa-MDR1- V185) containing valine instead of 185 glycines and found that 21 restored resistance formed by vinblastine and colchicine in both cells. In addition, 21 was able to reverse P-gp-mediated MDR in HeLa cells transmitted by MDR1-V185 with increased Rhodamine 123 accumulation. The analysis showed that 21 joined sites G185 and V185 P- gp, and thus, this compound is able to reverse P-gp mutations [31-32].

4.3. P-gp Inhibitors from Corals

Octocoral, or *Isis hippuris*, is a major producer of several polyoxygenated steroids, including gorgosterol, hippuristanol, hippuristerone, and hippuristerol [33]. A number of the first type have been tested against KB-C2 overexpressing P-gp and against protein-1 cells, the KB-CV60 overexpressing resistance of multiple proteins. Multiple steroids reported moderate activity against KB-C2 cells (inhibition of average growth of 68.0, 70.0, 87.8, 89.2, 87.4 and 82.1, respectively, at a concentration of 3 μg/mL), but not against KB-CV60 cells (there was an increase percentage inhibition of 2.1, 16, 0, 35, 7, 41.0, 18.9 and 16.6, respectively, at a concentration of 3 μg/mL). This confirms the specificity of this type of compound in the overexpression P-gp cell lines [34].

The infection *Nocardiopsis* sp. CMB-M0232 was isolated from a drug sample collected in Australia. The saline liquid culture of the bacterium yielded non-saline diketopiperazines (DKP): nocardioazine A and nocardioazine B. Compound 28 restored the resistance discussed to SW620AD cells -300 and provided verapamil to the cells. However, nocardioazine B did not report inhibitory activity against P-gp, which could mean that the unique DKP receptor was formed between one of the nitrogens, and an external isoprene unit may be involved in biological activity [35].

Another red alga, *Jania rubens*, has also been explored for the presence of diterpenes, isoparguerenes, and parguerenes, as well as its antimicrobial and anticancer potential. A noncytotoxic derivative of bromoditerpenes inhibits a P-gp-mediated efflux of cyclosporine and verapamil. Moreover, these compounds have also been reported to inhibit the overexpression of P-gp induced by paclitaxel vinblastine and doxorubicin by distinctly damaging the antibody-binding epitope as shown by previously known inhibitors [23].

Carboline-β type alkaloids like harmine have been isolated from insects, mammalian, and marine alga such as *Melanothamnus afaghusainii.* Harmine is reported to have antifungal, antibacterial, antioxidant, antiproliferative, cytotoxic, antimutagenic, antiplasmodial, and anticancer biological potential. It inhibits cyclin-dependent kinases, monoamine oxidase, topoisomerase 1, and cross-links with DNA. Moreover, it also offers MDR reversal by inhibiting the expression of breast cancer receptor proteins in breast cancer cell lines MDA-MB-123; it also reduces the resistance camptothecin and mitoxantrone without affecting the growth of cell overexpressing the MDR-1. Clinically, the neurotoxicity and weaker pharmacological effects limit its therapeutic use [36-37].

Lamellarins are a group of polyaromatic alkaloids originally separated from Lamellaria sp. This segment of compounds undertakes a variety of biological functions, including cytotoxicity, vaccine activity, inhibition of HIV and the supposed ability to supply other lines of MDR cancer cells found in the fight against anti-cancer treatment [38-43]. Lamellarin 1 introduced more chemo activity than verapamil (nine to 16 in height) in a doxorubicin cell line that is not associated with human colon adenocarcinoma (LoVo/Dx). In addition, 2 increased the cytotoxicity of doxorubicin, vinblastine, and daunorubicin in the form of stress dependence on MDR cells. Compound 2 exerts this effect by direct inhibition of P-gp pump activity, as demonstrated by the accumulation of Rhodamine 123 in LoVo/Dx cells [3, 42].

Another marine compound, phenylpropanoid piperazines, from an Australian marine fish-derived fungus, *Chrysosporium sp* [43]. CMB-F294, reported inhibitory properties against P- glycoprotein (Osama et al., 2020). Chemical analysis of the fungus Chrysosporium sp. CMB-F294 isolated from the gastrointestinal tract of a market-purchased specimen of *Mugil* mullet contained eight specific alkaloids, related to a rare and important class of phenylpropanoid piperazines. Chrysosporazines F–M (1–8) perform as a balanced solution of acetamide rotamers and exceptional carbocyclic and heterocyclic scaffolds. Biosynthetic considerations and spectroscopic analysis have supported the presence of many configurations that confirmed the influence of P-gp activity. The differential structural orientation of various functional groups was present in the structure of molecules. Moreover, selected chrysosporazine isomers have been reported as nontoxic inhibitors of the MDR efflux pump P-gp and reversing doxorubicin resistance by affecting the expression of P-gp in human colon carcinoma cells (SW620 Ad300). Chrysosporazine F induced more than double the sensitivity of doxorubicin at a concentration of 2.5 μM, compared to the positive verapamil (GS 6.1) [43].

Amathia convoluta and *Bugula neritina* are well-known marine bryozoans enriched with highly oxygenated and poly acetate-rich macrolides known as bryostatin. Some bryostatins have been reported to induce apoptosis and reverse MDR and drug efflux inhibition by up-regulation of the BAX gene, and yet downregulate the BCL-2 and MDR 1. The macrolides polymer, halichondrin B has also been purified from *Halichondria okadai* [44].

4.4. P-gp Inhibitors from Algae

The marine organisms, mostly sponge and micro-algae and bacteria, spark much interest for pharmaceutical organizations and research institutes. *Ascophyllum nodosum, for example,* is a brown alga that belongs to the *Phaeophyceae* family and is the only species in the genus *Ascophyllum* which produces bioactive compounds with anti-oxidants and bioactive compounds that stimulate the properties. An important, red marine sponge, *Haliclona* sp. produces alkaloids, macrolides, peptides, polyketides, polyacetylenes, steroids, and halogenated derivatives as bioactive compounds. The *Halicona* sp. yields *salicylihalamide* A and *salicylihalamide* B which comes under the same family and species; they are, however, both structurally and functionally different. These compounds have suggested anti-cancerous characteristics. Ascorbic acid that decreases the probability of cardiovascular disease, cancer, and Alzheimer's disease could be found in all green red and brown seaweeds. Furthermore, frigocyclinone extracted and obtained from *Streptomyces griseus strain* NTK 97 have antibacterial and anti-tumor properties [45].

Alkaloids such as welwitindolinones have been isolated and evaluated as P-gp inhibitors. Many marine bacteria like *Fischerella muscicola, Westiella intracta, F. major*. The extracts rich in *N*-methylwelwitindolinone suggested larvicidal, antibacterial, antifungal, and antiprotozoal activities. The alkaloids have also been reported to mediate P-gp MDR and cytotoxicity anticancer drugs, including taxol, colchicine, vinblastine, daunomycin, and actinomycin D, as well as in MDR breast carcinoma cell lines. The derivatives of alkaloids methylwelwitindolinone have an affinity with P-gp and increase the accumulation of anticancer drugs like paclitaxel vinblastine by blocking the P-gp in SK-VLB-1 cell lines [46-47]. Marine actinomycetes Z039-2 is known to produce alkaloids with anticancer and other broad-spectrum pharmacological activities. It has been suggested, furthermore, that such alkaloids have the potential to mediate the reversal of MDR. The most well-known examples of these alkaloids are arcyriaflavin and indolocarbazole K-252. They reduce the resistance of drugs by potentially inhibiting the BCRP in BCRP-transferred HEK-293 cell lines [48].

4.5. P-gp Inhibitors from Bacteria and Fungi

The marine fungal strain, fungal A-f-11, BM939, *Aspergillus fumigatus* (YK-7), and *Aspergillus sydowii,* are both known to produce indolyl diketopiperazine type alkaloids known as fumitremorgins. The alkaloid also produced tremorgenic mycotoxins which inhibits the cell cycle. Moreover, a derivative of fumitremorgins could reverse the BCRP-mediated resistance effect of topotecan, mitoxantrone, and doxorubicin in cell lines [49]. A cyclic depsipeptide, Hapalosin, was purified by using the hydrophobic fraction of the extract of a cyanobacterium *Hapalosiphon welwitschii* W & G.S West and indicated a higher P-gp inhibitor inhibitory effect than verapamil. It reversed the MDR in P-gp, expressing vinblastine-resistant human ovarian adenocarcinoma cells [50].

Patellamides are thiazole- and oxazoline-containing cyclic octapeptides that are isolated from the *Lissoclinum patella* that demonstrated several biological functions, including cytotoxicity and restoring resistance in the human MDR cell line (Cuc/VLB100) when compared with vinblastine colchicine and adriamycin. The cytotoxicity of patellamide-type compounds may be the cause of synchronization limits set by the presence of the heterocycles and their ability to differentiate DNA. In this composite family, patellamide D indicated efficacy in reversing MDR; it developed the activity of vinblastine, adriamycin, and colchicine by 66, 2.8, and 1.4 respectively. Activity 3 is similar to verapamil, a well-known P-gp inhibitor [51-53].

Discodermia dissolute, a marine sponge, has been used to purify a polyketide, discodermolide, which has been reported to induce apoptosis by arresting the cell cycle G2/M. The P-gp-mediated drug influence of drug efflux has been explored with a derivative of discodermolide, and reduced drug efflux susceptibility of MDR in tumor cell lines, but is more potent against several cancer cell types [54-56]. Typically, MDR ovarian carcinoma (A2780AD) and paclitaxel resistance to colon carcinoma (SW620AD-300) 25-9 cell lines are more resistant to uncontrolled drugs than their parental lines. Compound 5 significantly reduced resistance to multidrug to taxol in both cell lines, with IC50 values of 70 nM for SW620AD-300 (compared to 260 nM for taxol) and 580 nM for A2780AD cells (compared to 3900 nM for taxol) [57-58].

4.6. P-gp Inhibitors from Mollusk

The chemical compounds of *Halichondria okadai* have antiproliferative, immunosuppressive properties and anticancer potential similar to taxol. Many organisms such as *Lamellaria sp.* of the marine mollusk, *Daphniphyllum chartaceum, Dendrilla cactos,* and unidentified ascidians have also been seen to produce alkaloids that have a common chromoindoles 1 scaffold and the potential to modulate the P-gp activity. The methoxy and hydroxyl are major functional groups that can be substituted with major scaffolds to produce its variants. However, derivatives are known to have various biological functions such as cytotoxicity, antiproliferative activities, and immunomodulating activities [59-62]. Furthermore, lamellarin or its derivatives have also been reported to kill the MDR cancer cell line and reverse the MDR in non-MDR cell lines, even at a weaker cytotoxic concentration. Moreover, a 7-methoxy, 2-hydroxyl derivative more significantly mediates the cytotoxic effect than that of verapamil in doxorubicin-resistant Lo Vo/Dx cell lines by directly reducing the function of P-gp which leads to the accumulation of drugs in cell lines and kills them. However, bromo- or mono-/dimethyl substituents containing indole rings (Aryl-R2) of lamellarin reduce the inhibitory activity of breast cancer-resistant proteins [63]. Boger et al. (1999) isolated and reported a safe MDR reversing agent known as ningalin B, from an ascidian of the genus *Didemnun*. The ningalin B tested in-vitro on human colorectal carcinoma cell lines sensitized the overexpression of P-gp [64]. This increased MDR sensitivity, a decrease in cytotoxicity, and an increase in a carbon chain of molecules. Furthermore, it suggested that the activity is due to the presence of N-alkylaryl substituent. However, derivatives which have free methyl esters and phenolic groups have been reported as more toxic, without MDR reversal properties. The highest MDR reversal has found with tetra- or penta-substituted pyrroles, derivatives of ningalin B [65]. Some synthetic derivatives of Ningalin has discussed the competitive binding with [3H]-azidopine molecules that bind to P-gp binding site, accumulated, retained and increased the 4000 times sensitivity of the vinblastine at 1-10 μM conc. Some amide derivatives but not amine derivative, have been discussed with significant MDR activity. A cytotoxic molecule from styelid ascidians *Botryllus* sp. has also been reported to produce derivatives of dehydrotyrosine which, is known as Botryllamides. Some derivatives of botryllamide exert an inhibitory effect on BODIPY FL prazosin transport facilitated by BCRP and inhibit the action of BCRP [66]. Kendarimide A is an oligopeptide isolated from the Indonesian sponge *Haliclona sp.* This oligopeptide of *Haliclona sp* sponge evalulated for potential of MDR reversal in KB-C2 and KB-3-1 human carcinoma cell lines over P-gp at the concentration of 6 μM. The molecules exerted significant inhibitory effect on KB-C2 cell line but not in KB-3 at the conc. of 6 μM [67-68].

4.7. Inhibitors from Tunicates

The cell, ecteinascidin 743 (ET-743, 1), recovered from the Caribbean stem, *Ecteinascidia turbinata*, has reported good resistance to *in vitro* activity against hemorrhocytic leukemia mice (L1210)) and half the high inhibitory (IC50) values of 0.5 ng/mL. ET-743 slightly modulates the resistance of doxorubicin and vincristine to MDR perermermal carcinoma (KB-C2 and KB-8-5) P-gp/multidrug resistance 1 (MDR1) cell lines of overexpression. Significant concentrations of doxorubicin and vincristine (up to 122 and 22 fold, respectively) were observed in both the cells when the non-toxic concentration was observed. However, photos affinity image labeling studies did not desribed that overdose of doxorubicin/vincristine did not result in direct inhibition of P-gp activity. Because of these beneficial effects on cancer treatment, it has found orphan drug appointments specifically for soft tissue treatment in the United States and treatment for ovarian cancer in the United States and Europe [40, 68-71].

Conclusion and Future Prospects

Exploring and searching the marine world is a challenging task for the scientific community. Natural resources like ponds, lakes and rivers could be explored easily but to search the sea for novel natural compounds are highly expensive and time taking process. However, many government and non-government organizations are providing support to explore more about marine species especially those have inhibitory activities against severe disease or targeting specific molecular targets. In the current modern era sudden challenges appears in front of the scientific community due to pandemic breakout and restricts to run the core laboratory experimentation on full flow. So, to resolve such issue computational approaches including artificial intelligence established as a major tool to help researchers through in silico screening of huge library of compounds such and plant and marine natural compounds. Defiantly, in coming decay the technology will increase rapidly and offer us better platform to use technology to design new inhibitors and analogs against p-gp.

A reasonable drug development system can be utilized for describing natural compounds as P-gp inhibitors/substrates/inducers as it gives a way to deal with better comprehend the puzzle of P-gp in drug development process improvement. Using the in silico, in vitro screening strategies understand the configuration and molecular mechanism of P-gp communication with lead to design better inhibitor against P-gp. The two phases of normal drug development system for the transformative plan and assessment of P-gp inhibitors can be delegated disclosure or screening. The screening stage includes in silico and in vitro investigations where the mixes or synthetic compounds are screened for their P-gp binding affinity. The in silico investigation includes the utilization of chemical and structural databases for screening. The in vitro tests used to recognize P-gp interfacing drugs incorporate cytotoxicity measures, efflux examinations (in light of fluorescent), transport tests and ATPase tests. In this way recognized compound structures can be built up as P-gp inhibitors/ substrates/inducers, in light of the tests did in the characterization stage which are in-situ, in vivo and human examinations. These examinations give a more profound understanding into the liking and explicitness of the P-gp inhibitors/substrates/inducers. By utilizing this consecutive procedure, the drg compounds can be totally described beginning from their degree of affectability to P-gp or their P-gp improving effectiveness to their medication connection and toxic effect profiles (Bansal et al., 2009b). This sort of a schematic methodology can legitimize the revelation and advancement of more up to date, more secure, non-toxic, and more productive, explicitly focusing on P-gp inhibitors.

We are currently seeing a renaissance of the enthusiasm for efflux carriers, because of administrative necessities as well as to the noteworthy job of these transporters in the adsorption, distribution, metabolism, excretion, and toxicity (ADMET) procedure of drug designing and their mechanistic revelation. Subsequently, P-gp and other ABC carriers that intervene drug efflux are known as a "group to beat". Marine species have demonstrated to be a significant source in the revelation and improvement of drug compounds, and specifically in the search of anticancer molecules. These marine-determined natural compounds, which can be collected primarily as alkaloids, polyoxygenated sterols, terpenoids, and peptides, have exhibited an inversion impact of MDR without anyone else. A few compounds were appeared to increment instead of reducing cytotoxicity towards MDR cell lines and can be characterized as improved compounds or this impact was appeared in combination with anticancer drugs, being non-cytotoxic MDR inversion agents. The significant origin of marine MDR inversion agents and systems has been barely considered, and next to no is thought about their molecular activity. A few marine compounds which have indicated strong and specific MDR action against malignancy cell lines have a place with the alkaloids; could have some toxic characters. MDR actions against malignant growth cell lines have a place with the alkaloids; in any case, they present some harmfulness. Among marine common items, trabectedin has end up being the most encouraging against MDR with in vitro and in vivo capability. Synthetically, engineered analogs of marine compounds working as inhibitors have been explored to accomplish higher action, less toxic and less pharmacokinetic properties, and to set up SAR. With this assorted variety of platforms, it is beyond the realm of imagination to expect to separate regular highlights basic for MDR inversion action; be that as it may, the greater part of the analogs and derivatives are profoundly lipophilic and contain melded rings and various chiral focuses, which thus mirror their hard synthesizing strategies. Among the manufactured analogs, eriburin has been demonstrated to be the most encouraging P-gp modulator, dynamic against MDR in vitro and with demonstrated safety in clinical patients. These highlights additionally open new difficulties for therapeutic scientists to achieve feasible engineered developments and new roads in the structure of analogs with reasonable drugs like properties that could deliver potential medication up-and-comers. Consolidating all the bits of the synthetic organic pharmaceutical mystery, we can foresee more compelling chemotherapies dependent on compounds from the marine resources.

REFERENCES

[1] Ferreira, M., Costa, J., & Reis-Henriques, M. A. (2014). ABC transporters in fish species: A review. *Frontiers in Physiology*, *5*(266). https://doi.org/10.3389/fphys.2014.00266.

[2] Pokharel, D., Roseblade, A., Oenarto, V., Lu, J. F., & Bebawy, M. (2017). Proteins regulating the intercellular transfer and function of P-glycoprotein in multidrug-resistant cancer. *ecancermedicalscience*, *11*. https://doi.org/10.3332/ecancer.2017.768.

[3] Lopez, D., & Martinez-Luis, S. (2014). Marine natural products with P-glycoprotein inhibitor properties. *Marine Drugs*, *12*(1), 525-546. https://doi.org/10.3390/md12010525.

[4] Wu, C., Calcagno, A., & Ambudkar, S. (2008). Reversal of ABC drug transporter-mediated Multidrug resistance in cancer cells: Evaluation of current strategies. *Current Molecular Pharmacology*, *1*(2), 93-105. https://doi.org/10.2174/1874467210801020093.

[5] Huang, X., Kumar, P., Anreddy, N., Xiao, X., Yang, D., & Chen, Z. (2014). P-GP inhibitory activity from marine sponges, tunicates and algae. *Handbook of Anticancer Drugs from Marine Origin*, 593-619. https://doi.org/10.1007/978-3-319-07145-9_28.

[6] Housman, G., Byler, S., Heerboth, S., Lapinska, K., Longacre, M., Snyder, N., & Sarkar, S. (2014). Drug resistance in cancer: an overview. *Cancers*, *6*(3), 1769–1792. https://doi.org/10.3390/cancers6031769.

[7] Long, S., Sousa, E., Kijjoa, A., & Pinto, M. (2016). Marine natural products as models to circumvent Multidrug resistance. *Molecules*, *21*(7), 892.

[8] Sachs, J., Döhl, K., Weber, A., Bonus, M., Ehlers, F., Fleischer, E., Klinger, A., Gohlke, H., Pietruszka, J., Schmitt, L., & Teusch, N. (2019). Novel 3,4-Dihydroisocoumarins inhibit human P-GP and

BCRP in Multidrug resistant tumors and demonstrate substrate inhibition of yeast Pdr5. *Frontiers in Pharmacology*, *10*. https://doi.org/10.3389/fphar.2019.00400.

[9] Sharom, F. J. (2014). Complex interplay between the P-glycoprotein Multidrug efflux pump and the membrane: Its role in modulating protein function. *Frontiers in Oncology*, *4*. https://doi.org/10.3389/fonc.2014.00041.

[10] Omote, H., & Al-Shawi, M. K. (2006). Interaction of transported drugs with the lipid Bilayer and P-glycoprotein through a solvation exchange mechanism. *Biophysical Journal*, *90*(11), 4046-4059. https://doi.org/10.1529/biophysj.105.077743.

[11] Esser, L., Zhou, F., Pluchino, K. M., Shiloach, J., Ma, J., Tang, W., Gutierrez, C., Zhang, A., Shukla, S., Madigan, J. P., Zhou, T., Kwong, P. D., Ambudkar, S. V., Gottesman, M. M., & Xia, D. (2016). Structures of the Multidrug transporter P-glycoprotein reveal asymmetric ATP binding and the mechanism of Polyspecificity. *Journal of Biological Chemistry*, *292*(2), 446-461. https://doi.org/10.1074/jbc.m116.755884.

[12] Ambudkar, S. V., Dey, S., Hrycyna, C. A., Ramachandra, M., Pastan, I., & Gottesman, M. M. (1999). Biochemical, cellular, and pharmacological aspects of the multidrug transporter. *Annual Review of Pharmacology and Toxicology*, *39*(1), 361-398. https://doi.org/10.1146/annurev.pharmtox.39.1.361.

[13] Martin, C., Berridge, G., Higgins, C. F., & Callaghan, R. (1997). The multi-drug resistance reversal agent SR33557 and modulation of vinca alkaloid binding to P-glycoprotein by an allosteric interaction. *British Journal of Pharmacology*, *122*(4), 765-771. https://doi.org/10.1038/sj.bjp.0701429

[14] Zhu, H., Liu, Z., Tang, L., Liu, J., Zhou, M., Xie, F., Wang, Z., Wang, Y., Shen, S., Hu, L., & Yu, L. (2012). Reversal of P-GP and MRP1-mediated multidrug resistance by H6, a gypenoside aglycon from Gynostemma pentaphyllum, in vincristine-resistant human oral cancer (KB/VCR) cells. *European Journal of Pharmacology*, *696*(1-3), 43-53. https://doi.org/10.1016/j.ejphar.2012.09.046

[15] Abdallah, H. M., Al-Abd, A. M., El-Dine, R. S., & El-Halawany, A. M. (2015). P-glycoprotein inhibitors of natural origin as potential tumor chemo-sensitizers: A review. *Journal of advanced research*, *6*(1), 45–62.

[16] Gomes, N., Lefranc, F., Kijjoa, A., & Kiss, R. (2015). Can some marine-derived fungal metabolites become actual Anticancer agents? *Marine Drugs*, *13*(6), 3950-3991. https://doi.org/10.3390/md13063950

[17] Bogman, K., Erne-Brand, F., Alsenz, J., & Drewe, J. (2003). The role of surfactants in the reversal of active transport mediated by multidrug resistance proteins. *Journal of pharmaceutical sciences*, *92*(6), 1250–1261. https://doi.org/10.1002/jps.10395.

[18] Hoffmann, K., Bekeredjian, R., Schmidt, J., Büchler, M. W., & Märten, A. (2008). Effects of the high-affinity Peptide reversin 121 on multidrug resistance proteins in experimental pancreatic cancer. *Tumour biology : the journal of the International Society for Oncodevelopmental Biology and Medicine*, *29*(6), 351–358.

[19] Zhang, G., Li, J., Zhu, T., Gu, Q., & Li, D. (2016). Advanced tools in marine natural drug discovery. *Current opinion in biotechnology*, *42*, 13–23.

[20] Stonik, V. A., & Fedorov, S. N. (2014). Marine low molecular weight natural products as potential cancer preventive compounds. *Marine drugs*, *12*(2), 636–671.

[21] Zhang, Y., Zhang, Y. K., Wang, Y. J., Vispute, S. G., Jain, S., Chen, Y., Li, J., Youssef, D. T., El Sayed, K. A., & Chen, Z. S. (2015). Esters of the marine-derived triterpene sipholenol A reverse P-GP-mediated drug resistance. *Marine drugs*, *13*(4), 2267–2286.

[22] Rochfort, S., & Capon, R. (1996). Parguerenes revisited: New Brominated Diterpenes from the southern Australian marine red alga Laurencia Filiformis. *Australian Journal of Chemistry*, *49*(1), 19. https://doi.org/10.1071/ch9960019

[23] Awad N. E. (2004). Bioactive brominated diterpenes from the marine red alga Jania Rubens (L.) Lamx. *Phytotherapy research : PTR*, *18*(4), 275–279. https://doi.org/10.1002/ptr.1273.

[24] Takeda, S., Kurosawa, E., Komiyama, K., & Suzuki, T. (1990). The structures of cytotoxic Diterpenes containing bromine from the marine red AlgaLaurencia obtusa(Hudson) Lamouroux. *Bulletin of the Chemical Society of Japan*, *63*(11), 3066-3072. https://doi.org/10.1246/bcsj.63.3066

[25] Abraham, I., Jain, S., Wu, C. P., Khanfar, M. A., Kuang, Y., Dai, C. L., Shi, Z., Chen, X., Fu, L., Ambudkar, S. V., El Sayed, K., & Chen, Z. S. (2010). Marine sponge-derived sipholane triterpenoids reverse P-glycoprotein (ABCB1)-mediated multidrug resistance in cancer cells. *Biochemical pharmacology*, *80*(10), 1497–1506.

[26] Akl, M. R., Foudah, A. I., Ebrahim, H. Y., Meyer, S. A., & El Sayed, K. A. (2014). The marine-derived sipholenol A-4-O-3',4'-dichlorobenzoate inhibits breast cancer growth and motility in vitro and in vivo through the suppression of Brk and FAK signaling. *Marine drugs*, *12*(4), 2282–2304.

[27] Smith, C. D., Zilfou, J. T., Stratmann, K., Patterson, G. M., & Moore, R. E. (1995). Welwitindolinone analogues that reverse P-glycoprotein-mediated multiple drug resistance. *Molecular pharmacology*, *47*(2), 241–247.

[28] Huang, X. C., Sun, Y. L., Salim, A. A., Chen, Z. S., & Capon, R. J. (2013). Parguerenes: Marine red alga bromoditerpenes as inhibitors of P-glycoprotein (ABCB1) in multidrug resistant human cancer cells. *Biochemical pharmacology*, *85*(9), 1257–1268. https://doi.org/10.1016/j.bcp.2013.02.005.

[29] Pettit, G. R. The Bryostatins. In *Fortschritte der Chemie organischer Naturstoffe/Progress in the Chemistry of Organic Natural Products*; Herz, W., Kirby, G. W., Steglich, W., Tamm, Ch., Eds.; Springer: Vienna, Austria, 1991; Volume 57, pp. 153–195.

[30] Mutter, R., & Wills, M. (2000). Chemistry and clinical biology of the bryostatins. *Bioorganic & medicinal chemistry*, *8*(8), 1841–1860.

[31] Kraft, A. S., Smith, J. B., & Berkow, R. L. (1986). Bryostatin, an activator of the calcium phospholipid-dependent protein kinase, blocks phorbol ester-induced differentiation of human promyelocytic

leukemia cells HL-60. *Proceedings of the National Academy of Sciences of the United States of America*, *83*(5), 1334–1338.

[32] Jetten, A. M., George, M. A., Pettit, G. R., & Rearick, J. I. (1989). Effects of bryostatins and retinoic acid on phorbol ester- and diacylglycerol-induced squamous differentiation in human tracheobronchial epithelial cells. *Cancer research*, *49*(14), 3990–3995.

[33] Chen, W. H., Wang, S. K., & Duh, C. Y. (2011). Polyhydroxylated steroids from the bamboo coral Isis hippuris. *Marine drugs*, *9*(10), 1829–1839. https://doi.org/10.3390/md9101829.

[34] Tanaka, J., Trianto, A., Musman, M., Issa, H. H., Ohtani, I. I., Ichiba, T., Higa, T., Yoshida, W. Y., and Scheuer, P. J. (2014). New polyoxygenated steroids exhibiting reversal of multidrug resistance from the gorgonian *Isis hippuris*. *Tetrahedron*, *58*, 6259–6266.

[35] Raju, R., Piggott, A. M., Huang, X. C., & Capon, R. J. (2011). Nocardioazines: a novel bridged diketopiperazine scaffold from a marine-derived bacterium inhibits P-glycoprotein. *Organic letters*, *13*(10), 2770–2773.

[36] Ma, Y., & Wink, M. (2010). The beta-carboline alkaloid harmine inhibits BCRP and can reverse resistance to the anticancer drugs mitoxantrone and camptothecin in breast cancer cells. *Phytotherapy research : PTR*, *24*(1), 146–149.

[37] Cao, R., Fan, W., Guo, L., Ma, Q., Zhang, G., Li, J., Chen, X., Ren, Z., & Qiu, L. (2013). Synthesis and structure–activity relationships of harmine derivatives as potential antitumor agents. *European Journal of Medicinal Chemistry*, *60*, 135-143. https://doi.org/10.1016/j.ejmech.2012.11.045

[38] Andersen, R. J., Faulkner, D. J., He, C. H., Van Duyne, G. D., & Clardy, J. (1985). Metabolites of the marine prosobranch mollusk Lamellaria Sp. *Journal of the American Chemical Society*, *107*(19), 5492-5495. https://doi.org/10.1021/ja00305a027

[39] Davis, R. A., Carroll, A. R., Pierens, G. K., & Quinn, R. J. (1999). New Lamellarin alkaloids from the Australian Ascidian, Didemnum

chartaceum. *Journal of Natural Products*, *62*(3), 419-424. https://doi.org/10.1021/np9803530

[40] Urban, S., Butler, M., & Capon, R. (1994). Lamellarins O and P: New aromatic metabolites from the Australian marine sponge Dendrilla cactos. *Australian Journal of Chemistry*, *47*(10), 1919. https://doi.org/10.1071/ch9941919

[41] Reddy, M. V., Rao, M. R., Rhodes, D., Hansen, M. S., Rubins, K., Bushman, F. D., Venkateswarlu, Y., & Faulkner, D. J. (1999). Lamellarin alpha 20-sulfate, an inhibitor of HIV-1 integrase active against HIV-1 virus in cell culture. *Journal of medicinal chemistry*, *42*(11), 1901–1907.

[42] Quesada, A., García Grávalos, M., & Fernández Puentes, J. (1996). Polyaromatic alkaloids from marine invertebrates as cytotoxic compounds and inhibitors of multidrug resistance caused by P-glycoprotein. *British Journal of Cancer*, *74*(5), 677-682. https://doi.org/10.1038/bjc.1996.421

[43] Mohamed, O. G., Salim, A. A., Khalil, Z. G., Elbanna, A. H., Bernhardt, P. V., & Capon, R. J. (2020). Chrysosporazines F-M: P-Glycoprotein Inhibitory Phenylpropanoid Piperazines from an Australian Marine Fish Derived Fungus, *Chrysosporium* sp. CMB-F294. *Journal of natural products*, *83*(2), 497–504.

[44] Ohmori, K., Ogawa, Y., Obitsu, T., Ishikawa, Y., Nishiyama, S., & Yamamura, S. (2000). Total Synthesis of Bryostatin 3 This work was supported by the Ministry of Education, Science, Sports, and Culture (Japan). K.O. is grateful to JSPS for a predoctoral fellowship. *Angewandte Chemie (International ed. in English)*, *39*(13), 2290–2294.

[45] Ponnusamy N., Odumpatta R., Damodharan P., and Arumugam M.(2019). Computational Investigation of Marine Bioactive Compounds Reveals Frigocyclinone as a Potent Inhibitor of Kaposi's Sarcoma Associated Herpesvirus (KSHV). *Targets. Biomed Pharmacol J,*12(3).

[46] Fu, T. H., McElroy, W. T., Shamszad, M., & Martin, S. F. (2012). Formal syntheses of naturally occurring welwitindolinones. *Organic letters*, *14*(15), 3834–3837.

[47] MacKay, J. A., Bishop, R. L., & Rawal, V. H. (2005). Rapid synthesis of the N-methylwelwitindolinoneskeleton. *ChemInform*, *36*(49).

[48] Sanchez, C., Mendez, C., & Salas, J. A. (2007). Indolocarbazole natural products: Occurrence, biosynthesis, and biological activity. *ChemInform*, *38*(18).

[49] Kato, N., Suzuki, H., Okumura, H., Takahashi, S., & Osada, H. (2013). A point mutation in ftmD blocks the fumitremorgin biosynthetic pathway in Aspergillus fumigatus strain Af293. *Bioscience, biotechnology, and biochemistry*, *77*(5), 1061–1067.

[50] Stratmann, K., Burgoyne, D. L., Moore, R. E., Patterson, G. M., & Smith, C. D. (1995). Hapalosin, a Cyanobacterial cyclic Depsipeptide with multidrug-resistance reversing activity. [Erratum to document cited in CA122:10658]. *The Journal of Organic Chemistry*, *60*(9), 2950-2950. https://doi.org/10.1021/jo00114a062

[51] Degnan, B. M., Hawkins, C. J., Lavin, M. F., McCaffrey, E. J., Parry, D. L., van den Brenk, A. L., & Watters, D. J. (1989). New cyclic peptides with cytotoxic activity from the ascidian Lissoclinum patella. *Journal of medicinal chemistry*, *32*(6), 1349–1354.

[52] Smith, C. D. (1995). New compounds from cyanobacteria to circumvent mdr. *Drug News Perspect.* 8, 423–425.

[53] Dinh, T. Q., Smith, C. D., Du, X., & Armstrong, R. W. (1998). Design, synthesis, and evaluation of the multidrug resistance-reversing activity of D-glucose mimetics of hapalosin. *Journal of medicinal chemistry*, *41*(6), 981–987.

[54] Kowalski, R. J., Giannakakou, P., Gunasekera, S. P., Longley, R. E., Day, B. W., & Hamel, E. (1997). The microtubule-stabilizing agent discodermolide competitively inhibits the binding of paclitaxel (Taxol) to tubulin polymers, enhances tubulin nucleation reactions more potently than paclitaxel, and inhibits the growth of paclitaxel-resistant cells. *Molecular pharmacology*, *52*(4), 613–622.

[55] Honore, S., Kamath, K., Braguer, D., Horwitz, S. B., Wilson, L., Briand, C., & Jordan, M. A. (2004). Synergistic suppression of microtubule dynamics by discodermolide and paclitaxel in non-small cell lung carcinoma cells. *Cancer research*, *64*(14), 4957–4964.

[56] Longley, R. E., Caddigan, D., Harmody, D., Gunasekera, M., & Gunasekera, S. P. (1991). Discodermolide—A new, marine-derived immunosuppressive compound. *Transplantation*, *52*(4), 650-655. https://doi.org/10.1097/00007890-199110000-00014

[57] Kowalski, R. J., Giannakakou, P., Gunasekera, S. P., Longley, R. E., Day, B. W., & Hamel, E. (1997). The microtubule-stabilizing agent discodermolide competitively inhibits the binding of paclitaxel (Taxol) to tubulin polymers, enhances tubulin nucleation reactions more potently than paclitaxel, and inhibits the growth of paclitaxel-resistant cells. *Molecular pharmacology*, *52*(4), 613–622.

[58] Towle, M. J., Salvato, K. A., Budrow, J., Wels, B. F., Kuznetsov, G., Aalfs, K. K., Welsh, S., Zheng, W., Seletsky, B. M., Palme, M. H., Habgood, G. J., Singer, L. A., Dipietro, L. V., Wang, Y., Chen, J. J., Quincy, D. A., Davis, A., Yoshimatsu, K., Kishi, Y., Yu, M. J., … Littlefield, B. A. (2001). In vitro and in vivo anticancer activities of synthetic macrocyclic ketone analogues of halichondrin B. *Cancer research*, *61*(3), 1013–1021.

[59] Bailly C. (2015). Anticancer properties of lamellarins. *Marine drugs*, *13*(3), 1105–1123.

[60] Imbri, D., Tauber, J., & Opatz, T. (2014). Synthetic approaches to the lamellarins–a comprehensive review. *Marine drugs*, *12*(12), 6142–6177.

[61] Ishibashi, F., Tanabe, S., Oda, T., & Iwao, M. (2002). Synthesis and structure-activity relationship study of lamellarin derivatives. *Journal of natural products*, *65*(4), 500–504.

[62] Facompré, M., Tardy, C., Bal-Mahieu, C., Colson, P., Perez, C., Manzanares, I., Cuevas, C., & Bailly, C. (2003). Lamellarin D: a novel potent inhibitor of topoisomerase I. *Cancer research*, *63*(21), 7392–7399.

[63] Huang, X. C., Xiao, X., Zhang, Y. K., Talele, T. T., Salim, A. A., Chen, Z. S., & Capon, R. J. (2014). Lamellarin O, a pyrrole alkaloid from an Australian marine sponge, Ianthella sp., reverses BCRP mediated drug resistance in cancer cells. *Marine drugs*, *12*(7), 3818–3837.

[64] Boger, D. L., Boyce, C. W., Labroli, M. A., Sehon, C. A., & Jin, Q. (1999). Total syntheses of Ningalin a, Lamellarin O, Lukianol a, and Permethyl Storniamide a utilizing heterocyclic Azadiene Diels− Alder reactions. *Journal of the American Chemical Society*, *121*(1), 54-62. https://doi.org/10.1021/ja982078

[65] Chou, T., Guan, Y., Soenen, D. R., Danishefsky, S. J., & Boger, D. L. (2005). Potent reversal of multidrug resistance by ningalins and its use in drug combinations against human colon carcinoma xenograft in nude mice. *Cancer Chemotherapy and Pharmacology*, *56*(4), 379-390. https://doi.org/10.1007/s00280-005-1019-y

[66] González-Lobato, L., Real, R., Prieto, J. G., Alvarez, A. I., & Merino, G. (2010). Differential inhibition of murine Bcrp1/Abcg2 and human BCRP/ABCG2 by the mycotoxin fumitremorgin C. *European journal of pharmacology*, *644*(1-3), 41–48.

[67] Aoki, S., Cao, L., Matsui, K., Rachmat, R., Akiyama, S., & Kobayashi, M. (2004). Kendarimide a, a novel peptide reversing P-glycoprotein-mediated multidrug resistance in tumor cells, from a marine sponge of Haliclona Sp. *Tetrahedron*, *60*(33), 7053-7059. https://doi.org/10.1016/j.tet.2003.07.020

[68] Kotoku, N., Cao, L., Aoki, S., Kobayashi, M. (2005). Absolute stereo-structure of kendarimide a, a novelmdr modulator, from a marine sponge. *Heterocycles*, 65, 563–578.

[69] Rinehart, K. L., Holt, T. G., Fregeau, N. L., Stroh, J. G., Keifer, P. A., Sun, F., Li, L. H., & Martin, D. G. (1990). Ecteinascidins 729, 743, 745, 759a, 759B, and 770: Potent antitumor agents from the Caribbean tunicate Ecteinascidia turbinata. *The Journal of Organic Chemistry*, *55*(15), 4512-4515. https://doi.org/10.1021/jo00302a007

[70] Kanzaki, A., Takebayashi, Y., Ren, X. Q., Miyashita, H., Mori, S., Akiyama, S., & Pommier, Y. (2002). Overcoming multidrug drug

resistance in P-glycoprotein/MDR1-overexpressing cell lines by ecteinascidin 743. *Molecular cancer therapeutics*, *1*(14), 1327–1334.

[71] Carter, N. J., & Keam, S. J. (2007). Trabectedin : a review of its use in the management of soft tissue sarcoma and ovarian cancer. *Drugs*, *67*(15), 2257–2276. https://doi.org/10.2165/00003495-200767150-00009.

In: An Introduction to P-Glycoprotein
Editors: M. Wahajuddin et al.
ISBN: 978-1-53619-488-3

Chapter 9

P-GLYCOPROTEIN AND ITS ASSOCIATION IN NEURODEGENERATIVE DISORDERS

Himani Panwar[1], Anushruti Ashok[2], Swati Chaturvedi[3,4], Ranjay Kumar Chaudhary[5], Arti Thakur[6] and Sadaf Jahan[5,*]

[1]Gurukul Kangri Vishwavidyalaya, Haridwar, Uttarakhand, India
[2]Case Western Reserve University, Cleveland, OH, US
[3]CSIR-Central Drug Research Institute, Lucknow, India
[4]Academy of Scientific and Innovative Research (AcSIR), Ghaziabad, India
[5]Medical Laboratories, College of Applied Medical Sciences, Majmaah University, Al Majma'ah, Saudi Arabia
[6]Chinmaya Degree College, Haridwar, Uttarakhand, India

[*] Corresponding Author's Email: jahan149@gmail.com.

Abstract

Multidrug transporters (MDRs) are not only restricted to myeloma tissues but manifest all over fit organelles and tissues counting kidney, liver, intestine and at the blood-brain barrier (BBB). The convoluted microstructure of the BBB is responsible for the modulation of the central nervous system (CNS). BBB occupied with efflux transporters in order to maintain normal brain activity by avoiding neuronal pathophysiological condition. Any interference to the BBB (corresponding with genetic defects or with local antigenic invasion) can be cause of neuronal impairment, which leads to neurodegenerative disorders (NDs). The involvement of p-glycoprotein (P-gp), a multi-drug resistance (MDR) protein (product of the *ABCB1* gene), facilitates healthy brain function through effluxion of virulence factors. In last decade, several reports have shown that ABCB1 or P-gp is actively involved in the movement of amyloid beta (Aβ) peptide from the brain. These Aβ accumulations in brain indicate the onset of Alzheimer's disease (AD). Thus, P-gp plays specific role in the protection of brain by Aβ transport across the BBB. This finding has opened up an entirely new pharmaceutical window for other NDs. Therefore, the purpose of this chapter is to shed light on the association of the activity of P-gp in NDs.

Keywords: blood-brain barrier, neurodegenerative disease, Alzheimer's disease, P-gp

Introduction

ATP-binding cassette (ABC) gene family is recognized as one of the most featured transporter for the administration or elimination of the drug from Central Nervous System (CNS) [1]. The P-glycoprotein (P-gp), a member of the ABC efflux transporter has been denoted as an important element of the brain blood barrier (BBB) which is engaged in actively transporting a wide variety of lipophilic drugs out of the endothelial cells of the blood capillary that form the BBB [2]. ABC efflux transporter in the BBB prevents the entry of neurotoxic drugs into the brain [3]. Multidrug transporters are not only limit to the cancerous cells but also found in the apical membranes of intestine, liver, kidney and brain, where they perform the function of absorption, distribution and excretion of drugs [4]. Some transporters are involved in multidrug resistance, among which P-gp or ABC-B1 is the best studied transporter [5]. P-gp was the first ABC transporter, identified in the endothelial cells of the blood brain barrier (BBB) in 1989 [6]. P-gp efflux pump can transport many of the structurally distinct hydrophobic amphipathic compounds at the expense of ATP hydrolysis [7]. P-gp is located at barriers such as BBB, blood cerebrospinal fluid (B-CSF) barrier and blood testis barrier (BTB) [5]. P-gp is one of the most plentiful drug transporter in nature and it is efficient in binding and removing large number of substrates out of the cell [8]. When the expression of P-gp across BBB is decreased, it permits the entry of toxic chemicals to brain, leading to the development of neurodegenerative disorders (NDs) [9] such as Alzheimer's disease (AD), Parkinson disease (PD), Huntington diseases (HD), Amyotrophic lateral sclerosis (ALS) and Stroke [10]. NDs are the severe and most common disease of human nervous system and can disrupt many body activities like balance, communication, breathing, movement and functioning of heart [11]. These are chronic pathological processes that are indicated by the hematomas, increasing loss of populations of neurons and existence of misfolded protein [12]. Verapamil, a Pgp inhibitor drug is extensively studied for examination of P-gp substrate molecules [13]. The excessive expression of P-gp makes the cancer tumor resistance to drugs used against cancer. The upregulation and downregulation of P-gp are having specific role in various diseases. In the coming section, we will discuss the P-gp and its association with the NDs. Prior to this, we will unravel the details of drug transporters, BBB and NDs respectively.

BLOOD BRAIN BARRIER AND P-GP LOCATION

BBB act as a physiological barrier between blood and brain which helps in protecting the brain from blood borne microorganisms and foreign substances that may cause harm to brain [14]. BBB is one of the protection models for CNS. It separates the CNS from blood and plays a key role in maintaining the exact proportion of ions, neurotransmitters, and nutrients, also restrict the entry of toxic substances. Although it selectively allows the transport of small lipid soluble molecules across brain while limits the entry of toxins, inhibitors both endogenous and exogenous in nature. It also limits the entry of drugs, which create a hinder in the path of therapeutic treatments. BBB protects the brain from damage and also from neurodegeneration [15].

This barrier mainly comprises of a single layer of tightly arranged endothelial cells of brain capillaries [16]. Beside this it also requires the presence of interaction with neuroglia as well as nerve cells, pericytes, and collagen extracellular matrix. This complex system between vascular and nerve cells make neurovascular unit (NVU) [17]. This NVU prevents the entrance of chemical compounds and pathogens from the circulating blood to brain through diffusion. Thus, BBB plays key role in maintaining homeostasis with the help of specific transporters. BBB allows the passage of oxygen, carbon dioxide, glucose, vitamins, amino acids, and nucleosides that are essential for normal functioning of brain through it [15]. The transportation of these substances across the barrier occur by using transporter proteins. BBB prevents the passage of large hydrophilic molecules while it allows hydrophobic molecules and small polar molecules passage. It has been recognized that BBB restrict the entry of drugs approximately 98% efficiently. BBB act as neuro-protectant, it restricts the delivery of most potential drugs to the brain that would be efficient against diseases. This is the major therapeutic challenge in treatment of diseases related to the brain.

Main components of BBB are ion channels and transporters which maintain homeostasis. There are two major kinds of transporters demonstrated by CNS endothelial cells: efflux transporter and nutrient transporter. Current studies explain the full arrangements of transporters and their substrates. Efflux transporters consist of MDR1, BCRP and MRPs [18]. They work by hydrolysing ATP to transport substrates up to concentration gradient. These transporters are widely expressed at BBB and provide an efficient barrier system. MDR1 or P-glycoprotein (P-gp), its overexpression has been associated with drug resistance therapies [19]. P-gp is a transmembrane transporter protein encoded by ABC B1 gene, it is found throughout the body on the apical surface of the epithelial cells primarily where they perform the function of excretion such as in the lining of colon, small intestine, bile ductules, kidney proximal tubules, pancreatic ductules and the adrenal gland [20]. It is also detected in the endothelial cells of BBB. An important means of entry of drugs is to make efficient drug delivery system or by making substrates that can enter into the brain without effluxion and thus used against diseases. Nutrient transporters make possible the movement of specific nutrients down the concentration gradient [21]. CNS endothelial cells also have wide variety of transporters that transports nutrients across CNS. Most of these nutrient transporters belongs to the family Solute Carrier like Slc2a1 transports glucose, Slc16a1 transports lactate and pyruvate, Slc7a1 transports cationic amino acids and Slc7a5 transports neutral amino acids. Among them Slc2a1 or Glu1 is largely studied group because it translocates glucose to CNS and if there is a deficiency of Glu1 it can lead to epilepsy [22].

Disturbance in the BBB is recognized in many neurodegenerative diseases including Alzheimer's disease, stroke, and traumatic injury [23]. Additionally, via imaging technology, the breakage of BBB is noted in dead brain during post-mortem which shows that breakage of the barrier is responsible for different neurological syndrome [24]. The reason behind the disruption of BBB includes tight junction disruption, transporters expressions, etc. BBB is slightly important because disruption of BBB can develop neuropathological condition and crossing of drugs through BBB is important for treatment of many neurological diseases [25].

Background Knowledge about P-gp

P-gp/Multidrug resistance protein 1 (MDR 1) or ABC B1 (170kDa) is an important transmembrane protein that pushes many substances out of the cells. In humans it is coded by mdr1 gene or abc b1 gene [26] while it is coded by mdr1a and mdrb2 in mice (Croop et al. 1989). The first mammalian ABC transporter which is crystallized and distinguished was mouse P-gp

[27]. P-gp excludes a wide variety of structurally different compounds out of the cells. It is an efflux pump that works by using energy from the hydrolysis of ATP and also have broad range of substrate specificity (Figure A). The substrates for P-gp are HIV protease inhibitors, steroid hormones, cardiac glycosides, calcium channel blockers and anti-cancer drugs of classes vinca alkaloid, anthracycline, taxane [28]. It is present mostly in all organisms and act as a natural defence mechanism against foreign substances. P-gp is localized on the apical membranes of various tissues or cells such as liver, kidney, pancreas, colon, intestine, kidney and also at the Blood Brain Barrier (BBB) (Figure B), Blood cerebrospinal fluid (B-CSF) barrier and Blood testis barrier (BTB) [29]. It actively pumps xenobiotics compounds across the membranes of various cells and wide variety of hydrophobic amphipathic drugs out of the cells, this contribute to the poor penetration into the brain and cause neurotoxicity. P-gp plays a key role in protecting tissues from xenobiotics and the adverse effect of drugs. P-gp act as an efflux pump for various endogenous and exogenous chemical compounds and reducing the load of harmful substances. The function of P-gp is greatly altered with age, thus it make ease the accumulation of toxic substances in the brain which generates the risk of neurodegenerative diseases with aging. In some condition, the expression of P-gp increases such as in cancerous cells that make the cancer cells resistant to drugs which is main obstacle in cancer treatment by chemotherapy [30]. P-gp shows resistance to various drugs including immuno-suppressive drugs, HIV protease inhibitors and antibiotics thus affecting the treatment procedure. A wide range of strategies have been developed to overcome the Multidrug resistant of cancerous cells. P-gp function could be prevented by using inhibitors such as Verapamil, cyclosporine A, elacridar, ritonavir, quinidine and sertraline, etc. [31]. These drugs act by blocking substrate binding site either competitively or non-competitively or by interfering in ATP hydrolysis and by making changes to the cell membrane permeability [32]. The main purpose of using inhibitors of P-gp is to enhance the uptake of drugs by targeted organs and for better therapeutic treatment as in case of cancer but only for a short period of time because long term use of P-gp inhibitors will result in imbalance in the normal homeostasis of brain. Any

kind of modulation in the activity of P-gp may upgrade the drug effectiveness but also causes the progression of neurodegenerative diseases such as Alzheimer's disease (AD), Parkinson's disease (PD), and Amyotrophic lateral sclerosis (ALS) [33, 34].

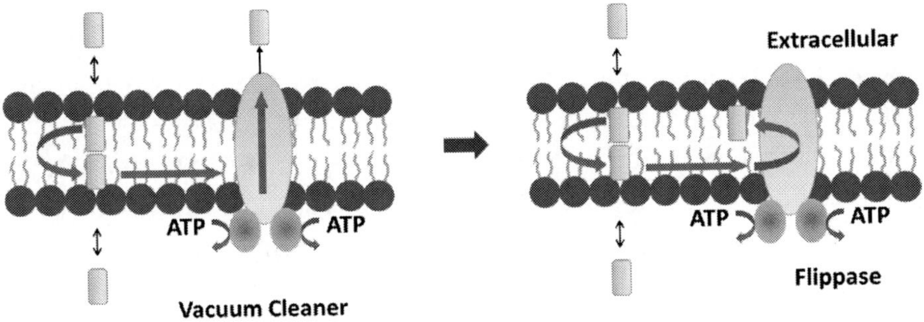

a

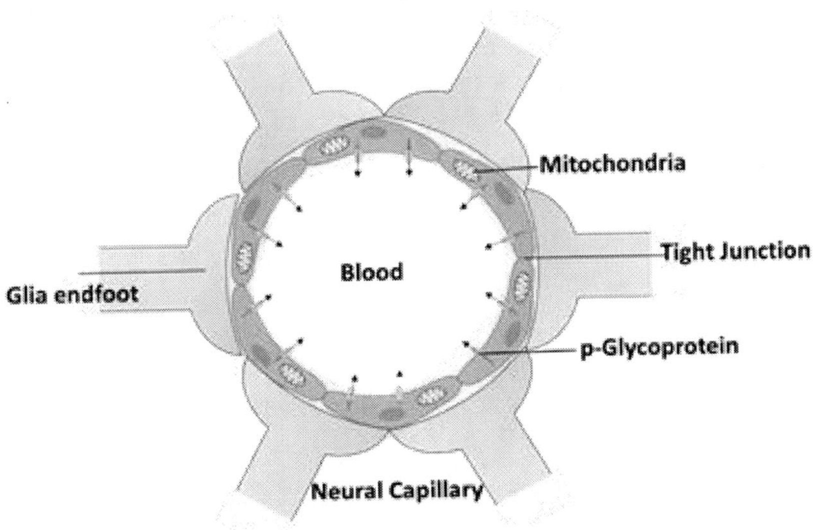

b

Figure A. Role of Pgp in substrate movement B. Location of Pgp on BBB.

Role of P-gp in Neurodegenerative Disorders

Blood-brain barrier plays an analytical role in maintaining homeostasis in CNS. Any kind of dysfunction in BBB can cause the development of neurodegenerative diseases including AD, PD, ALS and stroke. The characteristics of BBB dysfunction are disruption, disturbance of transporters and production of neurotoxic substance by BBB. P-gp, an efflux transporter present at BBB actively engaged in transporting several compounds across BBB. Disturbance in BBB P-gp transporter can result in accumulation of aggregated protein in neurological disorders [35]. Reduction in function of P-gp is associated with many neurodegenerative disorders. AD is the most chronic form of Dementia, which is caused by the deposition of Aβ peptide and tau protein in the brain because of the downregulation of P-gp [36]. PD is the second common neurodegenerative disease which causes the depigmentation of substantia nigra cells, misfolding of alpha-synuclein protein and accumulation of Lewy bodies. ALS is another fatal degenerative disease of nervous system which weakens our muscles and may face paralysis and disability. Stroke is another deadliest disease caused by thrombus formation which leads to the development of life-threatening obstructive blood clots, which further initiates secondary events including BBB damage.

Alzheimer Disease (AD)

AD is the most common neurodegenerative disease and a common form of dementia among aging population [37]. The major hallmarks of AD is the accumulation of amyloid beta (Aβ) plaque in the brain [38]. There are two major hypothesis which explains the deposition of Aβ: (i) overproduction of Aβ in the brain and (ii) reduction in clearance of Aβ from the brain. Familial AD, subtype of AD comprises approximately 5% of cases which is due to the mutation in the amyloid precursor protein (APP) and APP processing gene, i.e., Presenilin 1 and 2 that results in the overproduction of Aβ [39]. On the other hand, more than 95% cases are of sporadic AD in which reduction in clearance of Aβ from the brain through BBB is reported. The Aβ is pumped out of the brain through endothelial cells of BBB by an efflux transporter, i.e., via P-gp. The inadequate clearance of Aβ plaques from the brain is an important cause of AD-pathogenesis. A positron emission tomography (PET) scanning for labelled P-gp substrate *(R)*-[^{11}C]-verapamil across the BBB in healthy volunteers aged 18-86 demonstrated that its clearance was significantly lower amongst older volunteers as compared to younger volunteers [52].

Approximately 50% of Aβ clearance is through direct transport across BBB [40]. Aβ and ApoE complex together may function as a ligand to the LRP-1 [41, 42]. LRP-1 localized at the abluminal surface of endothelial cells of BBB also contribute to the export of Aβ into peripheral circulation. LRP-1 facilitates Aβ uptake into endothelial cells, but it is insufficient to promote transcytosis, suggesting the necessity of other transporters for Aβ efflux into the peripheral circulation [43]. In one mechanistic study, it was estimated that Aβ40 promotes the P-gp degradation via ubiquitination, internalization, and proteasome associated pathways in examined brain capillaries. This mechanistic approach would be found effective to search out the therapeutic ways to block the P-gp mortification in AD in order to clearance of Aβ from brain [44]. P-gp is present in various organs that act as excretory and/or barrier function such as intestine, liver, kidney and at Blood Brain Barrier. There is an inverse correlation between endothelial P-gp expression and cerebral Aβ deposition, both Aβ40 and Aβ42 isoforms were implicated but the significant inverse relationship is with Aβ40 [45]. Aging is the major risk factor for AD, P-gp expression declines with aging and with AD progression [46]. A recent study demonstrated that LRP-1 and P-gp are functionally linked via phosphatidylinositol-binding clathrin assembly protein (PICALM), a cytosolic protein that regulate intracellular trafficking to facilitate Aβ transcytosis and clearance [47]. P-gp, LRP-1 and PICALM has been reported to co-localise with each other within the brain endothelial cells. In mouse model of AD, knocking out of P- gp expression at BBB increases the deposition of Aβ in the brain [48] and by restoring BBB, P-gp expression increases the transport activity and thus reduces the Aβ level in the brain.

Parkinson Disease (PD)

PD is another common neurodegenerative disorder after AD that mainly affects the dopamine producing neurons in a particular area of the brain called substantia nigra [49]. Researchers noticed that the mutation in gene of the protein alpha-synuclein causes a rare form of Autosomal-dominant PD and some changes occur in the brain of parkinsonian patients which includes the presence of Lewy bodies and presence of α-synuclein in Lewy body [50]. The cause of PD is still unknown, but it has been suggested that some risk factors are responsible for this disease such as age, sex, heredity and exposure of toxins. Age is the most common factor in PD. It has also been suggested that environmental factors (use of chemicals such as pesticides, insecticide, etc.) also increases the chances of developing PD. Lower expression of P-gp transporter system at BBB could ease the entry of these toxic chemical compounds in the brain that would lead the chances of developing PD. It is believed that the neurotoxic substances also act as a substrate for P-gp and exposure of these may cause NDs. In one study, role of P-gp at damaged BBB was demonstrated in the brain of Parkinson patients as compared with healthy controls, estimated by (^{11}C)-verapamil PET that defines the role of P-gp in preventing the accumulation of toxic substances [51]. In both advanced PD and advanced PSP (Progressive supranuclear palsy), the frontal region of brain is decreased which possibly affected fronto-striatal neuronal projections [52]. PSP is a neurodegenerative disorder comprises with parkinsonism and cognitive decline, showing midbrain, striatal and frontal cell loss and tau protein inclusion bodies [53]. It was found that decreased cerebrovascular P-gp could impair the ability of the brain to expel excess proteins, and the resulting accumulation of protein, i.e., α-synuclein and Aβ [54, 53]. Downregulation of P-gp function lead to increased accumulation of insoluble α-synuclein in PD [55, 56].

Amyotrophic Lateral Sclerosis (ALS)

Amyotrophic lateral sclerosis (ALS) is a developing and deadly NDs that cause the degeneration of motor neurons in the brainstem, cerebral cortex and spinal cord. Motor neuron mainly controls all the voluntary muscle activity which produce movement like chewing, walking and talking. The symptoms of this disease get worse with time [57]. Any dysfunction in the transporters of Blood Brain Barrier (BBB), cerebral blood flow (CBF) and blood spinal cord barrier breakdown have been recognized earlier to degeneration of motor neuron [58]. Genetics and environmental factors are equally responsible for ALS. 90% of the ALS are considered sporadic in nature. Therefore, it occurs randomly with no family history of the disease and it is also reported that about 5-10% ALS cases are familial. Moreover, it is inherited from his or her parents. 12-20% of familial cases occurs due to the mutations in the gene SOD1 responsible for giving command for the production of the enzyme copper-zinc superoxide dismutase 1. Researchers suggested that the exposure of toxins may increase the risk of developing ALS [59]. ALS pathogenesis involves misfolding and aggregation in the cell of superoxide dismutase 1 (SOD1), a protein produced by mitochondria which converts the superoxide anion to H_2O_2. A role of P-gp in ALS treatment has been suggested.

Stroke

Stroke is the major cause of long-term disability worldwide and the third-leading cause of death in the United States. It is also known as cerebrovascular accident (CVA) or brain attack, patients may rapidly experience paralysis, impaired speech, or loss of vision due to interruption of cerebral blood flow (CBF) caused by thrombosis or embolism. Stroke comprises more than 80% cases of ischemic/hypoxic injury, as compared with hemorrhage or cardiac arrest, which includes 15% cases. Interrupted supply of oxygen and nutrients via blood stream exacerbate secondary biochemical events and other downstream mechanism like reactive oxygen species (ROS) generation through oxidative damage, inflammation, glutamate excitotoxicity and blood-brain barrier (BBB) damage [60] that further culminates into infarcts in different brain regions and ultimately neuronal degeneration. Elevated expression of P-gp at the BBB and decreased concentration of P-gp substrates in the ischaemic brain tissues were observed within 4 h after middle cerebral artery occlusion [61]. In another report, P-gp expression increases in brain and liver following 90-minute MCAO, as well as in cultured rat brain endothelial (RBE4) cells after 16-hour hypoxia and low glucose (HLG) treatment [62]. Upregulation of P-glycoprotein (P-gp) is also reported in rat brain microvessel endothelial cells (rBMECs) under oxygen glucose deprivation (OGD) [63]. However, it has been reported that the increase in P-gp expression could significantly reduce the bioavailability and efficacy of neuroprotective drugs.

Future Aspects

AD and other NDs are multifaceted diseases that involved an intricate mechanism. This chapter strengthen our understanding on recent investigation on Aβ transporter P-gp and its targeting approach for therapeutic strategies in the amelioration of AD and other NDs. Furthermore, substantial research is required to explore and validate this aspect.

Conclusion

BBB dysfunction is associated with accumulation of different vasculotoxic and neurotoxic macromolecules in the brain, which can further initiate neuronal injury that ultimately lead to NDs. P-gp transporter are present at the BBB and has been involved in the clearance of Aβ from the brain to the blood stream. BBB damage altered P-gp functioning which results in faulty Aβ clearance from the brain which is one of the key events during AD-pathogenesis. Apart from AD, role of P-gp has been also described in other NDs. This book chapter summarized the recent investigation on P-gp in the prevention and/or treatment of AD and other NDs which provide a novel targeted approach against these disorders.

ACKNOWLEDGMENTS

The authors are thankful to Deanship of Scientific Research for supporting this work.

CONFLICT OF INTEREST

The authors declare that there are no conflicts of interest.

REFERENCES

[1] Shen, S. and W. Zhang, ABC transporters and drug efflux at the blood-brain barrier. *Reviews in the Neurosciences*, 2010. 21(1): p. 29.

[2] Seelbach, M. J., *Acute Regulation of P-glycoprotein at the Blood-Brain Barrier by Peripheral Inflammatory Pain.* 2007.

[3] Löscher, W. and H. Potschka, Role of drug efflux transporters in the brain for drug disposition and treatment of brain diseases. *Progress in neurobiology*, 2005. 76(1): p. 22-76.

[4] Szakács, G., et al., The role of ABC transporters in drug absorption, distribution, metabolism, excretion and toxicity (ADME-Tox). *Drug Discovery Today*, 2008. 13(9-10): p. 379-393.

[5] Colabufo, N. A., et al., Perspectives of P-glycoprotein modulating agents in oncology and neurodegenerative diseases: pharmaceutical, biological, and diagnostic potentials. *Journal of Medicinal Chemistry*, 2010. 53(5): p. 1883-1897.

[6] Eisenblätter, T. and H. J. Galla, A new multidrug resistance protein at the blood-brain barrier. *Biochemical and Biophysical Research Communications*, 2002. 293(4): p. 1273-1278.

[7] Silva, R., et al., Modulation of P-glycoprotein efflux pump: induction and activation as a therapeutic strategy. *Pharmacology & Therapeutics*, 2015. 149: p. 1-123.

[8] Chufan, E. E., et al., Multiple transport-active binding sites are available for a single substrate on human P-glycoprotein (ABCB1). *PloS One*, 2013. 8(12): p. e82463.

[9] Palmer, A. M., The role of the blood brain barrier in neurodegenerative disorders and their treatment. *Journal of Alzheimer's Disease*, 2011. 24(4): p. 643-656.

[10] Paganoni, S. and M. A. Schwarzschild, Urate as a marker of risk and progression of neurodegenerative disease. *Neurotherapeutics*, 2017. 14(1): p. 148-153.

[11] Choonara, Y. E., et al., Improving drug delivery technology for treating neurodegenerative diseases. *Expert Opinion on Drug Delivery*, 2016. 13(7): p. 1029-1043.

[12] Fricker, M., et al., Neuronal cell death. *Physiological Reviews*, 2018. 98(2): p. 813-880.

[13] Mesraoua, B., et al., Novel therapies for epilepsy in the pipeline. *Epilepsy & Behavior*, 2019. 97: p. 282-290.

[14] Abbott, N. J., et al., Structure and function of the blood-brain barrier. *Neurobiology of Disease*, 2010. 37(1): p. 13-25.

[15] Sweeney, M. D., A. P. Sagare, and B. V. Zlokovic, Blood-brain barrier breakdown in Alzheimer disease and other neurodegenerative disorders. *Nature Reviews Neurology*, 2018. 14(3): p. 133.

[16] Campisi, M., et al., 3D self-organized microvascular model of the human blood-brain barrier with endothelial cells, pericytes and astrocytes. *Biomaterials*, 2018. 180: p. 117-129.

[17] Muoio, V., P. Persson, and M. Sendeski, The neurovascular unit-concept review. *Acta Physiologica*, 2014. 210(4): p. 790-798.

[18] Choudhuri, S. and C. D. Klaassen, Structure, function, expression, genomic organization, and single nucleotide polymorphisms of human

ABCB1 (MDR1), ABCC (MRP), and ABCG2 (BCRP) efflux transporters. *International Journal of Toxicology*, 2006. 25(4): p. 231-259.

[19] Picchianti-Diamanti, A., et al., P-glycoprotein and drug resistance in systemic autoimmune diseases. *International Journal of Molecular Sciences*, 2014. 15(3): p. 4965-4976.

[20] Zhou, S. F., Structure, function and regulation of P-glycoprotein and its clinical relevance in drug disposition. *Xenobiotica*, 2008. 38(7-8): p. 802-832.

[21] Marschner, H., Marschner's mineral nutrition of higher plants. 2011: Academic press.

[22] Klepper, J. and T. Voit, Facilitated glucose transporter protein type 1 (GLUT1) deficiency syndrome: impaired glucose transport into brain - a review. *European Journal of Pediatrics*, 2002. 161(6): p. 295-304.

[23] Hay, J. R., et al., Blood-brain barrier disruption is an early event that may persist for many years after traumatic brain injury in humans. *Journal of Neuropathology and Experimental Neurology*, 2015. 74(12): p. 1147-1157.

[24] Adams, S., H. Brown, and G. Turner, Breaking down the blood-brain barrier: signaling a path to cerebral malaria? *Trends in Parasitology*, 2002. 18(8): p. 360-366.

[25] Banks, W. A., From blood-brain barrier to blood-brain interface: new opportunities for CNS drug delivery. *Nature Reviews Drug Discovery*, 2016. 15(4): p. 275.

[26] Nies, A. T., et al., Vectorial transport of the plant alkaloid berberine by double-transfected cells expressing the human organic cation transporter 1 (OCT1, SLC22A1) and the efflux pump MDR1 P-glycoprotein (ABCB1). *Naunyn-Schmiedeberg's Archives of Pharmacology*, 2008. 376(6): p. 449-461.

[27] Borst, P. and R. O. Elferink, Mammalian ABC transporters in health and disease. *Annual Review of Biochemistry*, 2002. 71(1): p. 537-592.

[28] Lee, C. G., et al., HIV-1 protease inhibitors are substrates for the MDR 1 multidrug transporter. *Biochemistry*, 1998. 37(11): p. 3594-3601.

[29] Tsuji, A. and I. Tamai, Blood-brain barrier function of P-glycoprotein. *Advanced Drug Delivery Reviews*, 1997. 25(2-3): p. 287-298.

[30] Liu, F. S., Mechanisms of chemotherapeutic drug resistance in cancer therapy - a quick review. *Taiwanese Journal of Obstetrics and Gynecology,* 2009. 48(3): p. 239-244.

[31] Jambroszyk, M., A. Tipold, and H. Potschka, Add-on treatment with verapamil in pharmacoresistant canine epilepsy. *Epilepsia*, 2011. 52(2): p. 284-291.

[32] Amin, M. L., *P*-glycoprotein inhibition for optimal drug delivery. *Drug Target Insights*, 2013. 7: p. DTI. S12519.

[33] Rapposelli, S., M. Digiacomo, and A. Balsamo, P-gp transporter and its role in neurodegenerative diseases. *Current Topics in Medicinal Chemistry*, 2009. 9(2): p. 209-217.

[34] Durães, F., M. Pinto, and E. Sousa, Old drugs as new treatments for neurodegenerative diseases. *Pharmaceuticals*, 2018. 11(2): p. 44.

[35] Qosa, H., et al., Regulation of ABC efflux transporters at blood-brain barrier in health and neurological disorders. *Brain Research*, 2015. 1628: p. 298-316.

[36] ME van Assema, D. and B. NM van Berckel, Blood-brain barrier ABC-transporter P-glycoprotein in Alzheimer's disease: still a suspect? *Current Pharmaceutical Design*, 2016. 22(38): p. 5808-5816.

[37] Praticò, D., Evidence of oxidative stress in Alzheimer's disease brain and antioxidant therapy: lights and shadows. *Annals of the New York Academy of Sciences*, 2008. 1147(1): p. 70-78.

[38] Chai, A. B., et al., P-glycoprotein: a role in the export of amyloid-β in Alzheimer's disease? *The FEBS Journal*, 2020. 287(4): p. 612-625.

[39] Kurt, M., et al., Neurodegenerative changes associated with β-amyloid deposition in the brains of mice carrying mutant amyloid precursor protein and mutant presenilin-1 transgenes. *Experimental Neurology*, 2001. 171(1): p. 59-71.

[40] Deane, R., et al., Clearance of amyloid-β peptide across the blood-brain barrier: implication for therapies in Alzheimer's disease. *CNS & Neurological Disorders-Drug Targets* (Formerly Current Drug Targets-CNS & Neurological Disorders), 2009. 8(1): p. 16-30.

[41] Xin, S. H., et al., Clearance of amyloid beta and tau in Alzheimer's disease: from mechanisms to therapy. *Neurotoxicity Research*, 2018. 34(3): p. 733-748.

[42] Tarasoff-Conway, J. M., et al., Clearance systems in the brain - implications for Alzheimer disease. *Nature Reviews Neurology*, 2015. 11(8): p. 457.

[43] Gali, C. C., et al., Amyloid-beta impairs insulin signaling by accelerating autophagy-lysosomal degradation of LRP-1 and IR-β in blood-brain barrier endothelial cells *in vitro* and in 3XTg-AD mice. *Molecular and Cellular Neuroscience*, 2019. 99: p. 103390.

[44] Hartz, A. M., et al., Aβ40 reduces P-glycoprotein at the blood-brain barrier through the ubiquitin-proteasome pathway. *Journal of Neuroscience*, 2016. 36(6): p. 1930-1941.

[45] Silverberg, G. D., et al., Amyloid efflux transporter expression at the blood-brain barrier declines in normal aging. *Journal of Neuropathology & Experimental Neurology*, 2010. 69(10): p. 1034-1043.

[46] Chiu, C., et al., P-glycoprotein expression and amyloid accumulation in human aging and Alzheimer's disease: preliminary observations. *Neurobiology of Aging*, 2015. 36(9): p. 2475-2482.

[47] Storck, S. E. and C. U. Pietrzik, Endothelial LRP1 - A Potential Target for the Treatment of Alzheimer's Disease. *Pharmaceutical Research*, 2017. 34(12): p. 2637-2651.

[48] Cirrito, J. R., et al., P-glycoprotein deficiency at the blood-brain barrier increases amyloid-β deposition in an Alzheimer disease mouse model. *The Journal of Clinical Investigation*, 2005. 115(11): p. 3285-3290.

[49] Hirsch, E. C., P. Jenner, and S. Przedborski, Pathogenesis of Parkinson's disease. *Movement Disorders*, 2013. 28(1): p. 24-30.

[50] Ozansoy, M. and A. N. Başak, The central theme of Parkinson's disease: α-synuclein. *Molecular neurobiology*, 2013. 47(2): p. 460-465.

[51] L Bartels, A., et al., 11C-verapamil to assess P-gp function in human brain during aging, depression and neurodegenerative disease. *Current Topics in Medicinal Chemistry*, 2010. 10(17): p. 1775-1784.

[52] Erro, R., et al., Progressive Parkinsonism, balance difficulties, and supranuclear gaze palsy. *Jama Neurology*, 2014. 71(1): p. 104-107.
[53] Bartels, A., et al., Decreased blood-brain barrier P-glycoprotein function in the progression of Parkinson's disease, PSP and MSA. *Journal of Neural Transmission*, 2008. 115(7): p. 1001-1009.
[54] Vogelgesang, S., et al., Cerebrovascular P-glycoprotein expression is decreased in Creutzfeldt-Jakob disease. *Acta Neuropathologica*, 2006. 111(5): p. 436.
[55] Zlokovic, B. V., The blood-brain barrier in health and chronic neurodegenerative disorders. *Neuron*, 2008. 57(2): p. 178-201.
[56] Hernández-Montiel, H. L., et al., Phytochemicals Effects on Neurodegenerative Diseases. *Fruit and Vegetable Phytochemicals*, 2017: p. 85-114.
[57] Van Vliet, E. A., et al., Expression and Cellular Distribution of P-Glycoprotein and Breast Cancer Resistance Protein in Amyotrophic Lateral Sclerosis Patients. *Journal of Neuropathology & Experimental Neurology*, 2020. 79(3): p. 266-276.
[58] Zlokovic, B. V., Neurovascular pathways to neurodegeneration in Alzheimer's disease and other disorders. *Nature Reviews Neuroscience*, 2011. 12(12): p. 723-738.
[59] Alaskar, H. and A. J. Hussain. Data mining to support the discrimination of amyotrophic lateral sclerosis diseases based on gait analysis. In: *International Conference on Intelligent Computing*. 2018. Springer.
[60] Ahad, M. A., et al., Insights into the neuropathology of cerebral ischemia and its mechanisms. *Reviews in the Neurosciences*, 2020. 31(5): p. 521-538.
[61] Fang, W., et al., Penetration of verapamil across blood brain barrier following cerebral ischemia depending on both paracellular pathway and P-glycoprotein transportation. *Neurochemistry International*, 2013. 62(1): p. 23-30.

[62] DeMars, K. M., et al., Spatiotemporal changes in P-glycoprotein levels in brain and peripheral tissues following ischemic stroke in rats. *Journal of Experimental Neuroscience*, 2017. 11: p. 1179069517701741.

[63] Ji, B. S., et al., Modulation of P-glycoprotein in rat brain microvessel endothelial cells under oxygen glucose deprivation. *Journal of Pharmacy and Pharmacology*, 2013. 65(10): p. 1508-1517.

In: An Introduction to P-Glycoprotein ISBN: 978-1-53619-488-3
Editors: M. Wahajuddin et al.

Chapter 10

P-GLYCOPROTEIN POLYMORPHISM: GENETIC AND EPIGENETIC CHANGES

Tarique Mahmood Ansari[1,*], Mohammad Haris Siddiqui[2], Malik Mobeen[3], Farogh Ahsan[1] and Arshiya Shamim[1]

[1]Faculty of Pharmacy, Integral University, Lucknow, Uttar Pradesh, India
[2]Department of Bioengineering, Integral University, Lucknow, Uttar Pradesh, India
[3]Integral Institute of Agricultural Sciences & Technology, Integral University, Lucknow, Uttar Pradesh, India

ABSTRACT

P-glycoprotein (Pgp) is an efflux transporter highly expressed in the apical (luminal) membrane lining the gut, with its high expression in the enterocytes of the small intestine. It reduces the oral availability of drugs that act as its substrates. Like the enzymes involved in drug metabolism, substrates of P-glycoprotein can potentially act as inhibitors or inducers of

* Corresponding Author's Email: ansaritariq79@yahoo.co.in.

its function. Inhibition of Pgp can result in increased bioavailability of the susceptible drug and induction of Pgp reduces the bioavailability, likewise. The gene MDR1 (ATP Binding Cassette-B1) is responsible to encode for specific amino acids that polymerise to form Pgp. This chapter focuses on intricacies of Pgp expression amounting to genetic as well as epigenetic changes, which can help in tackling the issue of drug resistance offered to several chemotherapeutic, immunosuppressive and hormonal drugs. Controlled Pgp expression is the key to manipulate pharmacokinetic profiles of drugs from different classes (Anti-neoplastic, Cardiac glycosides, Antihistaminics, Anti-Thyroid, etc.) making pharmacotherapy more patient compliant and effective.

Keywords: bioavailability, drug absorption, drug elimination, inhibitors, multidrug resistance, substrates

Introduction

P-glycoprotein or permeability glycoprotein (abbreviated as Pgp or P-gp) is a significant drug transporter protein found in plasma membrane of the cells which decides the in and out of a variety of drugs and steroids from cells (Uhr et al., 2002). P-gp is an associate of the highly conserved superfamily of ATP-binding cassette (ABC) transporter proteins [1]. Depending upon the role as functional barrier and as an efflux transporter in different tissues, it has a number of other names like multidrug resistance protein 1 (MDR1) or ATP binding cassette sub-family B member 1 (ABCB1) [2] or cluster of differentiation 243 (CD243) or ABC20, CLCS, GP170, PGY1. It is basically an ATP-dependent transmembrane efflux pump with broad-range specificity, pumping its drug molecules from inside to outside the cell, thereby affecting the drug concentration in cytoplasm and finally their effect on cells. Due to its defensive mechanism against detrimental substances, almost all the living organisms like animals, fungi and bacteria also carried this gene.

Victor Ling discovered the P-glycoprotein, one of the proteins responsible for multidrug resistance, while studying drug resistance in cancer. The ABCB1 or MDR1 gene, encoding the P-glycoprotein, is located on chromosome 7q21.1 [3], consists of both 28 introns and exons. ABCB1 mRNA is of 4.7 kb in size with a coding region of 120 kb which further gets translated into 1280 aa arranged in two tandem repeats of 610 aa, attached with a linker region of 60 amino acids [4] having a molecular weight of 170 kDa (Pauli-Magnus and Kroetz, 2004). Pgp is a well-characterized and studied ATP-binding cassette (ABC)-transporter of the MDR/TAP subfamily [5]. The first mammalian P-glycoprotein structure was reported by Aller et al. (2009) which was derived from the mouse MDR3 gene product heterologously and expressed in *Pichia* spp. Functional studies recommend that different domains of P-glycoprotein must work together with each other for transport to take place. This means that coupling of ATPase activity to drug binding involves both homologous halves of the molecule [6]. In humans, the ABCB1 protein is extensively localized in liver, kidney, intestine and endothelial cells of the blood-brain barrier [7]. The apical or luminal epithelial Pgp effluxes the hydrophobic substrates including drugs such as colchicine, Adriamycin, etoposide (VP16) and vinblastine as well as steroids, lipids, peptides and xenobiotics [8, 9] back into the gastrointestinal tract, in liver cells which in turn pumps to bile ducts, then into proximal tubules of the kidney and then into and urine which further restricts the entrance of certain drugs into CNS. Its usual excretion back into the gut lumen by Pgp pharmacokinetically decreases the efficacy of foreign substances. Additionally, some cancerous cells also express Pgp in significant amount which further amplifies the effect and provide resistant for several drugs.

The *PGP* gene has comprehensively been studied for distinguishing polymorphisms and almost 50 SNPs for *PGP* genes have been recognized [10]. Out of these SNPs, the most commonly studied polymorphisms of the *ABCB1* gene are C1236T (rs1128503), G2677T/A (rs2032582) and C3435T (rs1045642). Genetic variants associated with a change in the amount or activity of transport proteins lead to the loss of the physiological role of these proteins and altered various drugs transporter's functions [11, 12].

These three most common *ABCB1* SNPs in the Caucasian population have been found to be in linkage disequilibrium. The allelic frequencies of these three SNPs are highly variable between ethnic groups. The most widely studied variant of *ABCB1* is a commonly synonymous C to T transition at nucleotide position 3435 in exon 26 (3435 C > T). Although this transition does not change its encoded amino acid with Ile at position 114522, TT variant has been significantly associated with the decreased mRNA expression and protein stability and may have reduced the drug transport capacity [13]. So far the effect of synonymous polymorphisms on the protein has not been fully understood. On the other hand, it is believed that they can influence the post-transcriptional processing of mRNA by interfering with the process of taking out introns or affect the process of alternative transcript splicing. In addition, as Kimchi-Sarfaty et al. (2007) pointed out, replacing as a result of silent polymorphisms often used in translation of codons into rare ones can affect the rate of protein folding, and thus change its function or change its substrate specificity. On the other hand, synonymous polymorphisms can modify the structure and/or function of a protein by coupling to non-synonymous polymorphisms that directly change the amino acid sequence of a protein [14, 15].

SNPs denote isolated nucleotide differences between individuals and represent the most common class of sequence variations throughout the human genome. On the basis of their location in the genome, SNPs can be classified as random SNPs (most common SNPs found in intergenic deoxyribonucleic acid region or in the introns of genes), coding SNPs (found in the exons representing the translated regions of a gene), and noncoding SNPs (found outside the translated regions of a gene such as the promoter and 5' and 3' untranslated regions). Of specific interest to pharmacogenetics are coding SNPs because they can result in encoded amino acid changes. Nonsynonymous SNPs refer to polymorphisms that result in amino acid changes, whereas synonymous SNPs do not lead to amino acid changes.

Genetic polymorphisms were first identified from *in vitro* studies with cancer cells. To date, 29 SNPs have been reported in the MDR1 gene. Nineteen SNPs are located in the exonic regions and 11 are nonsynonymous. Interestingly, SNPs at exon 21 in position 2677 can result in 2 distinct amino acid changes, namely, Ala893Ser (G2677T) and Ala893Thr (G2677A). However, a synonymous SNP in exon 26 (C3435T) was the first variant to be associated with altered protein expression, although the SNP does not change the encoded amino acid (Ile).89 In the same study P-gp expression in the duodenum of individuals with the homozygous T allele (variant) was noted to be decreased when compared with that in individuals with the C allele (wild type). Other studies have shown that SNPs at exon 21 (G2677T/A) and at exon 1b (T129C) may be associated with altered transporter function or expression. Studies from this laboratory demonstrated that a linkage disequilibrium exists between SNPs in exon 26 (C3435T) and exon 21 (G2677T/A), suggesting that the observed functional differences in P-gp, initially attributed to the exon 26 synonymous SNP, may be the result of the associated nonsynonymous polymorphism in exon 21. The existence of such distinct haplotypes has been further confirmed by several groups. Three common haplotype combinations appear to be observed across all ethnic groups. These haplotype combinations are found in more than 70% of the individuals reported in most studies, confirming the strong linkage disequilibrium between exon 26 and 21. It has also been recently shown that a synonymous SNP in exon 12 (C1236T) is linked to the exon 26 (C3435T) and 21 (G2677T/A) SNPs. Similarly, when the possible genotypic combinations of MDR1 polymorphisms in exons 26, 21, and 12 were examined, more than 50% of the studied individuals appeared to have strong linkage disequilibrium at the 3 loci.

P-glycoprotein, the most extensively studied ATP-binding cassette (ABC) transporter, functions as a biological barrier by extruding toxins and xenobiotics out of cells. *In vitro* and *in vivo* studies have demonstrated that P-glycoprotein plays a significant role in drug absorption and disposition. Because of its localization, P-glycoprotein appears to have a greater impact on limiting cellular uptake of drugs from blood circulation into brain and from intestinal lumen into epithelial cells than on enhancing the excretion of drugs out of hepatocytes and renal tubules into the adjacent luminal space. However, the relative contribution of intestinal P-glycoprotein to overall drug absorption is unlikely to be quantitatively important unless a very small oral dose is given, or the dissolution and diffusion rates of the drug are very slow. This is because P-glycoprotein transport activity becomes saturated by high concentrations of drug in the intestinal lumen.

Because of its importance in pharmacokinetics, P-glycoprotein transport screening has been incorporated into the drug discovery process, aided by the availability of transgenic *mdr* knockout mice and *in vitro* cell systems. When applying *in vitro* and *in vivo* screening models to study P-glycoprotein function, there are two fundamental questions: (i) can *in vitro* data be accurately extrapolated to the *in vivo* situation; and (ii) can animal data be directly scaled up to humans? Current information from our laboratory suggests that *in vivo* P-glycoprotein activity for a given drug can be extrapolated reasonably well from *in vitro* data. On the other hand, there are significant species differences in P-glycoprotein transport activity between humans and animals, and the species differences appear to be substrate-dependent.

Inhibition and induction of P-glycoprotein have been reported as the causes of drug-drug interactions. The potential risk of P-glycoprotein-mediated drug interactions may be greatly underestimated if only plasma concentration is monitored. From animal studies, it is clear that P-glycoprotein inhibition always has a much greater impact on tissue distribution, particularly with regard to the brain, than on plasma concentrations. Therefore, the potential risk of P-glycoprotein-mediated drug interactions should be assessed carefully. Because of overlapping substrate specificity between cytochrome P450 (CYP) 3A4 and P-glycoprotein, and because of similarities in P-glycoprotein and CYP3A4 inhibitors and inducers, many drug interactions involve both P-glycoprotein and CYP3A4. Unless the relative contribution of P-glycoprotein and CYP3A4 to drug interactions can be quantitatively estimated, care should be taken when exploring the underlying mechanism of such interactions [16].

P-glycoprotein was first identified by Juliano and Ling as a surface phosphoglycoprotein expressed in drug-resistant Chinese hamster ovary cells [17]. This discovery led to the finding that P-glycoprotein is an energy-dependent efflux transporter driven by ATP hydrolysis. In humans, two members of the P-glycoprotein gene family (*MDR1* and *MDR3*) exist, while three members of this family (*mdr1a*, *mdr1b* and *mdr2*) are found in mice [18]. The P-glycoprotein encoded by the human *MDR1* and mouse *mdr1a/1b* genes functions as a drug efflux transporter, whereas human *MDR3* P-glycoprotein and mouse *mdr2* P-glycoprotein are believed to be functional in phospholipid transport [19]. However, the involvement of human *MDR3* P-glycoprotein in drug transport has been recently reported. An increased directional transport of digoxin, paclitaxel and vinblastine across polarised monolayers of *MDR3*-transfected cells has recently been reported by Smith et al. [20]. These results suggest that *MDR3* P-glycoprotein is also able to transport a range of drugs in addition to phospholipids.

In addition to the expression in tumour cells, human P-glycoprotein is also highly expressed in normal tissues. This transporter is localised on the canalicular surface of hepatocytes in liver, the apical surface of epithelial cells of proximal tubules in kidneys, columnar epithelial cells of intestine, epithelial cells of placenta, and the luminal surface of capillary endothelial cells in brain in humans [21]. The anatomical localisation of P-glycoprotein expression suggests that the efflux transporter can functionally protect the body against toxic xenobiotics by excreting these compounds into bile, urine and the intestinal lumen, and by preventing their accumulation in brain. Because of its localisation, it is believed that P-glycoprotein may play a significant role in the processes of absorption, distribution, metabolism and excretion of drugs in humans and animals. Indeed, the role of P-glycoprotein in drug absorption and disposition has been demonstrated *in vivo* using *mdr1a* and *mdr1a/1b* knockout mice [22]. A lack of either one of the two murine P-glycoproteins (*mdr1a* or *mdr1b*) results in significant changes in drug absorption and disposition.

The purpose of this review is to briefly summaries the current knowledge regarding the structure and mechanism of drug-transporting P-glycoprotein and its role in drug absorption, distribution, metabolism and excretion. In addition, the potential for P-glycoprotein-mediated drug-drug interactions and its clinical implications will be discussed.

ROLE OF MDR1 GENE IN PGP POLYMORPHISM

The drug metabolism is majorly influenced by two important factors: the Multidrug resistance 1 (MDR1) and the metabolic enzyme CYP3A. The

MDR1 gene polymorphism, encodes a protein that affects the expression and function of Pgp [23]. More than 50 single nucleotide polymorphisms in MDR1, and the two common gene polymorphisms affecting MDR1 gene function in exon 26 (C3435T) and exon 12 (C1236T) [24] respectively, have been studied. The C1236T is a synonymous mutation that does not cause amino acid change [25]. Although, the C3435T is the only codon change discovered in MDR1 gene affecting the expression of Pgp in varying organs and tissues as well as in population of different ethnicities [26]. Pgp, being one of the most important causes of drug resistance [27, 28] is touted to be the main reason of steroid resistance in hormone-resistant Systemic lupus erythematosus (SLE) patients [29]. Many drugs commonly used to treat SLE, such as methotrexate, glucocorticoids, etc. are Pgp substrates, which could be pumped out of the cell by Pgp, thereby reducing their intracellular concentrations [30, 31]. Some drugs can inhibit the function of Pgp, such as cyclosporine [32].

Some drugs have been identified that suppress the expression of Pgp from major expression sites like intestinal lumen and hepato-canalalicular cells. In order to minimise this drug resistance towards varied chemotherapeutic agents by Pgp, these agents could be therapeutically explored. Studies advocate that by use of Pgp inhibitors, the drug resistance could be reversed. However, these claims have their own set of repercussions as down regulation of Pgp expression can affect the detoxification process of human system and amplify the adverse events of anticancer drugs. Cyclosporine, for example, serves as a transport substrate of Pgp competitively inhibiting the expression and reversing steroid resistance in a cancer patient [33]. Likewise, mycophenolic acid has been also reported to show inhibitory effects on Pgp activity of lymphocyte cell lines, but its effect is significantly weaker than Pgp specific blocking agents like cyclophosphamide [34]. Based on the mentioned study, hormones and some immunosuppressive agents are classified as substrates of Pgp, which can be clinically explored in the formation of MDR in SLE patients. Therefore, it is important to explore the role of MDR1 genotype and Pgp in patients with refractory SLE. Table 1, given in the latter section of chapter summarises few drugs that act as substrates or inhibitors for Pgp. The drugs whose metabolism and elimination is increased by expression of Pgp are termed as Pgp substrates and the ones who inhibit the Pgp expression are called Pgp inhibitors [35, 36].

Role of ATP-Binding Cassette-B1 (ABCB1) in Pgp Polymorphism

Pgp/ABCB1 is a glycosylated 170-kDa transmembrane protein that is encoded by the MDR1 gene [37] and is the best studied drug efflux pump of the family of ABC transporters. Pgp is composed of two hydrophobic domains which include 12 transmembrane α-helices that make up the drug binding domains (DBD) and are involved in transporting toxins and xenobiotics out of the cell. Although the ABCB1-polymorphisms (messenger RNA and protein expression) in various tissues (e.g., the liver, gut and heart) is very low quantitatively but these polymorphisms and subsequent haplotypes of ABCB1formed have been found to be associated with alterations in drug disposition and drug response. Such drugs are referred as ABCB1 substrates. The adverse events with various ABCB1 substrates in different ethnic populations are also attributed to be associated with ABCB1-Pgp polymorphism. However, the results have been highly conflicting, with confined clinical relevance at hand. Pgp may also have a role in the distribution of certain endocrine hormones, for example the thyroid hormones (T_3 & T_4) resulting in resistance to drugs used for treatment of hypo and hyperthyroidism. The relationship between Pgp and the high levels of serum free T3 in hyperthyroidism patients, requires further research to set the facts straight. ABCB1 expression is particularly elevated in cancerous cells of normal Pgp expressing tissues, such as the liver, kidney and adrenal gland as well as the colorectal epithelium, and these tumors are intrinsically resistant to most drugs. The expression of Pgp and levels of *ABCB1* mRNA correlate with pathological grading of colorectal tumors; high levels are observed in advance stage tumors and lower levels in early stage tumors. In recent years, an association between Pgp expression levels in different tissues and genetic polymorphisms of the ABCB1 gene has been reported [38].

The increased expression of ATP-binding cassette (ABC) transporters is sometimes associated with multidrug resistance (MDR) in cancer chemotherapies. There are currently no approved drugs available for clinical use in cancer chemotherapies to reverse MDR by inhibiting Pgp. Simulation studies have previously identified several compounds that inhibit Pgp by targeting its nucleotide binding domain (Table 1). Out of these compounds, many are reported to means successful MDR reversal when tested on a selected cell line. Despite advances in chemotherapies against cancer, multidrug resistance (MDR) remains a heavy obstacle to positive therapeutic outcomes in adult furthermore as pediatric cancers [39]. ABCB1 family Pgp (Pgp/ABCB1) is that the foremost typical explanation for MDR. The overexpression of this efflux pump (Pgp), reduces the intracellular accumulation of the various anticancer drugs to sub-therapeutic levels, thereby, decreasing or abolishing chemotherapeutic efficacy [40]. Two nucleotide binding domains within the cytoplasmic region are guilty for coupling ATP hydrolysis to the transport processes [41]. Pgp is expressed in an exceedingly very very reasonably normal tissues, almost like the intestine, brain, liver, placenta, kidney, and others and is protective against xenobiotic substances and toxic compounds. It absolutely was noted near 40 years ago that the expression of P-gp is correlated with MDR in many alternative varieties of cancers10, moreover because the dearth of response to chemotherapies and poor prognoses in breast and ovarian cancers [42]. Overexpression of P-gp in cancers ends up in reduced accumulation of chemotherapeutics and ends up in resistance against many of the currently available anti-cancer drugs like taxanes (paclitaxel), vinca alkaloids (vinblastine), and anthracyclines (daunorubicin). The flexibleness of P-gp to maneuver such diverse chemical classes is additionally a minimum of partly due to multiple transport pathways through the protein which are recently visualized using molecular dynamics simulations14. Studies show that overexpression of P-gp in cancers is either intrinsic or acquired upon drug treatment, looking forward to the tissue of origin [43]. Clinical trials using MDR-inhibitors have had only limited successbut the potential of the approach is appreciated from a trial that used cyclosporine to inhibit P-gp in patients with poor-risk acute leucaemia [44]. Inclusion of the inhibitor with therapy resulted in significant gains in relapse-free and overall survival [45-47]. The difficulties in clinical trials as discussed in were mainly thanks to inhibitor toxicities, drug-interactions, and trial design problems [48, 49]. Many of the initial inhibitors were P-gp transport substrates requiring relatively high systemic concentrations for efficacy; others lacked specificity for P-gp and led to drug interactions [50]. None of these complications, however, diminish the impact or significance that employing effective P-gp inhibitors in cancer chemotherapies would wear patient outcomes of the P-gp inhibitors studied here make them attractive leads for further development. While chemotherapy resistances may have a variety of causes, multidrug resistance is usually caused by the overexpression of P-gp or closely related members of the ABC-transporter family [51]. Unfortunately, up to now none of the P-gp inhibitors previously identified and pursued as potential co-therapeutics for treatment of MDR diseases has been successful in clinical trials [52]. the foremost recent trials employing the P-gp inhibitor, tariquidar, suffered from toxicities and kind of other clinical test|phase III|clinical trial|clinical test} run trials are abandoned [53]. A test trial with another P-gp inhibitor, zosuquidar-54, was recently completed, but didn't show improved outcomes in older leukaemia patients. The authors of the study speculated that resistances unrelated to P-gp were the cause for the negative outcomes. Despite these set-backs, the potential of P-gp inhibition to spice up cancer patient outcomes was demonstrated in an earlier randomized test trial with poor-risk, acute cancer of the blood patients [54]. These data indicated that positive effects from inhibitors were most prominent in patients with increased P-gp expression. Despite limited success within the clinic, P-gp still seems a very important and relevant target for drug discovery and development. More moderen advances within the knowledge of the structure and mechanism of P-gp yet because the related drug pumps will likely help discovery of specific inhibitors of specific pumps in an exceedingly more rational way [55]. Many of the inhibitors previously pursued are thought to bind to the drug binding domains and inhibit chemotherapeutic export by functioning as P-gp transport substrates and competing for transport cycles. This characteristic likely led to the requirement for relatively high systemic concentrations causing astray toxicities.

EPIGENETIC ROLE OF P-GLYCOPROTEIN IN ALTERATION OF PHARMACOKINETICS

Although the physiological function for P-glycoprotein is still not fully understood, the role of this efflux transporter in pharmacokinetics is becoming increasingly appreciated. In humans, P-glycoprotein is found on the apical surface of columnar epithelial cells of small and large intestines, the biliary canalicular membrane of hepatocytes, the apical surface of epithelial cells of the proximal tubules of kidney, the apical surface of epithelial cells of placenta and the apical surface of endothelial cells in blood capillaries of the brain [56]. Because of its strategic localisation, the P-glycoprotein transporter functionally can limit cellular uptake of drugs from the blood circulation into the brain and placenta, and from the gastrointestinal lumen into the enterocyte. On the other hand, this transporter can also enhance the elimination of drugs from hepatocytes, renal tubules and intestinal epithelial cells into the adjacent luminal space. Therefore, it is very important to distinguish the localisation of P-glycoprotein in cells in relation to drug movement — either uptake of drugs into cells or excretion of drugs out of cells. As will be discussed later, there is a tendency for P-glycoprotein to have a greater impact on drug uptake than on drug excretion.

Perhaps the most important milestone in P-glycoprotein research was the development of *mdr* knockout mice. Since *mdr* knockout mice became available, our understanding of the role of P-glycoprotein in pharmacokinetics has increased exponentially. As discussed above, mice have two types of drug-transporting P-glycoprotein (mdr1a and mdr1b), which are expressed in a tissue-specific manner [57]. For example, only mdr1a P-glycoprotein is expressed in the brain and intestine of mice, while both mdr1a and mdr1b P-glycoprotein are expressed in the liver and kidney. Interestingly, mdr1a and mdr1b P-glycoprotein together appear to cover the same tissues as the single human MDR1 P-glycoprotein, suggesting that mdr1a and mdr1b together fulfil the same function as the single P-glycoprotein in humans. Because of tissue-specific expression, it is expected that genetic disruption of the *mdr1a* gene would have a greater impact on drug uptake into the brain and intestine than drug excretion from the liver and kidney.

Table 1. Substrates and Inhibitors of Pgp

Gene (Protein)	Substrates	Inhibitors	Reference
MDR1-Gut/Apical ABCB1 (Pgp)	Digoxin,	GG918, verapamil, Progesterone, Gomisin A, Valspodar, Elacridar	Overview of P-glycoprotein inhibitors: a rational outlook Kale Mohana Raghava Srivalli, P. K. Lakshmi* Department of Pharmaceutics, G.
	Fexofenadine		
	Indinavir		
	Vincristine		
	Colchicine		
	Topotecan		
	Paclitaxel		
	Cimetidine		
	Bromocriptine		

In addition, it should be noted that genetic disruption of one or both of the *mdr* genes might affect the expression and function of other transporter systems or even drug-metabolising enzyme systems in mice. For example, it is known that the *mdr1b* gene is upregulated in *mdr1a* knockout mice [58]. Recently, Schuetz et al. [59] have reported that both the protein expression and catalytic activity of CYP is significantly increased in the *mdr*1a, *mdr*1b and *mdr*1a/1b knockout mice housed in The Netherlands. However, for the genetically identical *mdr1a* and *mdr1a/1b* knockout mice housed in the US, there were no significant changes in their protein expression and catalytic activity of CYP. Because of the possible existence of unrecognized factors that are associated with the genetic disruption, data derived from *mdr1a* single knockout mice or from *mdr1a/1b* double knockout mice have to be interpreted with caution.

COMPOUNDS THAT EPIGENETICALLY INTERACT WITH P-GP

P-gp recognizes and effluxes a multitude of structurally and biochemically unrelated substrates (cyclic, linear, basic, uncharged, zwitterionic, negatively charged, hydrophobic, aromatic, nonaromatic, amphipathic) from 250 to 4000 molecular weight [60], sufficiently indeterminate to predict in drug design. Substrates include xenobiotics, endogenous compounds [e.g., peptides (including β-amyloids), steroid hormones, lipids, phospholipids, cholesterol, and cytokines] [61], pharmaceuticals [62], nutraceuticals (e.g., St John's wort), dietary compounds (e.g., grapefruit juice, green tea) [63], and other compounds, which may also modulate P-gp activity [64]. P-gp compounds can act as substrates, inhibitors, inducers, and repressors; and citations refer to P-gp compounds as being in more than one category, depending on the circumstance. Modulation of *ABCB1* gene expression and/or P-gp activity by various mechanisms consequently influences P-gp-mediated drug disposition.

Repressors of P-gp, including certain antineoplastic agents that act at nuclear receptors [65], or endotoxin [66], cobalamin [67], and atorvastatin [68], potentiate the action of substrates; whereas rifampin (rifampicin) [69] and cell stress signals induce P-gp-mediated drug resistance. Another mechanism for P-gp-related pharmacoresistance to cytotoxic agents is hypothesized to relate to the cell stress signals they induce. Upregulation of *ABCB1* gene expression can occur at gene promoter sequences through transactivation, for example, by the pregnane X receptor (*NR1I2*) gene in response to substrates that may have overlapping specificity for P-gp; or induction can occur independent of nuclear receptors. Alternatively, epigenetic inactivation of P-gp can occur by DNA methylation at specific nucleotide sequences within the promoter sequence, called CpG islands, as has been observed in some cancer tissues; or downregulation of P-gp can also occur by mechanisms other than by DNA methylation, for example, in response to cobalamin, a vitamin B-12 derivative [70].

DRUG INTERACTIONS

P-glycoprotein is an important mediator of drug-drug interactions. The pharmacokinetics of a drug may be altered when co-administered with compounds which inhibit or induce P-glycoprotein. Inhibitors include clarithromycin, erythromycin, ritonavir and verapamil. Inducers include rifampicin and St John's wort.

P-glycoprotein has a very wide substrate spectrum similar to CYP3A4. It is involved in the transport of drugs from different drug classes including:

(a) Antineoplastic Drugs e.g., Docetaxel, Etoposide, Vincristine
(b) Calcium Channel Blockers e.g., Amlodipine
(c) Calcineurin Inhibitors e.g., Cyclosporin, Tacrolimus
(d) Digoxin
(e) Macrolide Antibiotics e.g., Clarithromycin
(f) Protease Inhibitors.

The substrates of P-glycoprotein can be further divided into drugs which are not metabolized in humans, such as digoxin, and those which are substrates of both P-glycoprotein and drug-metabolizing enzymes, particularly CYP3A4. As many P-glycoprotein substrates are alsosubstrates of CYP3A4 and because P-glycoprotein inhibitors are also inhibitors of CYP3A4, many drug-drug interactions are related to inhibition or induction of both P-glycoprotein and CYP3A4. Drugs which are 'objects' of such interactions include cyclosporin, tacrolimus and rivaroxaban [71]. Enterocytes, like hepatocytes, simultaneously express the major drug-metabolizing enzyme CYP3A4 and the efflux transporter P-glycoprotein. This creates a drug efflux–metabolism 'alliance', which increases the exposure of the drug to metabolism by CYP3A4 through repeated cycles of absorption and efflux. Modification of this active barrier function by concomitantly administered drugs contributes to altered absorption, increased interindividual differences in systemic drug concentrations and probably an increased risk of toxicity [72].

Accurate prediction of potential drug-drug interactions through P-glycoprotein is complicated by pronounced interindividual differences in bioavailability. This also affects drugs that are not metabolised in humans (fexofenadine, digoxin). A better knowledge of the role of genetics in transporter expression and function will contribute to a better understanding of interindividual and interethnic differences in drug disposition and effects [73].

Drug Interactions Leading to Epigenetic Changes

Many studies have characterized the interactions among P-gp compounds, as concomitant administration can substantially alter the pharmacokinetics of the compounds involved [74]. Research has focused on both the deleterious and beneficial effects of interactions among P-gp compounds: (i) interactions that potentially affect drug safety and efficacy [75], and (ii) interactions exploited to optimize drug delivery (see MDR).

Drug safety and efficacy are major health concerns, particulary for drugs with a narrow therapeutic index and/or large clinical effect [76]. A number of drug interactions of clinical relevance are cited as warnings in the drug labels by the Federal Drug Administration. For example, the drug label for the contraceptive, Trinessa (Watson Pharma, Inc.), warns against potential drug inefficacy when coadministered with compounds that induce P-gp (e.g., rifampin, St John's wort, protease inhibitors, carbamazepine, and barbiturates). The drug label for the antidiarrheal, loperamide (Imodium, McNeil Consumer Healthcare), warns against neurotoxic side effects when coadministered with P-gp inhibitors (e.g., quinidine, ritonavir) as this gut-targeted optiate relies upon P-gp to prohibit intestinal absorption and entry into the central nervous system [77].

Interactions between compounds are substrate-specific, concentration-dependent [78], and tissue-specific [79] For example, unlike the drug-potentiating interaction between quinine or ritonavir [80] on loperamide, the potent P-gp inhibitor, tariquidarr, does not produce the same analgesic effects, despite its efficient inhibition of P-gp in lymphocytes. This is presumably because of tissue-specific factors [81]. Concentration is another important determinant of drug interactions. For example, at the therapeutic concentration for the β blocker and P-gp substrate, propranolol (Innopran Xl, Reliant Pharmaceuticals Inc.), modulation of P-gp by other compounds does not affect propranolol disposition. Other influences include key pharmacokinetic genes that affect the disposition of substrates for P-gp. For example, P-gp and cytochrome P450 3A4 metabolizing enzyme (*CYP3A4*) overlap in tissue distribution and specificity for a substantial number of substrates, inducers, and inhibitors [82-83]. Furthermore, genes responsible for the disposition of a drug can act synergistically [84]. Marchetti et al. cite clinically relevant drug interactions influenced by the interplay of *ABCB1* with other genes in the disposition of P-gp compounds, such as paclitaxel and cyclosporine A (CsA) (through *CYP3A4* inhibition), digoxin and rifampin (through *CYP3A4* induction), and topotecan and elacridar (through *ABCG2* inhibition) [85].

Conclusion

The multidrug resistance (MDR1) gene product P-glycoprotein is a membrane protein that functions as an ATP-dependent efflux pump, transporting exogenous and endogenous substrates from the inside of cells to the outside. Physiological expression of P-glycoprotein in tissues with excretory or protective function is a major determinant of drug disposition and provides a cellular defense mechanism against potentially harmful compounds. Therefore, P-glycoprotein has significant impact on therapeutic efficacy and toxicity as it plays a key role in absorption of oral medications from the intestinal tract, excretion into bile and urine, and distribution into protected tissues such as the brain and testes. There is increasing interest in the possible role of genetic variation in MDR1 in drug therapy. Numerous genetic polymorphisms in MDR1 have been described, some of which have been shown to determine Pglycoprotein expression levels and substrate transport. Furthermore, some of these polymorphisms have an impact on pharmacokinetic and pharmacodynamic profiles of drug substrates and directly influence outcome and prognosis of certain diseases.

REFERENCES

[1] Ambudkar, Suresh V; Saibal Dey, Christine A. Hrycyna, Muralidhara Ramachandra, Ira Pastan, Michael M. Gottesman. "Biochemical, cellular, and pharmacological aspects of the multidrug transporter." *Annual review of pharmacology and toxicology*, 39, no. 1, (1999), 361-398.

[2] Callen, DF; Baker, E; Simmers, RN; Seshadri, R; Roninson, IB. "Localization of the human multiple drug resistance gene, MDR1, to 7q21. 1." *Human genetics*, 77, no. 2, (1987), 142-144.

[3] Uhr, M; Holsboer, F; Müller, MB. "Penetration of endogenous steroid hormones corticosterone, cortisol, aldosterone and progesterone into the brain is enhanced in mice deficient for both mdr1a and mdr1b P-glycoproteins." *Journal of neuroendocrinology*, 14, no. 9, (2002), 753-759.

[4] Ieiri, Ichiro, Hiroshi Takane, Kenji Otsubo. "The MDR1 (ABCB1) gene polymorphism and its clinical implications." *Clinical pharmacokinetics*, 43, no. 9, (2004), 553-576.

[5] Pauli-Magnus, Christiane, Deanna L. Kroetz. "Functional implications of genetic polymorphisms in the multidrug resistance gene MDR1 (ABCB1)." *Pharmaceutical research*, 21, no. 6, (2004), 904-913.

[6] Pauli-Magnus, Christiane, Deanna L. Kroetz. "Functional implications of genetic polymorphisms in the multidrug resistance gene MDR1 (ABCB1)." *Pharmaceutical research*, 21, no. 6, (2004), 904-913.

[7] Chen, Wen-Hsiang, Shivali M. Chag, Mohan V. Poongavanam, Amadeo B. Biter, Ebe A. Ewere, Wanderson Rezende, Christopher A. Seid; et al. "Optimization of the production process and characterization of the yeast-expressed SARS-CoV recombinant receptor-binding domain (RBD219-N1), a SARS vaccine candidate." *Journal of pharmaceutical sciences*, 106, no. 8, (2017), 1961-1970.

[8] Gottesman, Michael M; Tito Fojo, Susan E. Bates. "Multidrug resistance in cancer: role of ATP–dependent transporters." *Nature Reviews Cancer*, 2, no. 1, (2002), 48-58.

[9] Ambudkar, Suresh V; John N. Abelson, Michael M. Gottesman, Melvin I. Simon. eds. *ABC Transporters: Biochemical, cellular, and molecular aspects*. Vol. 292. Gulf Professional Publishing, 1998.

[10] Chen, Chang Jie, Douglas Clark, Kazumitsu Ueda, Ira Pastan, Michael M. Gottesman, Igor B. Roninson. "Genomic organization of the human multidrug resistance (MDR1) gene and origin of P-glycoproteins." *Journal of Biological Chemistry*, 265, no. 1, (1990), 506-514.

[11] Loo, Tip W; Clarke, DM. "Reconstitution of drug-stimulated ATPase activity following co-expression of each half of human P-glycoprotein as separate polypeptides." *Journal of Biological Chemistry*, 269, no. 10, (1994), 7750-7755.

[12] Aller, Stephen G., Jodie Yu, Andrew Ward, Yue Weng, Srinivas Chittaboina, Rupeng Zhuo, Patina M. Harrell; et al. "Structure of P-glycoprotein reveals a molecular basis for poly-specific drug binding." *Science*, 323, no. 5922, (2009), 1718-1722.

[13] Hamidovic, Alma, Kristine Hahn, Jill Kolesar. "Clinical significance of ABCB1 genotyping in oncology." *Journal of Oncology Pharmacy Practice*, 16, no. 1, (2010), 39-44.

[14] Liu, Hai, Zhong-Kun Yang, Yan Li, Wen-Jia Zhang, Ying-Ting Wang, Xuan-Chu Duan. "ABCB1 variants confer susceptibility to primary open-angle glaucoma and predict individual differences to latanoprost treatment." *Biomedicine & Pharmacotherapy*, 80, (2016), 115-120.

[15] Au, Anthony, Abdul Aziz Baba, Ai Sim Goh, S. Abdul Wahid Fadilah, Alan Teh, Hassan Rosline, Ravindran Ankathil. "Association of genotypes and haplotypes of multi-drug transporter genes ABCB1 and ABCG2 with clinical response to imatinib mesylate in chronic myeloid leukemia patients." *Biomedicine & Pharmacotherapy*, 68, no. 3, (2014), 343-349.

[16] Lin, Jiunn H; Masayo Yamazaki. "Role of P-glycoprotein in pharmacokinetics." *Clinical pharmacokinetics*, 42, no. 1, (2003), 59-98.

[17] Juliano, R. Lâ, Ling, V. "A surface glycoprotein modulating drug permeability in Chinese hamster ovary cell mutants." *Biochimica et Biophysica Acta (BBA)-Biomembranes*, 455, no. 1, (1976), 152-162.

[18] Gottesman, Michael M; Ira Pastan. "Biochemistry of multidrug resistance mediated by the multidrug transporter." *Annual review of biochemistry*, 62, no. 1, (1993), 385-427.

[19] Gottesman, Michael M; Ira Pastan. "Biochemistry of multidrug resistance mediated by the multidrug transporter." *Annual review of biochemistry*, 62, no. 1, (1993), 385-427.

[20] Smith, Alexander J., Ardy Van Helvoort, Gerrit Van Meer, Katalin Szabó, Ervin Welker, Gergely Szakács, András Váradi, Balázs Sarkadi, Piet Borst. "MDR3 P-glycoprotein, a phosphatidylcholine translocase, transports several cytotoxic drugs and directly interacts with drugs as judged by interference with nucleotide trapping." *Journal of Biological Chemistry*, 275, no. 31, (2000), 23530-23539.

[21] Thiebaut, Franz, Takashi Tsuruo, Hirofumi Hamada, Michael M. Gottesman, Pastan, IRA; Mark, C. Willingham. "Cellular localization of the multidrug-resistance gene product P-glycoprotein in normal human tissues." *Proceedings of the National Academy of Sciences*, 84, no. 21, (1987), 7735-7738.

[22] Schinkel, AH; Smit, JJM; mO van Tellingen, Beijnen, JH; Wagenaar, E; Van Deemter, L; Mol, CAAM. et al. "Disruption of the mouse mdr1a P-glycoprotein gene leads to a deficiency in the blood-brain barrier and to increased sensitivity to drugs." *Cell*, 77, no. 4, (1994), 491-502.

[23] Subhani, Syed, Archana Jayaraman, Kaiser Jamil. "Homology modelling and molecular docking of MDR1 with chemotherapeutic agents in non-small cell lung cancer." *Biomedicine & pharmacotherapy*, 71, (2015), 37-45.

[24] Kong, Ling-Lei, Hai-Ying Yang, Mei Yuan, Liang Xu, Hua Li. "Inhibition of P-glycoprotein gene expression and function enhances triptolide-induced hepatotoxicity in mice." *Scientific reports*, 5, (2015), 11747.

[25] Aydos, SE; Karadag, A; Ozkan, T; Altınok, B; Bunsuz, M; Heidargholizadeh, S. "Association of MDR1 C3435T and C1236T single nucleotide polymorphisms with male factor infertility." *Genet Mol Res*, 14, no. 2, (2015), 6330-9.

[26] Andersen, Vibeke, Katrine Svenningsen, Lina Almind Knudsen, Axel Kornerup Hansen, Uffe Holmskov, Allan Stensballe, Ulla Vogel. "Novel understanding of ABC transporters ABCB1/MDR/P-glycoprotein, ABCC2/MRP2, and ABCG2/BCRP in colorectal pathophysiology." *World Journal of Gastroenterology*, 21, no. 41, (2015), 11862.

[27] Kreisl, William C., Jeih-San Liow, Nobuyo Kimura, Nicholas Seneca, Sami S. Zoghbi, Cheryl L. Morse, Peter Herscovitch, Victor W. Pike, Robert B. Innis. "P-glycoprotein function at the blood–brain barrier in humans can be quantified with the substrate radiotracer 11C-N-desmethyl-loperamide." *Journal of Nuclear Medicine*, 51, no. 4, (2010), 559-566.

[28] Wang, GY; Zheng, HH; Zhang, KY; Yang, F; Kong, T; Zhou, B; Jiang, ShX. "The roles of cytochrome P450 and P-glycoprotein in the pharmacokinetics of florfenicol in chickens." *Iranian Journal of Veterinary Research*, 19, no. 1, (2018), 9.

[29] Ge, Chun, Bei Cao, Dong Feng, Fang Zhou, Jingwei Zhang, Na Yang, Siqi Feng, Guangji Wang, Jiye Aa. "The down-regulation of SLC7A11 enhances ROS induced P-gp over-expression and drug resistance in MCF-7 breast cancer cells." *Scientific reports*, 7, no. 1, (2017), 1-11.

[30] García-Carrasco, M; Mendoza-Pinto, C; Macias Díaz, S; Vera-Recabarren, M; Vázquez de Lara, L; Méndez Martínez, S; Soto-Santillan, P; Gonzalez-Ramirez, R; Ruiz-Arguelles, A. "P-glycoprotein in autoimmune rheumatic diseases." *Autoimmunity reviews*, 14, no. 7, (2015), 594-600.

[31] Llaudó, Inés, Helena Colom, Pepita Giménez-Bonafé, Joan Torras, Anna Caldés, Maria Sarrias, Josep Mª Cruzado; et al. "Do drug transporter (ABCB 1) SNP s and P-glycoprotein function influence cyclosporine and macrolides exposure in renal transplant patients? Results of the pharmacogenomic substudy within the symphony study." *Transplant International*, 26, no. 2, (2013), 177-186.

[32] Rocha-Pereira, Carolina, Carolina I. Ghanem, Renata Silva, Alfredo G. Casanova, Margarida Duarte-Araújo, Salomé Gonçalves-Monteiro, Emília Sousa, Maria de Lourdes Bastos, Fernando Remião. "P-glycoprotein activation by 1-(propan-2-ylamino)-4-propoxy-9H-thioxanthen-9-one (TX5) in rat distal ileum: ex vivo and *in vivo* studies." *Toxicology and Applied Pharmacology*, 386, (2020), 114832.

[33] Vesel, M; Rapp, J; Feller, D; Kiss, E; Jaromi, L; Meggyes, M; Gy Miskei; et al. "ABCB1 and ABCG2 drug transporters are differentially expressed in non-small cell lung cancers (NSCLC) and expression is modified by cisplatin treatment via altered Wnt signaling." *Respiratory research*, 18, no. 1, (2017), 1-11.

[34] Hensing, Thomas, Apoorva Chawla, Rishi Batra, Ravi Salgia. "A personalized treatment for lung cancer: molecular pathways, targeted therapies, and genomic characterization." In *Systems Analysis of Human Multigene Disorders*, pp. 85-117. Springer, New York, NY, 2014.

[35] Srivalli, Kale Mohana Raghava, Lakshmi, PK. "Overview of P-glycoprotein inhibitors: a rational outlook." *Brazilian Journal of Pharmaceutical Sciences*, 48, no. 3, (2012), 353-367.

[36] Schmoll, Hans-Joachim, Daniel Sargent. "Single agent fluorouracil for first-line treatment of advanced colorectal cancer as standard?." *The Lancet*, 370, no. 9582, (2007), 105-107.

[37] Houlston, Richard S; Ian PM Tomlinson. "Polymorphisms and colorectal tumor risk." *Gastroenterology*, 121, no. 2, (2001), 282-301.

[38] de Jong, Mirjam M; Ilja M. Nolte, Gerard J. te Meerman, Winette TA van der Graaf, Elisabeth GE de Vries, Rolf H. Sijmons, Robert MW Hofstra, Jan H. Kleibeuker. "Low-penetrance genes and their involvement in colorectal cancer susceptibility." *Cancer*

Epidemiology and Prevention Biomarkers, 11, no. 11, (2002), 1332-1352.

[39] Potočnik, Uroš, Metka Ravnik Glavač, Rastko Golouh, and Damjan Glavač. "The role of P-glycoprotein (MDR1) polymorphisms and mutations in colorectal cancer." *Pflügers Archiv* 442, no. 1 (2001): r182-r183.

[40] Choudhuri, Supratim, Curtis D. Klaassen. "Structure, function, expression, genomic organization, and single nucleotide polymorphisms of human ABCB1 (MDR1), ABCC (MRP), and ABCG2 (BCRP) efflux transporters." *International journal of toxicology*, 25, no. 4, (2006), 231-259.

[41] Cordon-Cardo, C; O'brien, JP; Boccia, J; Casals, D; Bertino, JR; Melamed, MR. "Expression of the multidrug resistance gene product (P-glycoprotein) in human normal and tumor tissues." *Journal of Histochemistry & Cytochemistry*, 38, no. 9, (1990), 1277-1287.

[42] Johnstone, Ricky W; Astrid A. Ruefli, Mark J. Smyth. "Multiple physiological functions for multidrug transporter P-glycoprotein?." *Trends in biochemical sciences*, 25, no. 1, (2000), 1-6.

[43] Weinstein, Ronald S., Shriram M. Jakate, Jose M. Dominguez, Miriam D. Lebovitz, George K. Koukoulis, Jerome R. Kuszak, Larry F. Klusens; et al. "Relationship of the expression of the multidrug resistance gene product (P-glycoprotein) in human colon carcinoma to local tumor aggressiveness and lymph node metastasis." *Cancer research*, 51, no. 10, (1991), 2720-2726.

[44] Sakaeda, Toshiyuki. "MDR1 genotype-related pharmacokinetics: fact or fiction?." *Drug metabolism and pharmacokinetics*, 20, no. 6, (2005), 391-414.

[45] Fellay, Jacques, Catia Marzolini, Emma R. Meaden, David J. Back, Thierry Buclin, Jean-Philippe Chave, Laurent A. Decosterd; et al. "Response to antiretroviral treatment in HIV-1-infected individuals with allelic variants of the multidrug resistance transporter 1: a pharmacogenetics study." *The Lancet*, 359, no. 9300, (2002), 30-36.

[46] Eichelbaum, Michel, Martin F. Fromm, Matthias Schwab. "Clinical aspects of the MDR1 (ABCB1) gene polymorphism." *Therapeutic drug monitoring*, 26, no. 2, (2004), 180-185.

[47] Aarnoudse, Albert LHJ; Ron HN van Schaik, Jeanne Dieleman, Mariam Molokhia, Melanie M. van Riemsdijk, Robert J. Ligthelm, David Overbosch, Ilse P. van der Heiden, Bruno H. Ch Stricker. "MDR1 gene polymorphisms are associated with neuropsychiatric adverse effects of mefloquine." *Clinical Pharmacology & Therapeutics*, 80, no. 4, (2006), 367-374.

[48] Osswald, Elena, Andreas Johne, Gabriele Laschinski, Farhad Arjomand-Nahad, Uwe Malzahn, Julia Kirchheiner, Thomas Gerloff; et al. "Association of MDR1 genotypes with susceptibility to colorectal cancer in older non-smokers." *European journal of clinical pharmacology*, 63, no. 1, (2007), 9-16.

[49] Komoto, Chiho, Tsutomu Nakamura, Toshiyuki Sakaeda, Deanna L. Kroetz, Toshio Yamada, Hideaki Omatsu, Tatsuya Koyama; et al. "MDR1 haplotype frequencies in Japanese and Caucasian, and in Japanese patients with colorectal cancer and esophageal cancer." *Drug metabolism and pharmacokinetics*, 21, no. 2, (2006), 126-132.

[50] Drozdzik, Marek, Monika Bialecka, Katarzyna Mysliwiec, Krystyna Honczarenko, Jan Stankiewicz, and Zbigniew Sych. "Polymorphism in the P-glycoprotein drug transporter MDR1 gene: a possible link between environmental and genetic factors in Parkinson's disease." *Pharmacogenetics and Genomics*, 13, no. 5, (2003), 259-263.

[51] Koyama, Tatsuya, Tsutomu Nakamura, Chiho Komoto, Toshiyuki Sakaeda, Mayuko Taniguchi, Noboru Okamura, Takao Tamura et al. "MDR1 T-129C polymorphism can be predictive of differentiation, and thereby prognosis of colorectal adenocarcinomas in Japanese." *Biological and Pharmaceutical Bulletin*, 29, no. 7, (2006), 1449-1453.

[52] Hinoshita, Eiji, Takeshi Uchiumi, Ken-ichi Taguchi, Naoko Kinukawa, Masazumi Tsuneyoshi, Yoshihiko Maehara, Keizo Sugimachi, Michihiko Kuwano. "Increased expression of an ATP-binding cassette superfamily transporter, multidrug resistance protein

2, in human colorectal carcinomas." *Clinical cancer research*, 6, no. 6, (2000), 2401-2407.

[53] Goff, Barbara A; Justin A. Ries, Lisa P. Els, Marc D. Coltrera, Allen M. Gown. "Immunophenotype of ovarian cancer as predictor of clinical outcome: evaluation at primary surgery and second-look procedure." *Gynecologic Oncology*, 70, no. 3, (1998), 378-385.

[54] Siu, Lillian L., Diponkar Banerjee, Reena J. Khurana, Xia Pan, Rafael Pflueger, Ian F. Tannock, Malcolm J. Moore. "The prognostic role of p53, metallothionein, P-glycoprotein, and MIB-1 in muscle-invasive urothelial transitional cell carcinoma." *Clinical Cancer Research*, 4, no. 3, (1998), 559-565.

[55] Yeh, Kun-Huei, Chi-Long Chen, Chia-Tung Shun, Jaw-Town Lin, Wei-Jei Lee, Po-Huang Lee, Yao-Chang Chen, Ann-Lii Cheng. "Relatively low expression of multidrug resistance-1 (MDR-1) and its possible clinical implication in gastric cancers." *Journal of clinical gastroenterology*, 26, no. 4, (1998), 274-278.

[56] Ralhan, Ranju, Rajeeb K. Swain, Sandhya Agarwal, Jasbir Kaur, Neera Nath, Gautam Sarkar, Meera Mathur, Nootan K. Shukla. "P-glycoprotein is positively correlated with p53 in human oral pre-malignant and malignant lesions and is associated with poor prognosis." *International journal of cancer*, 84, no. 1, (1999), 80-85.

[57] Pirker, R; Wallner, J; Gsur, A; Götzl, M; Zöchbauer, S; Scheithauer, W; Depisch, D. "MDR1 gene expression in primary colorectal carcinomas." *British journal of cancer*, 68, no. 4, (1993), 691-694.

[58] Faivre, J; Lemmens, VEPP; Quipourt, V; Bouvier, AM. "Management and survival of colorectal cancer in the elderly in population-based studies." *European Journal of Cancer*, 43, no. 15, (2007), 2279-2284.

[59] Debri, Khadija, Alan R. Boobis, Donald S. Davies, Robert J. Edwards. "Distribution and induction of CYP3A1 and CYP3A2 in rat liver and extrahepatic tissues." *Biochemical pharmacology*, 50, no. 12, (1995), 2047-2056.

[60] Watkins, Paul B; Scott A. Murray, Paul E. Thomas, Steven A. Wrighton. "Distribution of cytochromes P-450, cytochrome b5, and NADPH-cytochrome P-450 reductase in an entire human liver." *Biochemical pharmacology*, 39, no. 3, (1990), 471-476.

[61] Hochman, Jerome H., Masato Chiba, Masayo Yamazaki, Cuyue Tang, Jiunn H. Lin. "P-glycoprotein-mediated efflux of indinavir metabolites in Caco-2 cells expressing cytochrome P450 3A4." *Journal of Pharmacology and Experimental Therapeutics*, 298, no. 1, (2001), 323-330.

[62] Koepsell, H; Gorboulev, V; Arndt, P. "Molecular pharmacology of organic cation transporters in kidney." *The Journal of membrane biology*, 167, no. 2, (1999), 103-117.

[63] Zhou, SF. "Structure, function and regulation of P-glycoprotein and its clinical relevance in drug disposition." *Xenobiotica*, 38, no. 7-8, (2008), 802-832.

[64] Miller, David S; Björn Bauer, Anika MS Hartz. "Modulation of P-glycoprotein at the blood-brain barrier: opportunities to improve central nervous system pharmacotherapy." *Pharmacological reviews*, 60, no. 2, (2008), 196-209.

[65] Litman, Thomas, Thomas Zeuthen, Torben Skovsgaard, Wilfred D. Stein. "Competitive, non-competitive and cooperative interactions between substrates of P-glycoprotein as measured by its ATPase activity." *Biochimica et Biophysica Acta (BBA)-Molecular Basis of Disease*, 1361, no. 2, (1997), 169-176.

[66] Takara, Kohji, Toshiyuki Sakaeda, Katsuhiko Okumura. "An update on overcoming MDR1-mediated multidrug resistance in cancer chemotherapy." *Current pharmaceutical design*, 12, no. 3, (2006), 273-286.

[67] Zhou, Shufeng, Lee Yong Lim, Balram Chowbay. "Herbal modulation of P-glycoprotein." *Drug metabolism reviews*, 36, no. 1, (2004), 57-104.

[68] Zhang, Wenxia, Yi Han, Siok Lam Lim, Lee Yong Lim. "Dietary regulation of P-gp function and expression." *Expert opinion on drug metabolism & toxicology*, 5, no. 7, (2009), 789-801.

[69] Hermann, Dirk M., Ertugrul Kilic, Annett Spudich, Stefanie D. Krämer, Heidi Wunderli-Allenspach, Claudio L. Bassetti. "Role of drug efflux carriers in the healthy and diseased brain." *Annals of Neurology: Official Journal of the American Neurological Association and the Child Neurology Society*, 60, no. 5, (2006), 489-498.

[70] Kalitsky-Szirtes, J; Shayeganpour, A; Brocks, DR; Piquette-Miller, M. "Suppression of drug-metabolizing enzymes and efflux transporters in the intestine of endotoxin-treated rats." *Drug Metabolism and Disposition*, 32, no. 1, (2004), 20-27.

[71] Marguerite, Véronique, Mylene Beri-Dexheimer, Sandrine Ortiou, Jean-Louis Guéant, Marc Merten. "Cobalamin potentiates vinblastine cytotoxicity through downregulation of mdr-1 gene expression in HepG2 cells." *Cellular Physiology and Biochemistry*, 20, no. 6, (2007), 967-976.

[72] Rodrigues, Alice Cristina, Rui Curi, Fabiana Dalla Vecchia GEnVIGIR, Mario Hiroyuki Hirata, Rosario Dominguez Crespo Hirata. "The expression of efflux and uptake transporters are regulated by statins in Caco-2 and HepG2 cells." *Acta Pharmacologica Sinica*, 30, no. 7, (2009), 956-964.

[73] Greiner, B; Eichelbaum, M; Fritz, P; Kreichgauer, HP; von Richter, O; Zundler, J; Kroemer, HK. "The interaction of digoxin and rifampin: role of intestinal P-glycoprotein." *J Clin Invest*, 104, (1999), 147-153.

[74] Hodges, Laura M; Svetlana M. Markova, Leslie W. Chinn, Jason M. Gow, Deanna L. Kroetz, Teri E. Klein, Russ B. Altman. "Very important pharmacogene summary: ABCB1 (MDR1, P-glycoprotein)." *Pharmacogenetics and genomics*, 21, no. 3, (2011), 152.

[75] Fromm, Martin F. "Importance of P-glycoprotein at blood–tissue barriers." *Trends in pharmacological sciences*, 25, no. 8, (2004), 423-429.

[76] Aszalos, Adorjan. "Drug–drug interactions affected by the transporter protein, P-glycoprotein (ABCB1, MDR1): II. Clinical aspects." *Drug discovery today*, 12, no. 19-20, (2007), 838-843.

[77] Litman, Thomas, Thomas Zeuthen, Torben Skovsgaard, Wilfred D. Stein. "Competitive, non-competitive and cooperative interactions between substrates of P-glycoprotein as measured by its ATPase activity." *Biochimica et Biophysica Acta (BBA)-Molecular Basis of Disease*, 1361, no. 2, (1997), 169-176.

[78] Yang, Xiao-Xia, Ze-Ping Hu, Wei Duan, Yi-Zhun Zhu, Shu-Feng Zhou. "Drug-herb interactions: eliminating toxicity with hard drug design." *Current pharmaceutical design*, 12, no. 35, (2006), 4649-4664.

[79] Seneca, Nicholas, Sami S. Zoghbi, Jeih-San Liow, William Kreisl, Peter Herscovitch, Kimberly Jenko, Robert L. Gladding, Andrew Taku, Victor W. Pike, Robert B. Innis. "Human brain imaging and radiation dosimetry of 11C-N-desmethyl-loperamide, a PET radiotracer to measure the function of P-glycoprotein." *Journal of Nuclear Medicine*, 50, no. 5, (2009), 807-813.

[80] Choo, Edna F., Daniel Kurnik, Mordechai Muszkat, Tadashi Ohkubo, Sheila D. Shay, James N. Higginbotham, Hartmut Glaeser, Richard B. Kim, Alastair JJ Wood, Grant R. Wilkinson. "Differential *in vivo* sensitivity to inhibition of P-glycoprotein located in lymphocytes, testes, and the blood-brain barrier." *Journal of Pharmacology and Experimental Therapeutics*, 317, no. 3, (2006), 1012-1018.

[81] Sadeque, Abu JM; Christoph Wandel, Hauibing He, Selina Shah, Alastair JJ Wood. "Increased drug delivery to the brain by P-glycoprotein inhibition." *Clinical Pharmacology & Therapeutics*, 68, no. 3, (2000), 231-237.

[82] Mukwaya, Geoffrey, Thomas MacGregor, David Hoelscher, Thomas Heming, Daniel Legg, Kelli Kavanaugh, Phillip Johnson, John P. Sabo, Scott McCallister. "Interaction of ritonavir-boosted tipranavir with loperamide does not result in loperamide-associated neurologic side effects in healthy volunteers." *Antimicrobial agents and chemotherapy*, 49, no. 12, (2005), 4903-4910.

[83] Wacher, Vincent J; Chi-Yuan Wu, Leslie Z. Benet. "Overlapping substrate specificities and tissue distribution of cytochrome P450 3A and P-glycoprotein: implications for drug delivery and activity in

cancer chemotherapy." *Molecular carcinogenesis*, 13, no. 3, (1995), 129-134.

[84] Liu, Yu, Anthony Hunt, C. "Mechanistic study of the cellular interplay of transport and metabolism using the synthetic modeling method." *Pharmaceutical research*, 23, no. 3, (2006), 493-505.

[85] Marchetti, Serena, Roberto Mazzanti, Jos H. Beijnen, Jan HM Schellens. "Concise Review: Clinical Relevance of Drug-Drug and Herb-Drug Interactions Mediated by the ABC Transporter ABCB1 (MDR1, P-glycoprotein)." *Oncologist*, 12, no. 8, (2007), 927-941.

In: An Introduction to P-Glycoprotein
Editors: M. Wahajuddin et al.
ISBN: 978-1-53619-488-3

Chapter 11

QUANTIFICATION AND ANALYSIS OF P-GLYCOPROTEIN: *IN VITRO*, *IN SITU*, AND *IN VIVO* MODELS

Deepak S. Chauhan, Meena Jaggi, Subhash C. Chauhan and Murali M. Yallapu*

Department of Immunology and Microbiology,
School of Medicine, University of Texas Rio Grande Valley,
McAllen, TX, US and
South Texas Center of Excellence in Cancer Research,
School of Medicine, University of Texas Rio Grande Valley,
McAllen, TX, US

ABSTRACT

The chemical homeostasis in the cells is maintained by the Adenosine triphosphate (ATP)-Binding Cassette (ABC) transporter. The important transporter is the multidrug resistance mutation 1 (MDR1) (also referred as ABCB1), which is the product of the permeability-glycoprotein (P-gp) gene expression. In cancer and other diseases, overexpression of P-gp leads

* Corresponding Author's Email: murali.yallapu@utrgv.edu.

to the elimination of therapeutic drugs. Also, the change in P-gp expression in gastrointestinal tract could affect drug-drug interaction. It might be responsible for drug resistance and impediment to the therapeutic concentration. There are several platforms available for the evaluation of P-gp expression like liquid chromatography coupled with mass spectrometry, flow cytometry, positron emission tomography (PET), and so on. It requires the technique like labeling with antibodies, quantification of effluxed fluorescent dye, and mRNA of MDR1 gene. This chapter reviews the currently used methods for quantifying the P-gp function at *in vitro*, *in situ*, and *in vivo* settings.

Keywords: P-glycoprotein, ABC transporters, blood-brain barrier, chemotherapy, multidrug resistance, oral bioavailability

INTRODUCTION

Permeability-glycoprotein (P-gp) is a 180 kDa glycoprotein functions as a multidrug efflux pump that is present in the plasma membrane of the cells (Figure 1). It is an ATP-Binding Cassette (ABC) and particularly located at the interface tissues such as intestinal, renal, hepatic, brain barriers, and responsible for efflux of drugs towards the body clearance and regulating the drug absorption in tumors and other specific organs like testes, placenta, and brain. It is overexpressed in cancer patients, especially those who have undergone chemotherapy. Also, the function of P-gp is altered during various diseases like epilepsy, Alzheimer's, depression, and Parkinson's, which affect the drug efficacy regimen.

Although the methods for the absolute quantification of P-gp are still under development, crystallography of P-gp with drug binding and ATP hydrolysis is being researched out actively. The surrogate mRNA expression and immunoreaction are other researching out methods. The exclusion of fluorescent dyes is commonly used for determining the P-gp expression. However, the lack of reproducibility, mismatching of data in different labs, and specificity place constraints on the fluorescent dyes and immunoaffinity methods. The fact is that these approaches are qualitative or semiquantitative, which does not allow the exact quantification of the

P-gp. It confounds the analysis of extrapolation or determining the effect of P-gp on the drug distribution in humans. Thus, reviewing the current methods of P-gp quantification and analysis will help in understanding the problem and finding out the solution for the absolute quantification of P-gp towards helping in organ targeting, drug disposition prediction, and drug resistance. Figure 2 presents the currently available methods for qualification and analysis of P-gp.

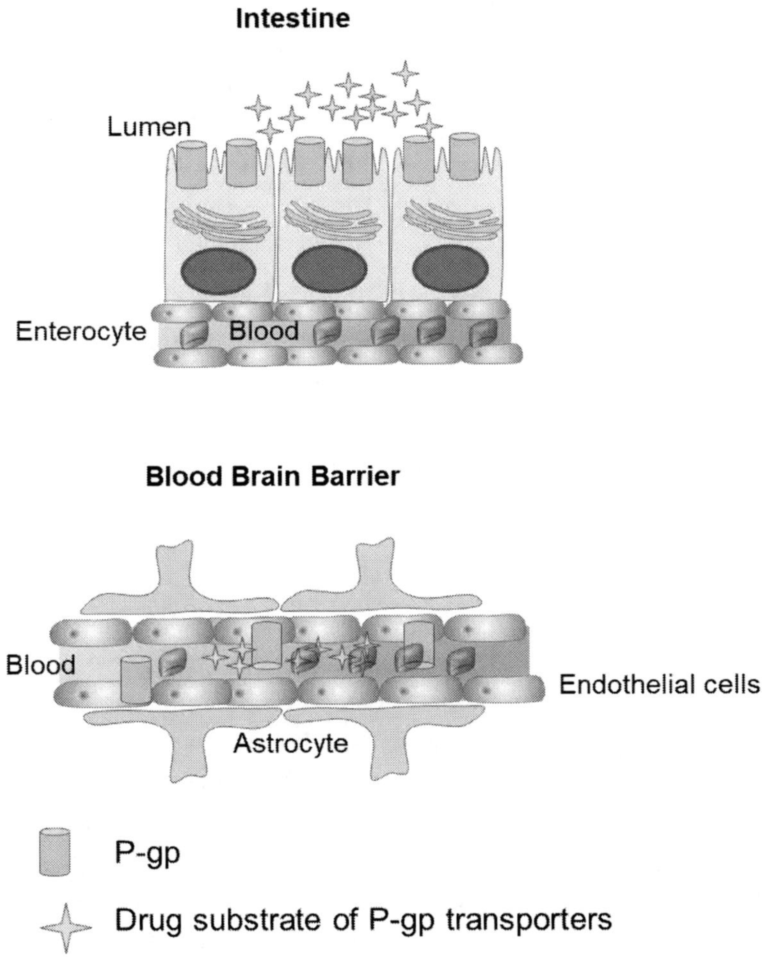

Figure 1.Schematic representation of P-gp presence in the intestine (at the apical surface in the intestinal enterocytes) and blood-brain barrier (brain capillary endothelial cells).

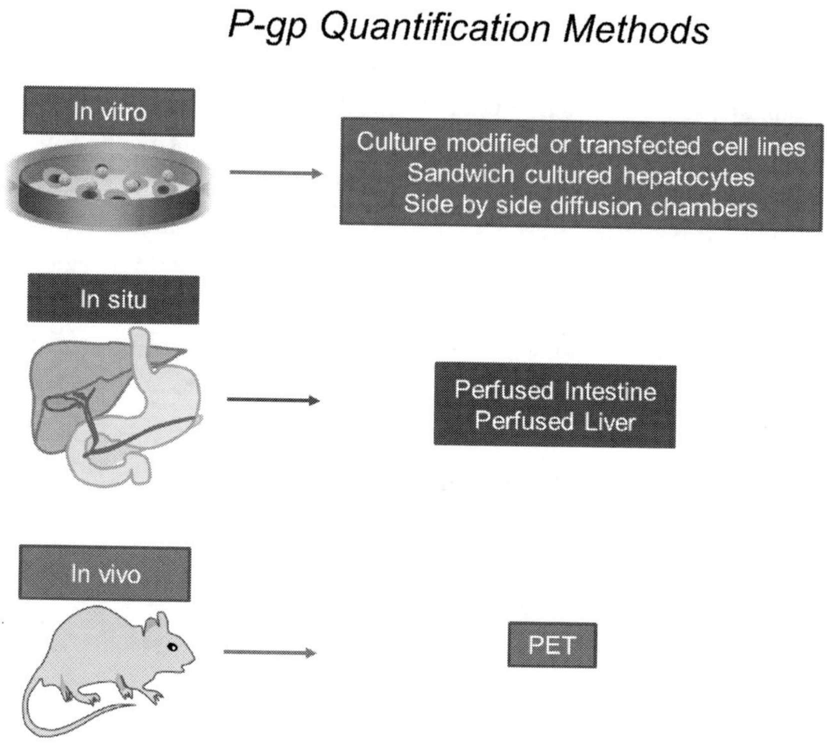

Figure 2. Currently available methods for quantification and analysis of P-gp.

In Vitro Methods

Human colorectal adenocarcinoma cells (Caco-2) is one of the widely used *in vitro* models employed as a reference point for the absorption studies of the human intestinal mucosa barrier. Another cell line is the Madin-Darby canine kidney (MDCK); it shares the epithelial characteristics with Caco-2 and also grows at a faster speed. There are also modified MDCK and Lewis lung carcinoma (LLC) cells (MDCK-BCRP, MDCK-MDR1, and LLC-PK1) available for the *in vitro* P-gp evaluation studies. These modified cell lines are engineered to overexpress a particular transporter protein to study their involvement in drug resistance. These cell lines share the common characteristics when grown on the transwell membrane inserts, even having a different origin. The common characteristics include the confluent membrane, polarized layer with the apical region expressing the P-gp. The efflux studies on these cell lines are a gold standard for determining the P-gp involvement. The barrier resistance (transepithelial electrical resistance (TEFR) value) measured for the Caco-2 and MDCK is determined to be 600 Ωcm^2 and 100 Ωcm^2, respectively. There are also several assays available to get the information of P-gp at the mRNA and protein level; however, these are skeptical for the *in vivo* studies.

During the *in vitro* bidirectional permeability study, the interaction of test compounds with P-gp is determined on the basis of efflux ratio (ER), which depends on the permeability of apical to basolateral and vice versa. The ER (>2) indicates the interaction of the compound with the P-gp and otherwise.

Zhang et al. [1] have compared the MDCK-MDR1 with the caco-2 cell lines for assessing the P-gp of the gut. After finding similar results, they concluded that MDCK-MDR1, which doesn't require extensive cell culture condition, can be a very well alternative for the P-gp study considering the half-maximal inhibitory concentration (IC50) value, which varies from cell lines to cell lines. Also, calcein-AM assay (inhibition assay) can be easily performed in MDCK-MDR1 in high throughput settings using the generic fluorescence lamp. The following are the common methods used for studying the P-gp in *in vitro* studies.

Culture Modified

Culture-modified or transfected cell lines are the most common *in vitro* method for evaluating P-gp function. The routine monitoring of transfected cells is very important as there is a high chance of heterogeneity and change in P-gp expression over time. This leads to the variability of results from lab to lab.

The Caco-2 and LLC-PK1 cell lines expressing the P-gp have been transduced with Adenovirus-P450 reductase and Adenovirus-3A4 vector for studying the interaction of drug-metabolizing enzyme (DME) and P-gp transporter. The virus transfection is advantageous in many ways, such as potential to infect several cell types, large cDNA accommodation, tolerability, and ability to perform multiple infections in the same cell. Cummins et al. [2] have also done remarkable work by transfecting the Caco-2 cells with the DMEs (CYP34A) and used the combination of inhibitors for the DME and P-gp interaction study towards reducing the assumptions. There are also reports which suggest determining the intracellular concentration in *in vitro* studies as it may saturate the enzyme, which may hamper the extraction rate [3].

A subclone of the Caco-2 named TC7 has also been characterized and isolated. It displays enhanced expression of DME (CYP3A4) and may represent a good model for studying the function of P-gp in reference to the CYP3A4. Also, this study determined the exact protein expression as many times the mRNA level doesn't represent very well the activity of enzymes and transporter protein. However, the results published appear more qualitative than quantitative in nature, which warrants caution in data analysis.

Sandwich Cultured Hepatocytes

It is a little expensive method for studying the P-gp transporter protein in the liver. Herein, the hepatocytes are grown in between the layer of collagen to improve the morphology, viability, as well as development of intact bile canalicular networks. Also, it helps in the improvement of polarized excretory function, albumin, and bile secretion towards simulating the *in vivo* conditions. This methodology can be easily followed even with the cryopreserved or plateable culture in getting the cohesive monolayer.

There are number of experiments have been conducted for understanding the relation between the transporter protein and drug-metabolizing enzymes. Drugs such as pafuramidine and furamide as well as terfenadine and fexofenadine, have been very helpful in studying the metabolism, biliary excretion, and basolateral transport in dexamethasone-treated hepatocytes and control. The *in vitro* studies are coupled with pharmacokinetic modeling for better understanding the P-gp activity.

Side by Side Diffusion Chambers

It is an intensive *in vitro* methodology for assessing the P-gp function. The transport data similar to the tissue can be achieved by studying the drug appearance rate in the receiver chamber and drug disappearance in the donor chamber. Johnson et al. [4] have worked on the consideration of enterocyte accumulation using the four-chamber kinetic model wherein the submucosal compartment was also included. When the P-gp specific inhibitor was used, there was minimal effect on the verapamil efflux; however, on the usage of midazolam (CYP3A4 inhibitor), the transport of verapamil increased by 2-fold. The impact of P-gp on the verapamil extraction in the intestinal model has also been assessed using the four-compartment model. In the simulation study, it was concluded that the drug's metabolization should be relatively low compared to the uptake for studying the P-gp function.

In Situ Methods

Today, it's important for the pharmaceutical scientist to understand the experimental models and the assumptions behind for closely defining the interplay between the DME and transporter proteins. It is required for efficacious, cost-effective, and safer drug therapies and better drug disposition and pharmacokinetics study.

The perfused organs offer the simultaneous study of the metabolism and transport of drug molecules. Although complicated to many *in vitro* models and high throughput limitation, *in situ* perfused organs give advantage of physiology and naturally occurring tissue structure. It also ensures the presence of all DME and transport proteins. However, this method might add further complexities and increase the assumptions that might affect the study's conclusion.

For example, the perfused organs are not only supposed to contain the P-gp or CYP3A but other DME and transporter proteins which could also act on the investigational substrate. Also, regional differences and non-specific binding should also be considered to determine the difference in expression and determine the transport kinetics. It should also be cautioned that the diseased animals' model results in altered expression of transporter proteins. For example, chronic renal failure and lipopolysaccharide induced inflammatory rat models to express lower P-gp protein and mdr1a mRNA in the intestine. A similar has been observed in other diseased models. It underscores the expression of transporter proteins in reference to control animals.

Perfused Intestine

There is number of evidence that correlates the effective intestine permeability (Peff) of humans with the Peff of the rat. The rat intestine is often deployed for the absorption hypothesis testing and complementing the *in vivo* data. However, certain factors like the expression difference between the species and different tissue within the same species must be considered. The regional difference should also be considered due to differences in expression, as well as non-specific binding during the determination of transport kinetics.

The intestinal mucosa is filled with transporter proteins like P-gp, Oatp3, Asbt, MRP3, and others. In the mammalian intestine, P-gp is relatively expressed more in the villus tip of the intestinal mucosa's brush border. The expression is low in the duodenum and increases towards the colon. The rate of efflux is highly dependent on the location and 3-4 fold to the length of the intestine. There has been a difference in the absorption of atenolol, metoprolol, and antipyrine, which are passively absorbed in the intact intestine study. This difference could be blamed on the tight junction pore and less surface area of the ileum and colon. Thus, it could be concluded that the variations (both physical and biochemical) persist throughout the length of the intestine which warrants the careful design of the study.

The methods like isolated or closed-loop systems, single-pass perfusion, and static perfusion method are widely used. Griffiths et al., [5] have done remarkable work in the single-pass method in rat intestinal model; their work has been recognized with each bit of detail of the experiment.

The intestinal segments (duodenum, jejuna, and ileum) are taken out after the midline incision of the anesthetized animal. The incision is made around (20 cm in rat) and flushed with phosphate buffer saline with due care of intestinal mucosa. The cannula is inserted, and the drug solution with or without inhibitor is injected at the pH 6-7 or could be low as 4, at the rate of 0.15-0.20 mL/min in rats and mice *in situ* models [6]. The perfusion efflux is collected via the distal cannula over time. The disappearance permeability is calculated as follow for finding the parent drug permeability [7].

$$P_{lumen} = \frac{Q_{in}}{2\pi rl} ln \frac{C(l) \times (\frac{Q_{out}}{Q_{in}})}{C(0)}$$

Wherein, perfusion buffer concentration (C(0)), sample effluent (C(l)), gravimetric analysis (Q_{out}/Q_{in}), measured proximal perfusion flow rate (Q_{in}), distal effluent flow rate (Q_{out}), luminal surface area (2πrl).

The intestinal perfusion is performed up to max 60 min., with the 20-30 min. interval to reach the equilibrium for the steady-state. In recent studies, after the 60 min of perfusion study, P-gp inhibitor was introduced, and the study was conducted for another 60 min. After the introduction of verapamil (150 μM) and 20-30 min of equilibrium, the apparent permeability (Papp) of the talinolol increased to 4-fold while ketoconazole (10 μM) caused 2-4 fold rise in the case of amprenavir [8]. However, in the absence of inhibitor there was no change in the permeability of amprenavir and other passive diffusion markers like atenolol and propranolol. It demands the alternative model for reducing the animal resources and conduct cross-over study in the case of highly variable subjects.

The most common constraint to these types of studies is the assumption of selective inhibition by the chemical method. The availability of intestine from the genetic knockout mice avoids the complexities of selective inhibition. For example, the apparent permeability of talinolol was 6.9-fold higher in the mdr1a/1b(-/-) mice compared with the wild type. Also, the administration of 150 μM verapamil leads to the 5 fold increase in the Paap of talinolol, while no effect was observed in the case of knockout mice [9]. Similar results have been observed in the case of darunavir administered with the intestinal fluid, wherein the inhibitor used was the verapamil and ritonavir [10]. Thus, these studies suggest that genetic knockout mice along with specific bioanalytical techniques and blood supply, give more advanced model for the study towards deconvoluting the transporter protein function.

Perfused Liver

P-gp is expressed in higher amount, particularly in the bile canalicular of the apical membrane. Several *in situ* perfusion studies have been done in the rat liver via the single pass or closed-loop methods. In single-pass method, the perfusion of beta-estradiol-17-(beta-D-glucuronide) mediated cholestasis was prevented on the inclusion of 1.5 μM daunorubicin, 1 μM paclitaxel, or 6 μM cyclosporin A [11]. However, in the closed-loop study, on the inclusion of 10 μM quinine, vinblastine, or verapamil, the biliary excretion of doxorubicin was significantly reduced [12]. Although in the case of paclitaxel and digoxin, biliary elimination is only moderately perturbed in mdr1a/mdr1b(-/-) or chemical inhibition mice in both the *in vivo* and *in situ* studies. It suggests the availability of other compensatory pathways whose assumptions should be carefully considered.

The detailed study of *in situ* perfusion wherein the liver was isolated and cannulated but remained in the animal has been done by Ballatori et al. [13]. This study details the required flow rate and recommended equipment (e.g., peristaltic pump, tubings, etc.) and other factors affecting the study. The two common methods used are the closed-loop (recirculating) and single pass. After the midline excision, liver is exposed in the animal (rats/mice). For the continuous sampling, the bile duct is connected to collecting tubes after cannulation, and the ascending portal vein is connected to perfusate lines, as shown in Figure 3.

The blood is flushed out using the composite Krebs-Henseleit or Ringer buffer containing the glucose (1% w/v), BSA (10-30 mg/ml), and heparin (2U units/ml) with the flow rate of 2-4 mL/min/g liver. Just after the perfusion start, the abdominal vena cava is cut to exit the system. At last, the thoracic inferior vena cava is connected to the collecting tube after cannulation, which is routed as per the single pass or closed-loop method. Similar to the intestine model, the assumptions can be reduced by following the genetic knockout model than the chemical inhibition.

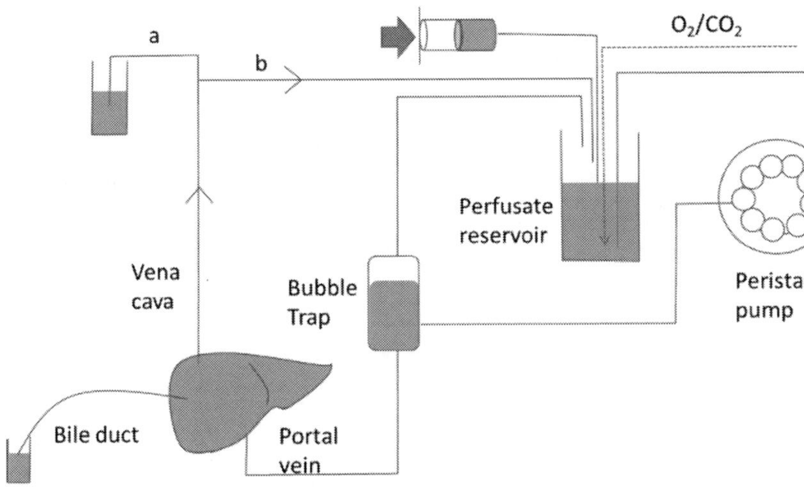

Figure 3. Isolated liver perfusion setup: (a) single-pass or (b) recirculating taurocholic acid.

The perfusate pH and pressure should be monitored in line, wherein pH should be around 7.35-7.45 and pressure 7.4 mmHg. After 15 min. of equilibrium, drugs and inhibitors can be introduced. The perfusate could be collected via thoracic vena cava or recirculated to the perfusate chamber. The single-pass method represents the zero-order kinetics with the steady-state pharmacokinetics by delivering constant conc. of parent drug over the duration of the experiment. The single-pass method requires relatively large volume of perfusate, i.e., 1.2-2.4 L/hr. While the recirculating method representing the first-order kinetics, the perfusate volume required is less, i.e., 0.2-0.3 L/hr. Also, the sampling of microliter volume can also be done without perturbing the kinetics. By the help of either type of study, the typical pharmacological parameters like the area under curve (AUC), elimination half-life, and clearance can be determined.

The perfusion study in the liver usually carried out up to 3 hr due to the requirement of tissue oxygenation (1.4-2 μmol/min/g of the liver) and supplementing the perfused media with red blood cells. However, recent development shows that the usage of gas respirators for bubbling 95% O_2 and 5% CO_2 could help in hemoglobin-free perfusion. The addition of taurocholic acid is preferred as per the requirement 258 ± 48 nmol/g liver for maintaining the bile (1-10 μl/min/rat liver). In the recirculating method, the taurocholic acid is injected into the perfused reservoir at the rate of (0.05 ml/min) by infusing in the saline (3.8 mg/ml). It should be noted that an inappropriate amount of taurocholic acid can impair the bile flow. However, even in optimized taurocholic acid amount, the bile flow could be reduced by 90% during the 2-3 h study.

In Vivo Methods

The recent understanding of positron emission tomography (PET) and positron tracer is helpful in studying the dynamic function of P-gp in *in vivo* setting. The study of transporters in *in vivo* model is a current requirement. The validation of such model is very important for the specific and accurate quantification, as rodents and humans are not the same; also, most of the animal models are limited by technical and ethical boundaries [14, 15]. For example, in humans, there is only one variant of transporter gene MDR1, while in mice, the two variants Mdr1a and Mdr1b are present to perform the same function [16]. Also, the problem is in the complete replacement of the mouse gene with the human one for accurate and specific studies, as the function of humans and mice overlaps significantly. However, recent developments in protein quantification allow us to specifically determine the difference in amino acids towards distinguishing the mouse and human proteins.

The first MDR1 model was developed in the 90s and contributed a lot to the P-gp function study [17]. In the humanized P-gp mouse model, both the Mdr1a and Mdr1b variants are replaced with the MDR1 gene. Recent studies show the difference in function between different species. For example, Cutler et al. [18] found that inhibitor (elacridar) is required in larger quantity for the guinea pig than in the mice and rats. Also, the [^{11}C]GR205171 and [^{18}F]altanserine penetration in the brain lining to be 8.6 and 4.5 times more than rodents [19]. These studies are also limited by the requirement of a specific substrate. The accumulation of the labeled substrate in the tissue and blood can affect the PET interpretation data. The different labeling positions also end up in different structures; thus, careful considerations are required [20, 21].

Although the P-gp pump study can be performed using PET *in vivo*, it has several limitations like unavailability of transporter-specific probes, interference of the probe metabolite, cost, and safety involved in the instrument and radioactive substance [22-24]. Further, the extrapolation of data from the primary cells to the other tissue is not a good approach as the net transport involves multiple transporters.

Earlier studies have shown the usage of verapamil for the measurement of P-gp function in resistant tumor and blood-brain barrier. Although higher lipophilicity of verapamil limits its application, thus new substrate carvedilol researched out having the log P value 2 instead of 3.8 (in case of verapamil), and also twice effectively modulate the P-gp than verapamil. Another compound is GR218231, which in a combination of modulator CsA, proved to be very impressive for the PET driven quantification as well as visualization of P-gp pump.

There are several other compounds explored for quantifying the P-gp *in vitro* and *in vivo* models, such as [^{64}Cu]copper (I) bis(diphosphine), [^{18}F]paclitaxel, [^{64}Cu]copper monocationic complex, and [^{11}C]Lopermide [25]. The molecules interacting with P-gp are classified into 3 categories: substrate, inhibitor, and modulators. The positron emitters are most frequently incorporated into the drugs act as the P-gp substrate for studying the P-gp function and multidrug resistance (MDR) such as [^{11}C]verapamil, [^{11}C]danurobuicin, [$^{11/F18}$C]paclitaxel,[^{11}C]colchicine,

[^{11}C]loperamide, [^{11}C]Desmethy loperamide, [^{11}C]Carvedilol, [^{11}C]D617, and [^{11}C]Docetaxel.

[^{11}C]Verapamil and [^{11}C]D617

It is one of the best characterized P-gp tracers and already being used in patients[20, 26]. At starting, the racemic mixtures were followed, but currently, pure enantiomer (R) is used for the best quantification. There are also limitations of extensive peripheral metabolism, which lead to the formation of radioactive metabolites themselves are substrates of the P-gp [27]. Also, the formation of polar radioactive metabolites causes non-P-gp mediated signals.

[^{11}C]D617 is one of the main metabolites of verapamil and has similar kinetics to it. However, it's a weak P-gp substrate with the increase of only 3-fold after the treatment of P-gp inhibitor tariquidar.

[^{11}C]Desmethy-Loperamide and[^{11}C]Loperamide

Loperamide is an opiate receptor agonist and substrate for the P-gp. The first synthesis of the tracer was reported in 2003 from the [C^{11}] methylation of N-desmethyl-loperamide [28]. The knockout mice showed 16 times higher metabolite presence and indicated the presence of dLop (degradation metabolites doesn't enter the brain), thus considered it to be superior to [C^{11}] loperamide [29]. A reliable synthesis of the dLop with high yield was achieved using amide precursor [30]. Recent studies on humans indicate that dLop generates negligible amount of metabolites that penetrate the brain [31].

[^{11}C]Colchicine

It is an alkaloid with anti-inflammatory properties and labeled using [^{14}C] and [^{11}C] for studying the P-gp function [32, 33]. It has been validated in the mice chemosensitive and chemoresistant tumor model. However, further studies need to be performed for translating it to the clinics.

[^{11}C]Daunorubicin

It is an anticancer drug and has been tested in A2780AD P-gp overexpressing ovarian cancer cells as well as in Wistar rats [34]. It is prepared by alkaline hydrolysis of [^{11}C]diazomethane reacting to formyl trifluroacetyl daunorubicin. It has very low specificity and yield (correct radiodecay, i.e., < 1%). The enzymatic reduction has not very successful, so no further studies have been documented [35].

[^{11}C]Paclitaxel

It is prepared using the [^{11}C]benzoyl chloride and taxane paclitaxel. The radiochemical yield with corrected decay is 7%, with a purity of > 99%. However, only [^{18}F] is reported for the *in vivo* studies, not [^{11}C] variant, probably due to the short half-life of [^{11}C] (i.e., 20 min.) and slow pharmacokinetics of paclitaxel [36].

[^{11}C]Docetaxel

It is a very known anticancer drug for several types of cancers. The [^{11}C] isotope is introduced into the tert-butoxycarbonyl (BOC) group of tertiary butanol during the synthesis [37]. Currently, no updated reports are available.

[^{11}C]Carvedilol

It is an adrenoceptor antagonist, and its uptake increases 3 fold after modulation with cyclosporine A (CsA). Also, proved to be more sensitive than verapamil on the kinetic graph in *in vivo* study [38]. However, due to the peripheral metabolism and unsuitable kinetics of metabolites, no further progress has been reported.

In the case of P-gp overexpression, uptake of the labeled substrate is reduced, which leads to poor statistics and unprecise PET measurements [39]. Thus, there are also labeled inhibitors for studying P-gp function, which in the overexpression of P-gp results in increase of PET signal instead of decrease. Some of the commonly used inhibitors are as follow:

[^{11}C]Laniquidar

It is a relatively stable inhibitor of P-gp with IC50 of 0.51 μM [40]. The yield of the radioactive [^{11}C] laniquidar is ~25%, which is sufficient for the preclinical studies. After the modulation with CsA, 5-fold uptake difference was observed in the study.

[^{11}C]Elacridar

It is a very potent inhibitor with IC50 of 0.02 μM; however, the corrected decay yield is meager (~5%) [41]. The signal was increased 5.4-fold in comparison to saline after the pretreatment of elacridar and then administration of [^{11}C]elacridar. Also, even after 20 min. of injection, 82% of compound was intact in the blood plasma. There was 2.5 fold increase in the Mdr1a/b(-/-)and 1.3-fold Bcrp(-/-) mice in comparison to wild type [42]. Although several studies show that [^{11}C]elacidar is an inhibitor, data also suggest it to be a weak substrate.

[11C]Tariquidar

The uptake of tariquidar in the brain is lower than [^{11}C]verapamil, and the metabolic activity is only 5% even after 60 min of injection [43]. Also, different to MC18, the brain uptake increases after the treatment of cold compound.

There are several other receptor ligands that have been studied for the P-gp after labeling with the positron emitter; however, none of them have reached the clinical studies, probably due to no significant advancement over the [^{11}C]verapamil. [^{11}C]verapamil is the only compound that has been thoroughly studied in human subjects. Also, some scanty reports of [^{11}C]dLop are also reported [31, 44]. Although the kinetics of R and S enantiomers of verapamil is similar, their metabolism is not [45]. R enantiomer is preferred over S due to slow metabolism. However, the major concern is the presence of metabolite [^{11}C]D617, which also binds with P-gp. Another is the generation of polar metabolites produced by the demethylation of [^{11}C]verapamil, which, although crosses the blood-brain barrier, but not the substrate of P-gp, hence cause the noise.

Most of the studies don't consider the effect of metabolites in studying the kinetics due to the assumption that in an initial 10 min, metabolites don't have significance in the brain [46]. However, Ikoma et al. [47] have shown that there is huge variation between the compartmental studies considering metabolite effect and graphical analysis (which don't consider the metabolite effect). But, some studies also showed the generation of erroneous results in epileptic patients after considering the metabolic effects [27]. It was suggested that metabolite consideration might not be relevant for the healthy patient; however, it should be considered in comparing the patients with control subjects. Also, the inclusion of metabolic consideration leads to a range of complexity to be analyzed by 60 min PET scan. Thus, following are the common assumption that [^{11}C]D617 metabolite is same as verapamil, and polar metabolites enter the BBB in a very little amount [20].

There are also questions on the measurement of verapamil uptake. Muzi and others have suggested the rate constant K1 (i.e., plasma to tissue), however, it is found to depend on the blood flow and sensitive to blood volume.[24] While Lubberink et al.[20] have suggested the usage of K2 (i.e., efflux from tissue to plasma). However, after the inhibition of P-gp, the K1 and volume of distribution (Vd) increased while K2 didn't, shows that K2 may not be a good option for studying the P-gp function.

The usage of Patlak plot involving the data of 3 min. and taking the Ki as the marker of P-gp function has been found to overcome the metabolite effect [47, 48]. Since in initial 3 min., the conc. of metabolite is negligible. In healthy volunteers, single compartment model has been preferred [20, 47]. However, there was no difference when considering it in the case of Parkinson patients on the calculation of Vd of [^{14}C]verapamil [49]. There is requirement of second compartment after inhibition of P-gp[24]. Although, in healthy tissue, such two-compartment model doesn't reflect the robust outcome [20].

There is concern whether the proposed model describes P-gp function accurately at the BBB. For example, the high hydrophobicity of [^{14}C]verapamil leads to the accumulation in the endothelium of the vessel wall, which can be distinguished from the actual uptake by the cerebral due to limited resolution of PET. It explains why the single compartment (verapamil present in endothelium) model suffices in the healthy controls, but not after the inhibition of P-gp, wherein second compartment is necessarily describing the verapamil uptake both by the cerebral tissue and endothelium.

There are some of the desired features for the ideal P-gp probes like easy and high selectivity, quick labeling, low metabolic product, high lipophilicity to pass BBB. The lipophilicity not only decides the plasma free fraction but also the level of specific binding [50]. The high lipophilicity helps in crossing the BBB via passive diffusion. However, the disadvantage of high lipophilicity is its non-specific binding in the target tissue, also high affinity towards the plasma proteins, which leads to low uptake of tracer [51]. The modification of verapamil to more polar has also been experienced by the O-demethylation of the methoxy group of the aromatic ring. However, there must be the reconsideration of specificity and transport kinetics [52].

[^{11}C]verapamil is the gold standard for measuring the P-gp function via PET and almost fill all the required criteria [20, 53, 54]. The synthesis of [^{11}C]verapamil is straightforward via the [^{11}C] methylation of norverapmil. It's has been automated for yield of 2.1 ± 0.5 GBq. Along with being the P-gp substrate, it's also a calcium channel antagonist. Thus the requirement of specificity becomes higher [34].

(R)-[^{11}C]verapamil is preferred over S enantiomer because of low affinity for the Ca2+ channels, and lower hepatic metabolism, helps in higher bioavalibity for the P-gp signal. In the (R) enantiomer, 57% radioactivity was detected in the plasma, while in the racemic mixture 37% radioactivity detected [26]. The radioactivity polar metabolite generated in the liver leads to non-P-gp related signal, which includes [^{11}C]formaldehyde, [^{11}C]carbon dioxide, and [^{11}C]formic acid [20, 27, 45].

In a study, there was a good correlation found in the Vd with or without the inclusion of polar metabolite compartment [55]. The omission caused the increase of Vd to 10%. As polar metabolite is not the substrate of P-gp, the alteration of P-gp function doesn't lead to much change in their Vd, and thus their omission does cause much change in the PET signal.

Considering the earlier discussion, it could be concluded that verapamil is the molecule of choice, although not being the ideal in terms of metabolite pattern and lipophilicity [55]. However, due to high specificity for the P-gp and ability to be test-retest, (R)-[^{11}C]verapamil remains the choice in clinical studies. However, in case of overexpression, (R)-[^{11}C]verapamil is not a preferred choice. Herein, the inhibitors labeled with [^{11}C] like MC-18 is preferred for the study. The binding and uptake of MC-18 is more in the overexpression and signals can be easily detected. Although MC-18 shows saturation in binding to the brain and peripheral organs, its modest affinity causes low target to non-target ratio.

CONCLUSION

P-glycoprotein is a membrane protein that can efflux many compounds across the plasma membrane, thus, competing its physiological role in protecting cells. P-gp is also widely implicated in the development of multidrug resistance in cancer and other disease cells. Many clinical investigations are devoted to block such efflux capability of cells or tissues for achieving improved therapeutic benefits. This chapter discussed progress made in recent years in developing and applying various methods that are commonly employed to quantify P-gp in serum (other biological liquids), cells, and tissues. This information may provide a standard how much P-gp modulators need to be administered along with chemotherapy to lower the required dose of chemotherapeutic agent.

REFERENCES

[1] Zhang, Y; Benet, LZ. Characterization of P-glycoprotein Mediated Transport of K02, a Novel Vinylsulfone Peptidomimetic Cysteine Protease Inhibitor, Across MDR1-MDCK and Caco-2 Cell Monolayers, *Pharmaceutical research*, 15(10), (1998), 1520-1524.

[2] Cummins, CL; Jacobsen, W; Christians, U; Benet, LZ. CYP3A4-transfected Caco-2 cells as a tool for understanding biochemical absorption barriers: studies with sirolimus and midazolam, *The Journal of pharmacology and experimental therapeutics*, 308(1), (2004), 143-55.

[3] Cummins, CL; Jacobsen, W; Benet, LZ. Unmasking the dynamic interplay between intestinal P-glycoprotein and CYP3A4, *The Journal of pharmacology and experimental therapeutics*, 300(3), (2002), 1036-45.

[4] Johnson, BM; Charman, WN; Porter, CJ. Application of compartmental modeling to an examination of *in vitro* intestinal permeability data: assessing the impact of tissue uptake, P-glycoprotein, and CYP3A, *Drug metabolism and disposition: the biological fate of chemicals*, 31(9), (2003), 1151-60.

[5] Griffiths, R; Lewis, A; Jeffrey, P. Models of drug absorption *in situ* and in conscious animals, *Pharmaceutical biotechnology*, 8, (1996), 67-84.

[6] Rogers, JD; Ho, NF; Morozowich, W. Physical model approach to gastrointestinal absorption of prostaglandins III: *In situ* rat intestinal absorption of dinoprostone, *Journal of pharmaceutical sciences*, 73(11), (1984), 1594-9.

[7] Taylor, DC. Animal models for oral drug delivery in man: *In situ* and *in vivo* approaches. Edited by William Crouthamel and Allen C. Sarapu. American Pharmaceutical Association, Academy of Pharmaceutical Sciences, 1983. 179 pp. 73(11), (1984), 1676-1676.

[8] Brouwers, J; Mols, R;Annaert, P; Augustijns, P.*Validation of a differential in situ perfusion method with mesenteric blood sampling in rats for intestinal drug interaction profiling*, 31(5-6), (2010), 278-285.

[9] Mols, R; Brouwers, J; Schinkel, AH; Annaert, P; Augustijns, P.*Intestinal perfusion with mesenteric blood sampling in wild-type and knockout mice: evaluation of a novel tool in biopharmaceutical drug profiling*, (2009).

[10] Holmstock, N; Mols, R;Annaert, P; Augustijns, P.*In situ* intestinal perfusion in knockout mice demonstrates inhibition of intestinal p-glycoprotein by ritonavir causing increased darunavir absorption, *Drug metabolism and disposition: the biological fate of chemicals*, 38(9), (2010), 1407-10.

[11] Liu, Y; Huang, L; Hoffman, T; Gosland, M; Vore, M. MDR1 substrates/modulators protect against beta-estradiol-17beta-D-glucuronide cholestasis in rat liver, *Cancer research*, 56(21), (1996), 4992-7.

[12] Smit, JW; Duin, E; Steen, H;Oosting, R; Roggeveld, J; Meijer, DK. Interactions between P-glycoprotein substrates and other cationic drugs at the hepatic excretory level, *British journal of pharmacology*, 123(3), (1998), 361-70.

[13] Ballatori, N. *Measurement of hepatobiliary transport, Current protocols in toxicology chapter*, 14, (2004), Unit14.5.

[14] Katoh, M; Suzuyama, N; Takeuchi, T; Yoshitomi, S; Asahi, S; Yokoi, T. Kinetic analyses for species differences in P-glycoprotein-mediated drug transport, *Journal of pharmaceutical sciences*, 95(12), (2006), 2673-83.

[15] Syvänen, S;Lindhe, Ö; Palner, M; Kornum, BR; Rahman, O; Långström, B; Knudsen, GM; Hammarlund-Udenaes, M. *Species Differences in Blood-Brain Barrier Transport of Three Positron*

Emission Tomography Radioligands with Emphasis on P-Glycoprotein Transport, 37(3), (2009), 635-643.

[16] Hsu, SI; Lothstein, L; Horwitz, SB. Differential overexpression of three mdr gene family members in multidrug-resistant J774.2 mouse cells. Evidence that distinct P-glycoprotein precursors are encoded by unique mdr genes, *The Journal of biological chemistry*, 264(20), (1989), 12053-62.

[17] Schinkel, AH; Smit, JJ; van Tellingen, O; Beijnen, JH; Wagenaar, E; van Deemter, L; Mol, CA; van der Valk, MA; Robanus-Maandag, EC; teRiele, HP; et al., Disruption of the mouse mdr1a P-glycoprotein gene leads to a deficiency in the blood-brain barrier and to increased sensitivity to drugs, *Cell*, 77(4), (1994), 491-502.

[18] Cutler, L; Howes, C; Deeks, NJ; Buck, TL; Jeffrey, P. Development of a P-glycoprotein knockout model in rodents to define species differences in its functional effect at the blood-brain barrier, *Journal of pharmaceutical sciences*, 95(9), (2006), 1944-53.

[19] Syvänen, S; Lindhe, O; Palner, M; Kornum, BR; Rahman, O; Långström, B; Knudsen, GM; Hammarlund-Udenaes, M. Species differences in blood-brain barrier transport of three positron emission tomography radioligands with emphasis on P-glycoprotein transport, *Drug metabolism and disposition: the biological fate of chemicals*, 37(3), (2009), 635-43.

[20] Lubberink, M; Luurtsema, G; van Berckel, BN; Boellaard, R; Toornvliet, R; Windhorst, AD; Franssen, EJ; Lammertsma, AA. Evaluation of tracer kinetic models for quantification of P-glycoprotein function using (R)-[11C]verapamil and PET, *Journal of cerebral blood flow and metabolism: official journal of the International Society of Cerebral Blood Flow and Metabolism*, 27(2), (2007), 424-33.

[21] Osman, S; Lundkvist, C; Pike, VW; Halldin, C; McCarron, JA; Swahn, CG; Farde, L; Ginovart, N; Luthra, SK; Gunn, RN; Bench, CJ; Sargent, PA; Grasby, PM. Characterisation of the appearance of radioactive metabolites in monkey and human plasma from the 5-HT1A receptor radioligand, [carbonyl-11C]WAY-100635--

explanation of high signal contrast in PET and an aid to biomathematical modelling, *Nuclear medicine and biology*, 25(3), (1998), 215-23.

[22] Eyal, S; Chung, FS; Muzi, M; Link, JM; Mankoff, DA; Kaddoumi, A; O'Sullivan, F; Hebert, MF; Unadkat, JD. Simultaneous PET imaging of P-glycoprotein inhibition in multiple tissues in the pregnant nonhuman primate, *Journal of nuclear medicine: official publication, Society of Nuclear Medicine*, 50(5), (2009), 798-806.

[23] Eyal, S; Ke, B; Muzi, M; Link, JM; Mankoff, DA; Collier, AC; Unadkat, JD. Regional P-glycoprotein activity and inhibition at the human blood-brain barrier as imaged by positron emission tomography, *Clinical pharmacology and therapeutics*, 87(5), (2010), 579-85.

[24] Muzi, M; Mankoff, DA; Link, JM; Shoner, S; Collier, AC; Sasongko, L; Unadkat, JD. Imaging of cyclosporine inhibition of P-glycoprotein activity using 11C-verapamil in the brain: studies of healthy humans, *Journal of nuclear medicine: official publication, Society of Nuclear Medicine*, 50(8), (2009), 1267-75.

[25] Vaalburg, W; Hendrikse, NH; Elsinga, PH; Bart, J; van Waarde, A. P-glycoprotein activity and biological response, *Toxicology and applied pharmacology*, 207(2 Suppl), (2005), 257-60.

[26] Sasongko, L; Link, JM; Muzi, M; Mankoff, DA; Yang, X; Collier, AC; Shoner, SC; Unadkat, JD. Imaging P-glycoprotein transport activity at the human blood-brain barrier with positron emission tomography, *Clinical pharmacology and therapeutics*, 77(6), (2005), 503-14.

[27] Abrahim, A; Luurtsema, G; Bauer, M; Karch, R; Lubberink, M; Pataraia, E; Joukhadar, C; Kletter, K; Lammertsma, AA; Baumgartner,C; Müller, M; Langer, O. Peripheral metabolism of (R)-[11C]verapamil in epilepsy patients, *European journal of nuclear medicine and molecular imaging*, 35(1), (2008), 116-23.

[28] Adams, ML; Lavasanifar, A; Kwon, GS. Amphiphilic block copolymers for drug delivery, *Journal of pharmaceutical sciences*, 92(7), (2003), 1343-1355.

[29] Zoghbi, SS; Liow, JS; Yasuno, F; Hong, J; Tuan, E; Lazarova, N; Gladding, RL; Pike, VW; Innis, RB. 11C-loperamide and its N-desmethyl radiometabolite are avid substrates for brain permeability-glycoprotein efflux, *Journal of nuclear medicine: official publication, Society of Nuclear Medicine*, 49(4), (2008), 649-56.

[30] Lazarova, N; Zoghbi, SS; Hong, J; Seneca, N; Tuan, E; Gladding, RL; Liow, JS; Taku, A; Innis, RB; Pike, VW. Synthesis and evaluation of [N-methyl-11C]N-desmethyl-loperamide as a new and improved PET radiotracer for imaging P-gp function, *Journal of medicinal chemistry*, 51(19), (2008), 6034-43.

[31] Seneca, N; Zoghbi, SS; Liow, JS; Kreisl, W; Herscovitch, P; Jenko, K; Gladding, RL; Taku, A; Pike, VW; Innis, RB. Human brain imaging and radiation dosimetry of 11C-N-desmethyl-loperamide, a PET radiotracer to measure the function of P-glycoprotein, *Journal of nuclear medicine: official publication, Society of Nuclear Medicine*, 50(5), (2009), 807-13.

[32] Mehta, BM; Rosa, E; Biedler, JL; Larson, SM.*In vivo* uptake of carbon-14-colchicine for identification of tumor multidrug resistance, *Journal of nuclear medicine: official publication, Society of Nuclear Medicine*, 35(7), (1994), 1179-84.

[33] Levchenko, A; Mehta, BM; Lee, JB; Humm, JL; Augensen, F; Squire, O; Kothari, PJ; Finn, RD; Leonard, EF; Larson, SM. Evaluation of 11C-colchicine for PET imaging of multiple drug resistance, *Journal of nuclear medicine: official publication, Society of Nuclear Medicine*, 41(3), (2000), 493-501.

[34] Elsinga, PH; Franssen, EJ; Hendrikse, NH; Fluks, L; Weemaes, AM; van der Graaf, WT; de Vries, EG; Visser, GM; Vaalburg, W. Carbon-11-labeled daunorubicin and verapamil for probing P-glycoprotein in tumors with PET, *Journal of nuclear medicine: official publication, Society of Nuclear Medicine*, 37(9), (1996), 1571-5.

[35] Eriks-Fluks, E; Elsinga, PH; Hendrikse, NH; Franssen, EJ; Vaalburg, W. Enzymatic synthesis of [4-methoxy-11C]daunorubicin for functional imaging of P-glycoprotein with PET, *Applied radiation and*

isotopes: including data, instrumentation and methods for use in agriculture, industry and medicine, 49(7), (1998), 811-3.

[36] Gangloff, A; Hsueh, WA; Kesner, AL; Kiesewetter, DO; Pio, BS; Pegram, MD; Beryt, M; Townsend, A; Czernin, J; Phelps, ME; Silverman, DH. Estimation of paclitaxel biodistribution and uptake in human-derived xenografts *in vivo* with (18)F-fluoropaclitaxel, *Journal of nuclear medicine: official publication, Society of Nuclear Medicine*, 46(11), (2005), 1866-71.

[37] van Tilburg, EW; Mooijer, MPJ; Brinkhorst, J; van der Meij, M; Windhorst, AD. Improved and semi-automated GMP-compliant radiosynthesis of [11C]docetaxel, *Applied Radiation and Isotopes*, 66(10), (2008), 1414-1418.

[38] Bart, J; Dijkers, EC; Wegman, TD; de Vries, EG; van der Graaf, WT; Groen, HJ; Vaalburg, W; Willemsen, AT; Hendrikse, NH. New positron emission tomography tracer [(11)C]carvedilol reveals P-glycoprotein modulation kinetics, *British journal of pharmacology*, 145(8), (2005), 1045-51.

[39] Marchi, N; Hallene, KL; Kight, KM; Cucullo, L; Moddel, G; Bingaman, W; Dini, G; Vezzani, A; Janigro, D. Significance of MDR1 and multiple drug resistance in refractory human epileptic brain, *BMC Medicine*, 2(1), (2004), 37.

[40] Luurtsema, G; Schuit, RC; Klok, RP; Verbeek, J; Leysen, JE; Lammertsma, AA; Windhorst, AD. Evaluation of [11C]laniquidar as a tracer of P-glycoprotein: radiosynthesis and biodistribution in rats, *Nuclear medicine and biology*, 36(6), (2009), 643-649.

[41] Hyafil, F; Vergely, C; Du Vignaud, P; Grand-Perret, T. *Reversal of Multidrug Resistance by GF120918, an Acridonecarboxamide Derivative*, 53(19), (1993), 4595-4602.

[42] Dörner, B; Kuntner, C; Bankstahl, JP; Bankstahl, M; Stanek, J; Wanek, T; Stundner, G; Mairinger, S; Löscher, W; Müller, M; Langer, O; Erker, T. Synthesis and small-animal positron emission tomography evaluation of [11C]-elacridar as a radiotracer to assess the distribution of P-glycoprotein at the blood-brain barrier, *Journal of medicinal chemistry*, 52(19), (2009), 6073-82.

[43] Bauer, F; Kuntner, C; Bankstahl, JP; Wanek, T; Bankstahl, M; Stanek, J; Mairinger, S; Dörner, B; Löscher, W; Müller, M; Erker, T; Langer, O.*Synthesis and in vivo evaluation of [11C]tariquidar, a positron emission tomography radiotracer based on a third-generation P-glycoprotein inhibitor, Bioorganic & medicinal chemistry*, 18(15), (2010), 5489-97.

[44] Kreisl, WC; Liow, JS; Kimura, N; Seneca, N; Zoghbi, SS; Morse, CL; Herscovitch, P; Pike, VW; Innis, RB. P-glycoprotein function at the blood-brain barrier in humans can be quantified with the substrate radiotracer 11C-N-desmethyl-loperamide, *Journal of nuclear medicine:official publication, Society of Nuclear Medicine*, 51(4), (2010), 559-66.

[45] Luurtsema, G; Molthoff, CF; Schuit, RC; Windhorst, AD; Lammertsma, AA; Franssen, EJ.*Evaluation of (R)-[11C]verapamil as PET tracer of P-glycoprotein function in the blood-brain barrier: kinetics and metabolism in the rat, Nuclear medicine and biology*, 32(1), (2005), 87-93.

[46] Kortekaas, R; Leenders, KL; van Oostrom, JC; Vaalburg, W; Bart, J; Willemsen, AT; Hendrikse, NH. *Blood-brain barrier dysfunction in parkinsonian midbrain in vivo, Annals of neurology, 57*(2), (2005), 176-9.

[47] Ikoma, Y; Takano, A; Ito, H; Kusuhara, H; Sugiyama, Y; Arakawa, R; Fukumura, T; Nakao, R; Suzuki, K; Suhara, T. Quantitative analysis of 11C-verapamil transfer at the human blood-brain barrier for evaluation of P-glycoprotein function, *Journal of nuclear medicine: official publication, Society of Nuclear Medicine*, 47(9), (2006), 1531-7.

[48] Lee, YJ; Maeda, J; Kusuhara, H; Okauchi, T; Inaji, M; Nagai, Y; Obayashi, S; Nakao, R; Suzuki, K; Sugiyama, Y; Suhara, T.*In vivo* evaluation of P-glycoprotein function at the blood-brain barrier in nonhuman primates using [11C]verapamil, *The Journal of pharmacology and experimental therapeutics*, 316(2), (2006), 647-53.

[49] Bartels, AL; van Berckel, BNM; Lubberink, M; Luurtsema, G; Lammertsma, AA; Leenders, KL.*Blood–brain barrier P-glycoprotein*

function is not impaired in early Parkinson's disease, *Parkinsonism & Related Disorders*, 14(6), (2008), 505-508.

[50] Miller, MM; Wasik, SP; Huang, GL; Shiu, WY; Mackay, D. Relationships between octanol-water partition coefficient and aqueous solubility, *Environmental Science & Technology*, 19(6), (1985), 522-529.

[51] Waterhouse, RN. Determination of lipophilicity and its use as a predictor of blood-brain barrier penetration of molecular imaging agents, *Molecular imaging and biology*, 5(6), (2003), 376-89.

[52] Toffoli, G; Simone, F; Corona, G; Raschack, M; Cappelletto, B; Gigante, M; Boiocchi, M. Structure-activity relationship of verapamil analogs and reversal of multidrug resistance, *Biochemical pharmacology*, 50(8), (1995), 1245-55.

[53] Bartels, AL; Willemsen, AT; Kortekaas, R; de Jong, BM; de Vries, R; de Klerk, O; van Oostrom, JC; Portman, A; Leenders, KL. Decreased blood-brain barrier P-glycoprotein function in the progression of Parkinson's disease, PSP and MSA, *Journal of neural transmission* (Vienna, Austria: 1996), 115(7), (2008), 1001-9.

[54] Toornvliet, R; van Berckel, BN; Luurtsema, G; Lubberink, M; Geldof, AA; Bosch, TM; Oerlemans, R; Lammertsma, AA; Franssen, EJ. Effect of age on functional P-glycoprotein in the blood-brain barrier measured by use of (R)-[(11)C]verapamil and positron emission tomography, *Clinical pharmacology and therapeutics*, 79(6), (2006), 540-8.

[55] Luurtsema, G; Verbeek, GL; Lubberink, M; Lammertsma, AA; Dierckx, R; Elsinga, P; Windhorst, AD; van Waarde, A. Carbon-11 labeled tracers for *in vivo* imaging P-glycoprotein function: kinetics, advantages and disadvantages, *Current topics in medicinal chemistry*, 10(17), (2010), 1820-33.

In: An Introduction to P-Glycoprotein
Editors: M. Wahajuddin et al.
ISBN: 978-1-53619-488-3

Chapter 12

RECENT ADVANCEMENTS AND FUTURE PERSPECTIVES

Nazneen Sultana[1], Swati Chaturvedi[1,2], Divya Chauhan[1] and M. Wahajuddin[1,2,*]

[1]Pharmaceutics and Pharmacokinetics Division,
CSIR - Central Drug Research Institute, Lucknow, Uttar Pradesh, India
[2]Academy of Scientific and Innovative Research (AcSIR),
Ghaziabad, India

ABSTRACT

P-glycoprotein (P-gp), an ATP binding cassette (ABC) efflux transporter is a transmembrane permeability glycoprotein that pumps out xenobiotics and toxic substances out of the cells. A Number of pharmaco-therapeutics falls under the category of P-gp substrate that consequently reduces the bioavailability of these drugs systemically. Moreover, overexpression of P-gp also leads to efflux of intracellular therapeutic agents, resulting in the induction of multi-drug resistance (MDR) and failure of chemotherapy. Hence, it is essential to explore the role of P-gp inhibitors with suitable formulation strategy to overcome the poor

* Corresponding Author's Email: wahajuddin@gmail.com.

bioavailability issue and to combat the multidrug resistance phenomenon of P-gp substrate. In recent years, researchers have discovered many lead molecules that function as P-gp inhibitors thereby increasing the concentration of drugs in blood and hence the therapeutic potency. This chapter emphasizes on the recent advances in the discovery of novel, inert, non-toxic, and highly efficient and target specific P-gp inhibitors such as third-generation inhibitors, emerging nanomaterial inhibitors and those obtained from the natural sources. The Application of nanomaterials to directly inhibit P-gp is emerging as new area of interest to overcome MDR. Therefore, we also emphasized on the recent advancements of nanomaterial inhibitors that has proven application in the treatment of P-gp mediated MDR and are currently under development. Furthermore, new thoughts have also been suggested to tackle the P-gp mediated disease therapy issues.

Keywords: P-glycoprotein, ABC transporters, nanomaterial, MDR, pharmaco-therapeutics

INTRODUCTION

P-glycoprotein a member of ATP-dependent efflux transporters, has a broad substrate specificity. It consists of two hydrophobic domains with twelve trans-membrane α-helices which works as a drug binding domain and transport xenobiotics and toxins outside the cells. The two nucleotide-binding domains present in the cytoplasmic region are involved in correlating hydrolysis of ATP to the transport processes [1, 2]. About 40 years back, the correlation of P-glycoprotein (P-gp) expression with multidrug resistance in different kinds of cancer cells [3] was established such as leukemia and adenocarcinoma [4, 5]. Eventually, it was noted that p-glycoprotein transporter is not only expressed in cancer cells, but also in a wide range of normal tissue including intestine [6, 7], liver [8], brain [9, 10], adrenal gland [11], and kidney [12], etc. P-glycoprotein receptors act as a protecting shield for these organs by regulating the transport of exogenous compounds out of the cells. It shows the protective action against toxic compounds and xenobiotic substances [13]. Consequently, P-glycoprotein serves as a barrier to intestinal drug absorption and drug distribution to the brain and cancer tissue.

The phenomenon of multidrug resistance (MDR) refers to the development of cross-resistance against multiple structurally and/or functionally irrelevant drug molecules by the tumor cells in the course of treatment. Several mechanisms contributes in the development of multidrug resistance such as overexpression of the efflux pump in the cell [14, 15], improvement in the DNA repair process, the progression of the cell cycle pathways [16], suppression of apoptosis [17] and cytochrome P450 hepatic enzyme system activation [16]. Since overexpression of efflux pumps plays a crucial role in the development of MDR to tumor cells, henceforth this mechanism is the common cause of frequent failure of chemotherapy. Among the efflux pumps, ATP-binding cassette transporters (ABC transporters) are majorly overexpressed transporter in the cancer cells and are responsible for the MDR development [18]. Efflux transporters such as multidrug resistance-associated protein (MRP/ABCC1), breast cancer resistance protein (ABCG2/BCRP), and P-glycoprotein (ABCB1/P-gp) play an important role in this affair.

Researchers have been extensively exploring a varying aspects of the P-gp function in the search for the compound that can significantly inhibit the P-gp function to combat MDR. In this regard, several novel P-gp inhibitors have been identified in the last few decades and many more are in the run. Recently a combination of docetaxel with P-gp inhibitor for oral administration used in the treatment of cancer has been patented. In Table 1, a list of patents related to the design and utilization of P-gp inhibitor in the last five years has been represented. While many approaches are under clinical trials and needed to pass it for clinical utility. In Table 2, a list of the clinical trials, either completed in last five years or undergoing currently, associated with P-gp expression and P-gp substrate/inhibitors/markers are summarized.

Table 1. List of patents (2015-2020) related to design and utilization of P-gp inhibitor

Patent	Date	Title	Condition	Inventors	Status
US2020/0188386A1	June 18 2020	Therapeutic combinations of orally administered docetaxel and a P-gp inhibitor for the treatment of cancer	Cancer	Min-Fun R. Kwan, et al.	Pending
US9744210B2	December 23 2019	Treatment of rhinosinusitis with P-glycoprotein inhibitor	Rhinosinusitis	Benjamin S. Bleier	Pending
US9561227B2	November 29 2018	Inhibitors of multidrug resistance transporter P-glycoprotein	MDR	John G. Wise, et al.	Active
WO2017/123933A1	July 20 2017	Secreted P-glycoprotein is a noninvasive biomarker of chronic rhinosinusitis	Chronic Rhinosinusitis	Benjamin S. Bleier and Angela Nocera	Application filling
WO2017/173509A1	October 12 2017	Anti-tumor cocktail comprising an antitumor agent selective for tumor acidity, an antioxidant, and a P-glycoprotein inhibitor	MDR	Gerson Silva Paiva	Application filling
US2016/0193237A1	July 07 2016	Method of increasing the bioavailability of an HIV drug	Bioavailability	Pradeep K. Karla	Active
WO2015/060812A1	April 30 2015	Treating ocular disease with efflux transporter inhibitor	Ocular disease	Pradeep K. Karla and Harpal S. Mangat	Application filling
US2015/0231069A	August 20 2015	Oral formulation of chemotherapeutic agents	MDR	Pankaj Modi	Abandoned

Table 2. List of clinical trial related to P-glycoprotein

S. No.	Drug	Condition	Study	Phase	Status	NCT number
1	Mifamurtide arm	Osteosarcoma	P-gp expression as biologic stratification factor	Phase 2 Phase 3	Active, not recruiting	NCT01459484
2	Methotrexate, cisplatin, and adriamycin	Osteosarcoma	Influence of P-gp expression on osteosarcoma	-	Recruiting	NCT04383288
3	Carvedilol-CR	Epilepsy	P-gp inhibition as adjunct treatment	Phase 2 Phase 3	Terminated	NCT00524134
4	Caffeine, tolbutamide, omeprazole, digoxin, dextromethorphan and midazolam	AOD Effects and Consequences	Evaluate the effect of acute alcohol consumption on P-gp transporter	-	Completed	NCT02515526
5	Dabigatran etexilate and Tepotinib	Healthy	Effect of tepotinib on pharmacokinetic of P-gp substrate (Dabigatran etexilate)	Phase 1	Completed	NCT03492437
6	[11C] desmethyl-loperamide, ritonavir and efavirenz	Drug Effects	Effects of ritonavir and efavirenz on the activity of P-glycoprotein in human brain	Phase 1 Phase 2	Completed	NCT01668147
7	Paclitaxel	Gastrointestinal Stromal Tumors	Efficacy of paclitaxel in advanced GIST with low P-gp expression	Phase 2	Recruiting	NCT03944304
8	(11C)N-desmethyl-loperamide	Healthy	Quantify the P-gp expression	-	Completed	NCT00605254
9	[11C] desmethyl-loperamide, ritonavir and efavirenz	Alzheimer, Parkinson, Fronto-temporal Lobar Degeneration	Measure the P-gp function in disease condition	-	Completed	NCT00677885

Table 2. (Continued)

S. No.	Drug	Condition	Study	Phase	Status	NCT number
10	Lenalidomide, Quinidine, Temsirolimus and Diphenhydramine	Healthy	Effect of P-gp inhibition on lenalidomide pharmacokinetics	Phase 1	Completed	NCT01712828
11	Enzalutamide, digoxin, and rosuvastatin	Prostate Cancer	Effect of enzalutamide on pharmacokinetics of P-gp substrate	Phase 1	Active, not recruiting	NCT04094519
12	(11C)N-desmethyl-loperamide	Low Grade Glioma, Glioblastoma Astrocytoma, Anaplastic Oligodendroglioma, Oligoastrocytoma	Quantify the P-gp expression and evaluate BBB	-	Terminated	NCT01281982
13	Ketoconazole	Healthy	Influence of simultaneous CYP3A4 and p-gp inhibition on lenvatinib pharmacokinetics	Phase 1	Completed	NCT02198170
14	Pimodivir and cyclosporine	Healthy	Evaluate effect of cyclosporine, a P-gp, on pharmacokinetics of pimodivir	Phase 1	Completed	NCT03768609
15	11C-JNJ-63779586	Alzheimer Disease	Investigate the regional brain kinetics of brain drug transporters using P-gp	Phase 1	Completed	NCT03089918
16	Daptomycin and Rifampin	Drug Interactions, Pharmacokinetics	Evaluate effect of polymorphisms in P-gp on the blood levels of daptomycin	Early Phase 1	Completed	NCT02097953
17	[11C]-verapamil PET	Epilepsy	To quantify the P-gp expression	Phase 2	Unknown status	NCT02144792

S. No.	Drug	Condition	Study	Phase	Status	NCT number
18	Ze 117	Drug Interaction Study	Effect of Ze 117 on P-gp transporter	Phase 1	Unknown status	NCT03482817
19	Ondansetron and tariquidar	Neuropathic Pain	Effect of P-gp inhibitor tariquidar on ondasetron	Phase 1 Phase 2	Not yet recruiting	NCT04603066
20	Trospium chloride, and clarithromycin	Drug interaction	Effect of P-gp inhibitor clarithromycin on trospium pharmacokinetic	Phase 1	Completed	NCT03011463
21	Orvepitant and itraconazole	Healthy	Effect of P-gp inhibitor itraconazole on orvepitant pharmacokinetics	Phase 1	Completed	NCT03535662
22	Tariquidar, doxorubicin, docetaxel and vinorelbine	Wilms' Tumor Sarcoma, coldrhood cancer	Effect of P-gp inhibitor tariquidar on doxorubicin, docetaxel or vinorelbine pharmacokinetics	Phase 1	Completed	NCT00011414
23	-	Breast Carcinoma Breast Cancer Medullary Thyroid Carcinoma	Identify and evaluate the roles of P-gp in mediating drug resistance.	-	Completed	NCT00880503
24	Rifampicin	Tuberculosis	Effect of high dose rifampicin on P-gp	Phase 1	Not yet recruiting	NCT04525235
25	Respiratory Syncytial Virus Infections	Itraconazole, verapamil, rifampicin and midazolam	P-gp and CYP3A4 mediated drug interaction study	Phase 1	Completed	NCT03782662

Reversal of MDR by Novel P-gp Inhibitors

Overexpression of P-gp in tumor cells lowers the concentration of chemotherapeutics and cause resistance against currently available many anti-tumor drugs like anthracyclines (daunorubicin), vinca alkaloids (vinblastine), and taxanes (paclitaxel) [19]. The capability of P-gp to transport such as diverse range of chemical classes is due to multiple transport pathways facilitated by protein [20]. Recent studies indicated that depending on the tissue of origin, overexpression of P-gp in tumor cells can be either acquired while drug treatment or it can be intrinsic [21-25]. Various drugs which were initially P-gp inhibitors, at higher systemic concentration act as P-gp substrate [26, 27] whereas many drugs do not have P-gp specificity and results in drug interaction [28]. Three new compounds were identified that have the potential to surpass the challenges of earlier generation P-gp inhibitors. They have the ability to specifically interact with the nucleotide-binding domains of the P-gp transporter pump, meanwhile significantly avoiding the binding at the drug binding domains [29]. These three identified compounds (compounds 29, 34, and 45) can caused a reversal of resistance of paclitaxel in a P-gp overexpresses cells in prostate cancer cell line [30, 31]. Biophysical and biochemical analyses showed that the nucleotide-binding site was affected by the compounds 34 and 45 whereas transport substrate activated ATP hydrolysis was inhibited by all the three compounds by purified P-gp. The results indicated the interaction of inhibitors with the nucleotide-binding domains with no interference with the drug binding domains. It also suggested that the inhibitors have the potential of not being substrate transporter for P-gp. Co-administration of these compounds with chemotherapeutics have led to a significantly increase in the penetration and accumulation of P-gp substrate in the microtumor cells. These inhibitors directly shut off the pumping action of P-gp. Out of three, two of the compounds are highly specific to P-gp, whereas the third inhibited P-gp with low specificity. They also strongly inhibited cell migration without down-regulating the expression of P-gp while re-sensitizing the MDR tumor cells [29].

Nanotechnology Strategy to Combat P-gp Mediated MDR

Nanotechnology-based drug delivery strategies have enabled the delivery of drugs to the targeted organ and even cells [32]. It can be designed to optimize the biodistribution and pharmacokinetics. In the case of cancer treatment, uptake of nanomedicine can also be done through phagocytosis or endocytosis, thereby bypassing the efflux pumps and avoiding the mechanism of MDR [33]. Nanomedicine based techniques used to combat the MDR includes co-delivery of P-gp inhibitors and chemotherapeutic drugs through nanocarriers, utilizing the process of endocytosis to deliver chemotherapeutic drugs, and using polymeric P-gp inhibitors as drug carriers. Nanomedicine has the ability to enter the cancer cells through endocytosis or phagocytosis and thus bypass the efflux pumps such as P-gp expressed on the cell membrane. Co-administration of P-gp inhibitors with chemotherapeutic drugs is a promising way to avoid MDR [34, 35], however, it might suffer from difficulties such as formulation challenges, premature release, or inconsistent delivery efficiency due to physical stability and low drug loading. Using polymeric inhibitors as drug carrier can also circumvent MDR significantly by interfering with P-gp function along with carrying therapeutics in nanocarriers such as nanoparticles, liposomes, and micelles. In this content, the nanomaterial with P-gp inhibitory property can be the marvelous nano-scale drug delivery and cancer targeting system. Self–assembly of nano platform facilitates the formulation with higher drug loading. In contrast to traditional P-gp inhibitors, nanomaterial with P-gp inhibition property can alter the pharmacokinetic parameter to promote accumulation and drug targeting. For an instant, d-alpha-tocopheryl polyethylene glycol-1000 succinate (TPGS) has been extensively utilized as a P-gp inhibitory nanomaterial in preclinical studies [36]. It can be used to prepare different nanocarriers such as micelles [37, 38], liposomes [39], hybrid inorganic nanoparticles [40], and nanoemulsions [41]. The commonly recognized P-gp inhibitory nanomaterials such as TPGS, PEG-PLGA/PLA polymers, and pluronics could combine the nanocarriers' superiorities and the P-gp inhibition into one and increase the anticancer efficacy in chemo-resistant drugs. With the development in the field of pharmaceutical science and, nanotechnology many P-gp inhibitory nanomaterials have been emerged such as stimuli-responsive nanomaterials, inorganic nanomaterials and, pharmaceutical excipient Soluplus [42].

Stimuli-responsive nanomaterials have the ability to offer noticeable physical and chemical changes with respect to the surrounding pathological environment [43]. They have been used in the various medical applications including drug delivery, tissue engineering, and diagnosis. The stimuli can be exogenous or endogenous such as light, temperature, hypoxia, pH, enzyme, reactive oxygen species (ROS), salt concentration, and other factors [44]. Drug carriers prepare from stimuli-responsive nanomaterials can smartly identify the structural or surface change and target the required site to overcome the biological barriers or promote on-site drug delivery. They have the potential to combat the MDR in cancer treatment. They enhance the drug uptake and intracellular concentration, thus increasing the drug efficacy in the resistant models. Generally, self-assembled nanomaterial carrier gets destabilize in the stimuli-rich targeted site which causes the accelerated and controlled release of drug in the intracellular region, thereby overcoming the drug efflux pumps like P-gp [45]. There are several stimuli-responsive nanomaterials that can interfere with the efflux process and enhance total cellular concentration. For an instant, in many studies, TPGS has been endorse with the stimuli-sensitivity such as pH-responsive [46], enzyme-responsive [47], redox-responsive [48], and even dual-responsive nanocarriers [47] to sensitize the resistant cells and enhance the drug targetability. One of the major enzymes which is involved in the tumor initiation, progression, and metastasis process and used in treatment and diagnosis of cancer is matrix metalloproteinases (MMPs). Drug carrier prepared from nanomaterial responsive to the MMP can be promising cancer targeted drug delivery system in an MMP-responsive manner [49]. MMP-sensitive nanomaterials composed of the polymer-drug conjugate was significantly able to inhibit the P-gp mediated efflux of doxorubicin in resistant cells. Further, a polymer-lipid copolymer, PEG-pp-PE, composed of different lengths of PEG chain and varying sequence of peptides inhibited the P-gp function through MMP2 responsiveness, as shown in Figure 1. P-gp inhibition efficacy of PEG-pp-PE is lower than its commercial analogue, PEG-PE copolymer, whereas it is higher than TPGS at the equivalent concentration. Alteration in the length of PEG chain and sequence of peptides can affect the capability of efflux modulation of polymers. Co-polymers inhibit the efflux of drugs by interfering with the ATPase activity, hindering the P-gp expression, and altering the fluidity of the cell membrane. The primary functions of stimuli-sensitivity, efflux inhibition, and self-assembly of stimuli-responsive nanomaterials might give a new direction for the design of cancer targeted therapy [50].

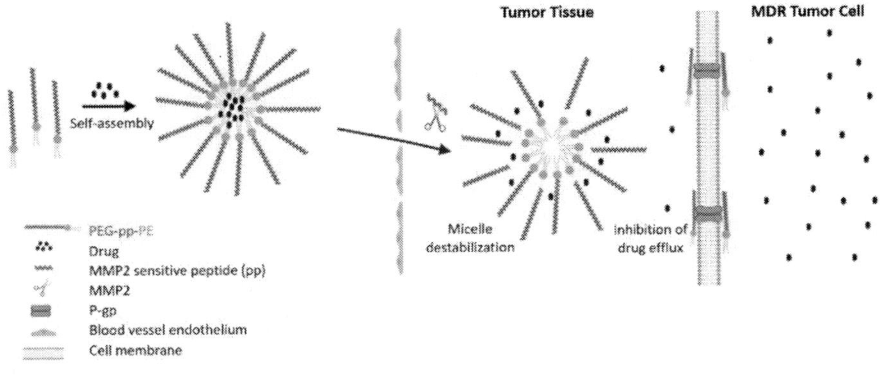

Figure 1. Schematic representation of MMP2 responsive P-gp inhibition mechanism of PEG-pp-PE.

Recently Inorganic nanomaterials have gained much interest in the field of biomedical. Metal oxide nanoparticles, carbon nanomaterials, and metal nanomaterials are emerging drug delivery vehicles in disease diagnosis and chemotherapy to combat drug resistance [51]. Fe_3O_4 magnetic nanoparticles, an inorganic nanomaterial, increases the intracellular accumulation of daunorubicin by modulating the efflux pump in the resistant cancer cell membrane [52]. Inorganic nanomaterials such as Fe_3O_4 can reverse the diaminedichloroplatinum resistance in the ovarian carcinoma cell membrane which is resistant to drugs. Diaminedichloro-platinum increases the apoptosis rate and cytotoxicity in the P-gp overexpressed human cell line

[53]. Fe_3O_4 nanoparticles decrease the expression of genes (such as B-cell lymphoma gene) and protein (such as MDR1, P-gp, and lung resistance-related protein) [54]. It also increases intracellular accumulation of drugs and induces apoptosis of cells to inhibit P-gp. It is also used to deliver MDR1 short hairpin RNA (shRNA) [55]. Apart from Fe_3O_4 magnetic nanoparticles, nano zinc oxide (ZnO), nano copper oxide (CuO), $CuSO_4$, $ZnSO_4$ nanoparticles, and multi-walled carbon nanotubes are other inorganic nanomaterials that can significantly inhibit the P-gp efflux transporter [56]. Though inorganic nanomaterials have been shown a potential to reverse the P-gp function their importance in the P-gp inhibition is still not clear. So there is the need to study the mechanism of reversal of P-gp function to facilitate the application of inorganic nanomaterials in combating MDR.

Several FDA approved pharmaceutical excipients possess the ability to inhibit the P-gp function. Cremophor EL, tween 80, and TPGS are some common examples of pharmaceutical excipients with P-gp inhibition property [57]. For an instant, cremophor EL increases the absorption of drugs in the gastrointestinal region through P-gp mediated inhibition. Recent advancement in the pharmaceutical industry has boosted the development of excipient with unique capabilities. One such excipient is Soluplus®, an amphiphilic graft copolymer, which is initially developed to enhance the solubility and bioavailability, can be an intrinsic P-gp inhibitor [58]. It interacts indirectly with P-gp transporter and alters the fluidity of the cell membrane [59]. Due to the P-gp inhibition property, Soluplus® can be used as tumor-targeting nanocarriers. For an instant, Soluplus micelles significantly enhance the intracellular concentration of doxorubicin in doxorubicinresistant cells [59]. However high effective inhibitory concentration is the big challenge faced by the Soluplus® [60]. Further sensitization of cancer cells to the delivered chemotherapeutics can be achieved by synergizing the cellular bioavailability and inhibition of efflux pumps through co-administration of Soluplus® and TPGS [61].

THIRD GENERATION SMALL MOLECULE P-GP INHIBITOR

First-generation P-gp inhibitors, which were initially P-gp substrates, are non-selective in nature. They are less potent and their concentration reaches to high toxicity level. Due to these reasons most of the first-generation P-gp inhibitors failed in the clinical trials [62]. Doxorubicin, verapamil, sertraline, vinblastine and erythromycin are some common first-generation P-gp inhibitors [63]. The second generation P-gp inhibitors are the structurally modified first generation inhibitors. They have a better pharmacological profile and lesser toxicity than first generation inhibitors. However, second-generation inhibitors suffer from unpredictable pharmacokinetic alteration which leads to difficulty in the adjustment of doses while chemotherapy [64]. The second generation inhibitors include tariquidar, dexverapamil, gallopamil, reversin 125 and valspodar, etc. [63]. To overcome the challenges related to first -generation and second-generation P-gp inhibitors, third-generation inhibitors came into action. Third-generation inhibitors were generated by the combination of quantitative structure-activity relationship (QSAR) with combinational chemistry method and high throughput screening techniques (HTS). The evolved third-generation inhibitors are 10 times more potent than a first and second generation and are highly specific in nature. They do not interact with CYP450 3A4 thus there is no need for dose adjustment while chemotherapy. Tariquidar (XR 9576), an anthranilamide derivatives, is a non-transported third-generation P-gp inhibitor. It can interact with the different modulatory binding site of the protein and inhibit the ATPase activity [65]. It increases the sensitivity of drug-resistant nematodes to various anthelmintics such as thiabendazole, levamisole, and ivermectin [66]. It has also the potential to significantly increase the intracellular concentration of drugs and overcome the bacterial multidrug resistance of antibiotic drug ciprofloxacin [67]. Tariquidar is supposed to be the most promising third-generation inhibitor, however, it needs to clear the unfavorable toxicity report of the Phase III clinical trial. The selectivity of tariquidar is also poor due to its interaction with other transporters like BCRP and MRP1 [68]. VX-710 (biricodar), a cyclopropyldibenzosuberane is another third-generation inhibitor developed by the same technique by Eli Lilly Inc. GF 120918 (elacridar) developed by GlaxoSmithKline is a derivative of acridonecarboxamide. Other example includes mitotane (NSC-38721), OC 144-093, ONT-093, annamycin, LY335979 (zosuquidar), and R101933 [63].

P-GP INHIBITORS FROM NATURAL PRODUCTS EXTRACTS

Recent discoveries in the natural resources are shifting the paradigm to plant-based drug discoveries due to their safe and non-toxic nature. Interaction of grapefruit with several drugs gave the first indication of herbal use in the inhibition of P-gp function [69]. Herbal constituents such as terpenoid derived from the red sea sponge, root extracts of *Stemona curtisii,* and Lathyrane obtained from the seeds of caper spurge are few P-gp inhibitors identified to have potent P-gp inhibitory activity. Though their efficacy has been proved effective in in-vitro studies, their clinical application is still a long way to go. A red ginseng saponin, ginsenoside Rg3 exhibits the ability to inhibit the P-gp in a competitive manner [70]. CBT-1 is bisbenzylisoquinoline which is isolated from plants and has the potential to alter the interaction of P-gp substrate, thereby acting as a P-gp inhibitor [71]. Jatrophane is a diterpenoid compound obtained from *Euphorbia sororia*. Ten known and five newly identified jatrophane diterpenoid compounds showed promising ability to reverse the MDR through P-gp inhibition activity. They stimulate P-gp ATPase activity and inhibit the transport of drugs in dose-dependent manner. Inhibition of drug transport leads to intracellular accumulation of the drug and finally resensitizing the resistant cell to the drug [72]. Three series of furan derivatives containing tetrahydroisoquinoline or tetrahydroquinoline are recently developed as P-gp inhibitors. They displayed a potent antiproliferative effect in malignant tumor cells with multi-drug resistance [73]. Glabridin is a flavonoid obtained from the root extract of licorice. It is widely used as an anti-inflammatory agent. It reverses the MDR by suppressing the overexpression of P-gp, downregulating the P-gp ATPase activity, and competitively inhibiting the

P-gp efflux pump. It has a strong binding ability as shown by simulation molecular docking modeling. It increases the apoptosis in a cancer cell and reverses the effect of MDR [74]. Novel diterpenoids, euphoroyleans A-H, isolated from whole plants of *Euphorbia royleana* can inhibit the transport activity of P-gp and reverse the effect of MDR in cancer cells [75]. Series of monoterpene indole alkaloids are isolated from *Tabernarmontana elegans.* These alkaloids have the ability to increase the multidrug resistance reversal in cancer cells. Their MDR reversal activity can be significantly enhanced when co-administered with anticancer therapeutics such as doxorubicin [76]. Isopetasin and S-isopetasin are novel herbal P-gp inhibitors. They are obtained from *Petasites formosanus*. These bioactive natural products act selectively against the resistant cancer cell. They increase the ATPase activity of P-gp in tumor cell and generate a pressure in mitochondria to produce ATP. The pressure generated by P-gp inhibition induces the production of reactive oxygen species (ROS) in mitochondria which are further followed by the cell apoptosis [77]. Apart from herbal inhibitors, marine origin inhibitors are also identified. Lamellarin D, an antineoplastic agent, is a pro-apoptosis alkaloid that exhibits insensitivity to P-gp mediated efflux of the drug [78].

CONCLUSION

P-gp efflux transporter radically affects the pharmacokinetics and bioavailability of P-gp substrates by reducing the concentration below the effective plasma level. Simultaneous administration of the P-gp inhibitors and the P-gp substrate can eliminate the substrate expulsion by P-gp and alter the expected therapeutic interest of the substrate drugs. Due to this reason, the exploration of this domain remains an ever-challenging task to scientists. Disease therapy with the therapeutic compound co-administered with P-gp reversal drugs need to be monitored carefully after evaluation of all the intended side effects and risk involve in it. Many effective P-gp transport inhibitors were discovered earlier with the aim of improving the bioavailability of essential therapeutic P-gp substrates but most of them suffered from the shortcomings like unpredictable pharmacokinetics, toxicities, and unwanted side effects that hamper their clinical application. Hence there has always been a need to fine-tune drugs to avoid these restraining challenges. The development of third-generation P-gp inhibitors is one such attempt by researchers. Extensive hard work of researchers in the last few decades has led to the recognition of several P-gp inhibitors among the formulations, natural product extracts, and inert pharmaceutical excipients. Novel P-gp inhibitors to reverse the multidrug resistance effect is gaining utmost importance at present. Several inhibitor candidates spotted out under these categories have been briefly discussed above. The inert, non-gut absorbent property of excipients and the safe, non-toxic nature of herbs make them stand out unique forever. Though future researches identify and develop numerous possibility P-gp inhibitors from these categories, their clinical utility can only be established after intended clinical trial reports. Many plant-based candidates can give insights into wide range of possibilities of utilizing diverse techniques to develop efficient P-gp inhibitors. However, some of the herb-based drugs are identified to be non-specific P-gp inhibitors, which could interfere with other protein and human enzymatic targets. Henceforth, it is essential that in the future development of effective P-gp inhibitors should be guided by particularly, mechanism and specificity, and lower side-effect. At this stage of research, a deeper understanding of the rational drug design becomes crucial to emerging out with more promising non-toxic and inert P-gp inhibitor candidates. Characterization of compounds as P-gp inhibitors/substrates/ inducers can give a better insight to understand the mystery of P-gp in drug delivery. It can be achieved by rational drug design strategies involving *in silico* screening technique followed by *in vitro* screening approaches and further *de-Novo* design to study P-gp interaction. The interaction of P-gp with other compound establish the structural basis of protein for recognize of substrate and modulator. Excavating the proximity of the P-gp expression, structure and interaction of substrate is likely to give a better understanding and unravel new perspective to identify novel inhibitory strategies. The attempt has been made to provide the emerging novel P-gp inhibitor candidate and possible strategies to reverse the P-gp mediated MDR. The development of further specific targeted P-gp inhibitor in the near future is foreseen.

ACKNOWLEDGMENTS

The authors are thankful to Director, CSIR-CDRI for continuous encouragement and support. Nazneen Sultana and Swati Chaturvedi acknowledges DST and CSIR, India for providing the research fellowship.

CONFLICT OF INTEREST

The authors declare that there are no conflicts of interest.

REFERENCES

[1] C. Chen, J. E. Chin, K. Ueda, D. P. Clark, I. Pastan, M. M. Gottesman, I. B. Roninson, Internal duplication and homology with bacterial transport proteins in the mdr1 (P-glycoprotein) gene from multidrug-resistant human cells, *Cell.* 47 (1986) 381-389. doi:10. 1016/0092-8674(86)90595-7.

[2] C. F. Higgins, Multiple molecular mechanisms for multidrug resistance transporters, *Nature*. 446 (2007) 749-757. doi:10.1038/nature05630.

[3] L. J. Goldstein, H. Galski, A. Fojo, M. Willingham, S. L. Lai, A. Gazdar, R. Pirker, A. Green, W. Crist, G. M. Brodeur, M. Lieber, J. Cossman, M. M. Gottesman, I. Pastan, Expression of Multidrug Resistance Gene in Human Cancers, *JNCI J. Natl. Cancer Inst.* 81 (1989) 116-124. doi:10.1093/jnci/81.2.116.

[4] H. Shi, D. Lu, Y. Shu, W. Shi, S. Lu, K. Wang, Expression of Multidrug Resistance-Related Proteins p-Glycoproteinglutathione-s-

Transferases, Topoisomerase-II and Lung Resistance Protein in Primary Gastric Cardiac Adenocarcinoma, *Cancer Invest.* 26 (2008) 344-351. doi:10.1080/07357900701788072.

[5] J. A. Holmes, R. R. West, The effect of MDR-1 gene expression on outcome in acute myeloblastic leukaemia, *Br. J. Cancer.* 69 (1994) 382-384. doi:10.1038/bjc.1994.70.

[6] T. Ogihara, M. Kamiya, M. Ozawa, T. Fujita, A. Yamamoto, S. Yamashita, S. Ohnishi, Y. Isomura, What Kinds of Substrates Show P-Glycoprotein-Dependent Intestinal Absorption? Comparison of Verapamil with Vinblastine, *Drug Metab. Pharmacokinet.* 21 (2006) 238-244. doi:10.2133/dmpk.21.238.

[7] L. M. S. Chan, S. Lowes, B. H. Hirst, The ABCs of drug transport in intestine and liver: efflux proteins limiting drug absorption and bioavailability, *Eur. J. Pharm. Sci.* 21 (2004) 25-51. doi:10.1016/j.ejps.2003.07.003.

[8] A. D. Mottino, V. A. Catania, Hepatic drug transporters and nuclear receptors: regulation by therapeutic agents, *World J. Gastroenterol.* 14 (2008) 7068-7074. doi:10.3748/wjg.14.7068.

[9] A. Tsuji, I. Tamai, A. Sakata, Y. Tenda, T. Terasaki, Restricted transport of cyclosporin A across the blood-brain barrier by a multidrug transporter, P-glycoprotein, *Biochem. Pharmacol.* 46 (1993) 1096-1099. doi:10.1016/0006-2952(93)90677-o.

[10] A. H. Schinkel, P-Glycoprotein, a gatekeeper in the blood-brain barrier, *Adv. Drug Deliv. Rev.* 36 (1999) 179-194. doi:10.1016/ s0169-409x(98)00085-4.

[11] M. Ichikawa-Haraguchi, T. Sumizawa, A. Yoshimura, T. Furukawa, S. Hiramoto, M. Sugita, S. Akiyama, Progesterone and its metabolites: the potent inhibitors of the transporting activity of P-glycoprotein in the adrenal gland, *Biochim. Biophys. Acta - Gen. Subj.* 1158 (1993) 201-208. doi:10.1016/0304-4165(93)90016-2.

[12] M. Demeule, J. Jodoin, É. Beaulieu, M. Brossard, R. Béliveau, Dexamethasone modulation of multidrug transporters in normal tissues, *FEBS Lett.* 442 (1999) 208-214. doi:10.1016/s0014-5793(98) 01663-9.

[13] I. Cascorbi, P-glycoprotein: Tissue Distribution, Substrates, and Functional Consequences of Genetic Variations, *Handb. Exp. Pharmacol.* (2010) 261-283. doi:10.1007/978-3-642-14541-4_6.

[14] S. Aly, D. Boothe, S. S. *J. of Antimicrobial*, undefined 2015, A novel alanine to serine substitution mutation in SoxS induces overexpression of efflux pumps and contributes to multidrug resistance in clinical Escherichia coli, Academic.Oup.Com. (n.d.). https://academic.oup.com/jac/article-abstract/70/8/2228/811902 (accessed December 9, 2020).

[15] A. Bergman, H. Pinedo, I. T. B. *Journal of undefined 2003*, Increased sensitivity to gemcitabine of P-glycoprotein and multidrug resistance-associated protein-overexpressing human cancer cell lines, Nature.Com. (n.d.). https://www.nature.com/articles/6601011/ (accessed December 9, 2020).

[16] M. Ghandadi, A. S. C. *Pharmaceutical Design*, undefined 2016, Interleukin-6: a critical cytokine in cancer multidrug resistance, Ingentaconnect.Com. (n.d.). https://www.ingentaconnect.com/content /ben/cpd/2016/00000022/00000005/art00002 (accessed December 9, 2020).

[17] R. Tang, A. Faussat, P. Majdak, J. Perrot, D. C. *Leukemia*, undefined 2004, Valproic acid inhibits proliferation and induces apoptosis in acute myeloid leukemia cells expressing P-gp and MRP1, Nature.Com. (n.d.). https://www.nature.com/articles/2403390 (accessed December 9, 2020).

[18] A. Dréan, S. Rosenberg, F. X. Lejeune, L. Goli, A. A. Nadaradjane, J. Guehennec, C. Schmitt, M. Verreault, F. Bielle, K. Mokhtari, M. Sanson, A. Carpentier, J. Y. Delattre, A. Idbaih, ATP binding cassette (ABC) transporters: expression and clinical value in glioblastoma, *J. Neurooncol.* 138 (2018) 479-486. doi:10.1007/s 11060-018-2819-3.

[19] F. J. Sharom, ABC multidrug transporters: structure, function and role in chemoresistance, *Pharmacogenomics*. 9 (2008) 105-127. doi: 10.2217/14622416.9.1.105.

[20] J. W. McCormick, P. D. Vogel, J. G. Wise, Multiple Drug Transport Pathways through Human P-Glycoprotein, *Biochemistry*. 54 (2015) 4374-4390. doi:10.1021/acs.biochem.5b00018.

[21] A. Fojo, M. Cornwell, C. Cardarelli, D. P. Clark, N. Richert, D. Shen, K. Ueda, M. Willingham, M. M. Gottesman, I. Pastan, Molecular biology of drug resistance, *Breast Cancer Res. Treat*. 9 (1987) 5-16. doi:10.1007/bf01806689.

[22] A. T. Fojo, D. W. Shen, L. A. Mickley, I. Pastan, M. M. Gottesman, Intrinsic drug resistance in human kidney cancer is associated with expression of a human multidrug-resistance gene., *J. Clin. Oncol*. 5 (1987) 1922-1927. doi:10.1200/jco.1987.5.12.1922.

[23] P. D. W. Eckford, F. J. Sharom, ABC Efflux Pump-Based Resistance to Chemotherapy Drugs, *Chem. Rev*. 109 (2009) 2989-3011. doi:10.1021/cr9000226.

[24] M. M. Gottesman, Mechanisms of Cancer Drug Resistance, *Annu. Rev. Med*. 53 (2002) 615-627. doi:10.1146/annurev.med.53.082901.103929.

[25] M. M. Gottesman, T. Fojo, S. E. Bates, Multidrug resistance in cancer: role of ATP-dependent transporters, *Nat. Rev. Cancer*. 2 (2002) 48-58. doi:10.1038/nrc706.

[26] Z. Binkhathlan, A. Lavasanifar, P-glycoprotein Inhibition as a Therapeutic Approach for Overcoming Multidrug Resistance in Cancer: Current Status and Future Perspectives, *Curr. Cancer Drug Targets*. 13 (2013) 326-346. doi:10.2174/15680096113139990076.

[27] R. J. Kathawala, P. Gupta, C. R. Ashby, Z. S. Chen, The modulation of ABC transporter-mediated multidrug resistance in cancer: A review of the past decade, *Drug Resist. Updat*. 18 (2015) 1-17. doi:10.1016/j.drup.2014.11.002.

[28] H. Thomas, H. M. Coley, Overcoming Multidrug Resistance in Cancer: An Update on the Clinical Strategy of Inhibiting P-Glycoprotein, *Cancer Control*. 10 (2003) 159-165. doi:10.1177/107327480301000207.

[29] F. K. Brewer, C. A. Follit, P. D. Vogel, J. G. Wise, In silico screening for inhibitors of p-glycoprotein that target the nucleotide binding

domains, *Mol. Pharmacol.* 86 (2014) 716-726. doi:10.1124/mol.114.095414.

[30] C. A. Follit, F. K. Brewer, J. G. Wise, P. D. Vogel, In silico identified targeted inhibitors of P-glycoprotein overcome multidrug resistance in human cancer cells in culture, *Pharmacol. Res. Perspect.* 3 (2015) e00170-e00170. doi:10.1002/prp2.170.

[31] M. Takeda, A. Mizokami, K. Mamiya, Y. Q. Li, J. Zhang, E. T. Keller, M. Namiki, The establishment of two paclitaxel-resistant prostate cancer cell lines and the mechanisms of paclitaxel resistance with two cell lines, *Prostate.* 67 (2007) 955-967. doi:10.1002/pros. 20581.

[32] L. Yan, Y. Yang, W. Zhang, X. Chen, Advanced Materials and Nanotechnology for Drug Delivery, *Adv. Mater.* 26 (2014) 5533-5540. doi:10.1002/adma.201305683.

[33] A. R. Kirtane, S. M. Kalscheuer, J. Panyam, Exploiting nanotechnology to overcome tumor drug resistance: Challenges and opportunities, *Adv. Drug Deliv. Rev.* 65 (2013) 1731-1747. doi:10. 1016/j.addr.2013.09.001.

[34] M. Q. Gong, J. L. Wu, B. Chen, R. X. Zhuo, S. X. Cheng, Self-Assembled Polymer/Inorganic Hybrid Nanovesicles for Multiple Drug Delivery To Overcome Drug Resistance in Cancer Chemotherapy, *Langmuir.* 31 (2015) 5115-5122. doi:10.1021/acs. langmuir.5b00542.

[35] A. Saneja, R. Dubey, N. Alam, V. Khare, P. Gupta, Co-formulation of P-glycoprotein Substrate and Inhibitor in Nanocarriers: An Emerging Strategy for Cancer Chemotherapy, *Curr. Cancer Drug Targets.* 14 (2014) 419-433. doi:10.2174/1568009614666140407112 034.

[36] C. Yang, T. Wu, Y. Qi, Z. Zhang, Recent Advances in the Application of Vitamin E TPGS for Drug Delivery, *Theranostics.* 8 (2018) 464-485. doi:10.7150/thno.22711.

[37] M. S. Muthu, R. V. Kutty, Z. Luo, J. Xie, S. S. Feng, Theranostic vitamin E TPGS micelles of transferrin conjugation for targeted co-delivery of docetaxel and ultra bright gold nanoclusters, *Biomaterials.* 39 (2015) 234-248. doi:10.1016/j.biomaterials.2014. 11.008.

[38] R. V. Kutty, S. L. Chia, M. I. Setyawati, M. S. Muthu, S. S. Feng, D. T. Leong, *In vivo* and *ex vivo* proofs of concept that cetuximab

conjugated vitamin E TPGS micelles increases efficacy of delivered docetaxel against triple negative breast cancer, *Biomaterials*. 63 (2015) 58-69. doi:10.1016/j.biomaterials.2015.06.005.

[39] A. G. Assanhou, W. Li, L. Zhang, L. Xue, L. Kong, H. Sun, R. Mo, C. Zhang, Reversal of multidrug resistance by co-delivery of paclitaxel and lonidamine using a TPGS and hyaluronic acid dual-functionalized liposome for cancer treatment, *Biomaterials*. 73 (2015) 284-295. doi:10.1016/j.biomaterials.2015.09.022.

[40] W. Cheng, C. Liang, L. Xu, G. Liu, N. Gao, W. Tao, L. Luo, Y. Zuo, X. Wang, X. Zhang, X. Zeng, L. Mei, Cancer Therapy: TPGS-Functionalized Polydopamine-Modified Mesoporous Silica as Drug Nanocarriers for Enhanced Lung Cancer Chemotherapy against Multidrug Resistance (Small 29/2017), *Small*. 13 (2017). doi:10. 1002/smll.201770160.

[41] D. Sun, X. Wei, X. Xue, Z. Fang, M. Ren, H. Lou, X. Zhang, Enhanced oral absorption and therapeutic effect of acetylpuerarin based on D-α-tocopheryl polyethylene glycol 1000 succinate nanoemulsions, *Int. J. Nanomedicine*. 9 (2014) 3413-3423. doi:10. 2147/IJN.S63777.

[42] R. Nieto Montesinos, A. Béduneau, Y. Pellequer, A. Lamprecht, Delivery of P-glycoprotein substrates using chemosensitizers and nanotechnology for selective and efficient therapeutic outcomes, *J. Control. Release*. 161 (2012) 50-61. doi:10.1016/j.jconrel.2012.04. 034.

[43] Z. Yan, Y. Yang, X. Wei, J. Zhong, D. Wei, L. Liu, C. Xie, F. Wang, L. Zhang, W. Lu, D. He, Tumor-Penetrating Peptide Mediation: An Effective Strategy for Improving the Transport of Liposomes in Tumor Tissue, *Mol. Pharm*. 11 (2013) 218-225. doi:10.1021/mp 400393a.

[44] M. A. C. Stuart, W. T. S. Huck, J. Genzer, M. Müller, C. Ober, M. Stamm, G. B. Sukhorukov, I. Szleifer, V. V. Tsukruk, M. Urban, F. Winnik, S. Zauscher, I. Luzinov, S. Minko, Emerging applications of stimuli-responsive polymer materials, *Nat. Mater*. 9 (2010) 101-113. doi:10.1038/nmat2614.

[45] C. M. J. Hu, L. Zhang, Therapeutic Nanoparticles to Combat Cancer Drug Resistance, 2009. https://www.ingentaconnect.com/content/

ben/cdm/2009/00000010/00000008/art00002 (accessed December 9, 2020).

[46] A. M. Butt, M. C. I. Mohd Amin, H. Katas, Synergistic effect of pH-responsive folate-functionalized poloxamer 407-TPGS-mixed micelles on targeted delivery of anticancer drugs, *Int. J. Nanomedicine.* 10 (2015) 1321-1334. doi:10.2147/IJN.S78438.

[47] Y. Bao, M. Kong, X. Gao, M. Yin, H. Deng, Q. Tan, Q. Wang, S. Tan, pH-, redox dual-sensitive poly(β-amino ester)-g-TPGS copolymer nanoparticles for drug delivery and inhibition of multidrug resistance in cancer, *React. Funct. Polym.* 120 (2017) 131-138. doi:10.1016/j.reactfunctpolym.2017.09.013.

[48] Y. Bao, Y. Guo, X. Zhuang, D. Li, B. Cheng, S. Tan, Z. Zhang, d-α-Tocopherol Polyethylene Glycol Succinate-Based Redox-Sensitive Paclitaxel Prodrug for Overcoming Multidrug Resistance in Cancer Cells, *Mol. Pharm.* 11 (2014) 3196-3209. doi:10.1021/mp500384d.

[49] Q. Yao, L. Kou, Y. Tu, L. Zhu, MMP-Responsive 'Smart' Drug Delivery and Tumor Targeting, *Trends Pharmacol. Sci.* 39 (2018) 766-781. doi:10.1016/j.tips.2018.06.003.

[50] Z. Dai, Q. Yao, L. Zhu, MMP2-Sensitive PEG-Lipid Copolymers: A New Type of Tumor-Targeted P-Glycoprotein Inhibitor, *ACS Appl. Mater. Interfaces.* 8 (2016) 12661-12673. doi:10.1021/acsami.6b 03064.

[51] R. Liang, M. Wei, D. G. Evans, X. Duan, Inorganic nanomaterials for bioimaging, targeted drug delivery and therapeutics, *Chem. Commun.* 50 (2014) 14071-14081. doi:10.1039/c4cc03118k.

[52] X. Wang, R. Zhang, C. Wu, Y. Dai, M. Song, S. Gutmann, F. Gao, G. Lv, J. Li, X. Li, Z. Guan, D. Fu, B. Chen, The application of Fe_3O_4 nanoparticles in cancer research: A new strategy to inhibit drug resistance, *J. Biomed. Mater. Res. Part A.* 80A (2006) 852-860. doi: 10.1002/jbm.a.30901.

[53] Z. Jiang, B. A. Chen, G. H. Xia, Q. Wu, Y. Zhang, T. Y. Hong, W. Zhang, J. Cheng, F. Gao, L. J. Liu, X. M. Li, X. M. Wang, The reversal effect of magnetic Fe_3O_4 nanoparticles loaded with cisplatin on

SKOV3/DDP ovarian carcinoma cells, *Int. J. Nanomedicine*. 4 (2009) 107-114. doi:10.2147/ijn.s5393.

[54] B. Chen, Q. Sun, X. Wang, F. Gao, Y. Dai, Y. Yin, J. Ding, C. Gao, J. Cheng, J. Li, X. Sun, N. Chen, W. Xu, H. Shen, D. Liu, Reversal in multidrug resistance by magnetic nanoparticle of Fe_3O_4 loaded with adriamycin and tetrandrine in K562/A02 leukemic cells, *Int. J. Nanomedicine.* 3 (2008) 277-286. doi:10.2147/ijn.s2714.

[55] B. Chen, P. Mao, J. Cheng, F. Gao, G. Xia, W. Xu, H. Shen, J. Ding, C. Gao, Q. Sun, W. Chen, N. Chen, L. Liu, X. Li, X. Wang, Reversal of multidrug resistance by magnetic Fe_3O_4 nanoparticle copolymerizating daunorubicin and MDR1 shRNA expression vector in leukemia cells, *Int. J. Nanomedicine*. 5 (2010) 437-444. doi:10. 2147/ijn.s10083.

[56] B. Wu, C. Torres-Duarte, B. J. Cole, G. N. Cherr, Copper Oxide and Zinc Oxide Nanomaterials Act as Inhibitors of Multidrug Resistance Transport in Sea Urchin Embryos: Their Role as Chemosensitizers, *Environ. Sci. Technol.* 49 (2015) 5760-5770. doi:10.1021/acs.est.5b 00345.

[57] Y. Shono, H. Nishihara, Y. Matsuda, S. Furukawa, N. Okada, T. Fujita, A. Yamamoto, Modulation of Intestinal P-Glycoprotein Function by Cremophor EL and Other Surfactants by an *In Vitro* Diffusion Chamber Method Using the Isolated Rat Intestinal Membranes, *J. Pharm. Sci.* 93 (2004) 877-885. doi:10.1002/jps. 20017.

[58] M. Linn, E. M. Collnot, D. Djuric, K. Hempel, E. Fabian, K. Kolter, C. M. Lehr, Soluplus® as an effective absorption enhancer of poorly soluble drugs *in vitro* and *in vivo*, *Eur. J. Pharm. Sci*. 45 (2012) 336-343. doi:10.1016/j.ejps.2011.11.025.

[59] X. Jin, B. Zhou, L. Xue, W. San, Soluplus® micelles as a potential drug delivery system for reversal of resistant tumor, *Biomed. Pharmacother.* 69 (2015) 388-395. doi:10.1016/j.biopha.2014.12. 028.

[60] M. Linn, *In vitro* characterization of the novel solubility enhancing excipient Soluplus R, 2011. https://scidok.sulb.uni-saarland.de/handle/20.500.11880/22827 (accessed December 9, 2020).

[61] J. Zhao, Y. Xu, C. Wang, Y. Ding, M. Chen, Y. Wang, J. Peng, L. Li, L. Lv, Soluplus/TPGS mixed micelles for dioscin delivery in cancer therapy, *Drug Dev. Ind. Pharm.* 43 (2017) 1197-1204. doi:10.1080/03639045.2017.1304956.

[62] A. Dantzig, D. de Alwis, M. B. A. drug delivery reviews, undefined 2003, Considerations in the design and development of transport inhibitors as adjuncts to drug therapy, Elsevier. (n.d.). https://www.sciencedirect.com/science/article/pii/S0169409X02001758 (accessed December 9, 2020).

[63] K. M. Raghava, P. K. Lakshmi, Overview of P-glycoprotein inhibitors: A rational outlook, *Brazilian J. Pharm. Sci.* 48 (2012) 353-367. doi:10.1590/S1984-82502012000300002.

[64] R. A. Darby, R. C. C. drug, undefined 2011, P-glycoprotein inhibition: the past, the present and the future, Ingentaconnect.Com. (n.d.). https://www.ingentaconnect.com/content/ben/cdm/2011/00000012/00000008/art00004 (accessed December 9, 2020).

[65] T. O. F. letters, undefined 2006, Mechanisms and strategies to overcome multiple drug resistance in cancer, Elsevier. (n.d.). https://www.sciencedirect.com/science/article/pii/S0014579306002079 (accessed December 9, 2020).

[66] A. Raza, S. R. Kopp, A. Jabbar, A. C. Kotze, Effects of third generation P-glycoprotein inhibitors on the sensitivity of drug-resistant and -susceptible isolates of Haemonchus contortus to anthelmintics *in vitro*, *Vet. Parasitol.* 211 (2015) 80-88. doi:10.1016/j.vetpar.2015.04.025.

[67] I. Leitner, J. Nemeth, T. Feurstein, A. Abrahim, P. Matzneller, H. Lagler, T. Erker, O. Langer, M. Zeitlinger, The third-generation P-glycoprotein inhibitor tariquidar may overcome bacterial multidrug resistance by increasing intracellular drug concentration, *J. Antimicrob. Chemother.* 66 (2011) 834-839. doi:10.1093/jac/dkq526.

[68] N. Colabufo, F. Berardi, M. Contino, M. Niso, R. Perrone, ABC Pumps and Their Role in Active Drug Transport, *Curr. Top. Med. Chem.* 9 (2009) 119-129. doi:10.2174/156802609787521553.

[69] D. Bailey, J. Spence, C. Munoz, J. A. T. Lancet, undefined 1991, Interaction of citrus juices with felodipine and nifedipine, Elsevier. (n.d.). https://www.sciencedirect.com/science/article/pii/0140673691 90872M (accessed December 9, 2020).

[70] S. Kim, H. Kwon, D. Chi, J. Shim, J. P. B., undefined 2003, Reversal of P-glycoprotein-mediated multidrug resistance by ginsenoside Rg3, Elsevier. (n.d.). https://www.sciencedirect.com/science/article/pii/S0 006295202014466 (accessed December 9, 2020).

[71] R. Robey, S. Shukla, E. Finley, R. O. B., undefined 2008, Inhibition of P-glycoprotein (ABCB1)-and multidrug resistance-associated protein 1 (ABCC1)-mediated transport by the orally administered inhibitor, CBT-1®, Elsevier. (n.d.). https://www.sciencedirect.com/ science/article/pii/S0006295207007964 (accessed December 9, 2020).

[72] R. Hu, J. Gao, R. Rozimamat, H. A. Aisa, Jatrophane diterpenoids from Euphorbia sororia as potent modulators against P-glycoprotein-based multidrug resistance, *Eur. J. Med. Chem.* 146 (2018) 157-170. doi:10.1016/j.ejmech.2018.01.027.

[73] Y. S. Li, D. S. Zhao, X. Y. Liu, Y. X. Liao, H. W. Jin, G. P. Song, Z. N. Cui, Synthesis and biological evaluation of 2,5-disubstituted furan derivatives as P-glycoprotein inhibitors for Doxorubicin resistance in MCF-7/ADR cell, *Eur. J. Med. Chem.* 151 (2018) 546-556. doi:10. 1016/j.ejmech.2018.04.012.

[74] J. Qian, M. Xia, W. Liu, L. Li, J. Yang, Y. Mei, Q. Meng, Y. Xie, Glabridin resensitizes p-glycoprotein-overexpressing multidrug-resistant cancer cells to conventional chemotherapeutic agents, *Eur. J. Pharmacol.* 852 (2019) 231-243. doi:10.1016/j.ejphar.2019.04. 002.

[75] S. Shaker, J. Sang, X. L. Yan, R. Z. Fan, G. H. Tang, Y. K. Xu, S. Yin, Diterpenoids from Euphorbia royleana reverse P-glycoprotein-mediated multidrug resistance in cancer cells, *Phytochemistry.* 176 (2020) 112395. doi:10.1016/j.phytochem.2020.112395.

[76] D. Cardoso, A. Kincses, M. Nové, G. S. E. J. of, undefined 2020, Alkylated monoterpene indole alkaloid derivatives as potent P-glycoprotein inhibitors in resistant cancer cells, Elsevier. (n.d.). https://www.sciencedirect.com/science/article/pii/S0223523420309570 (accessed December 9, 2020).

[77] S. Abdelfatah, M. Böckers, M. Asensio, O. Kadioglu, A. Klinger, E. Fleischer, T. Efferth, Isopetasin and S-isopetasin as novel P-glycoprotein inhibitors against multidrug-resistant cancer cells, *Phytomedicine*. (2020) 153196. doi:10.1016/j.phymed.2020.153196.

[78] M. Vanhuyse, J. Kluza, C. Tardy, G. Otero, C. C. C. letters, undefined 2005, Lamellarin D: a novel pro-apoptotic agent from marine origin insensitive to P-glycoprotein-mediated drug efflux, Elsevier. (n.d.). https://www.sciencedirect.com/science/article/pii/S0304383504007311 (accessed December 9, 2020).

About the Editors

Dr. M. Wahajuddin

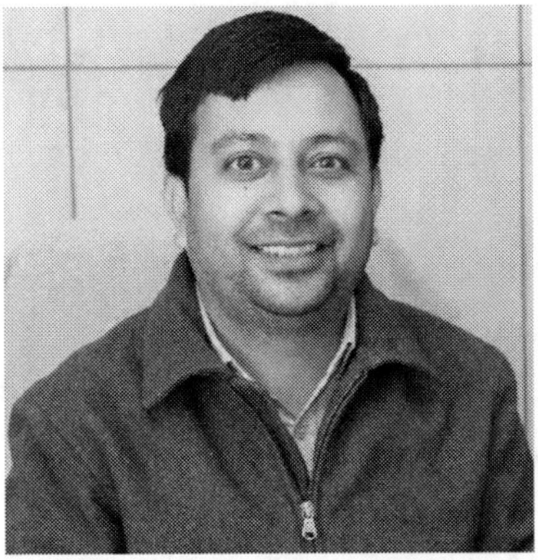

Dr. M. Wahajuddin is serving as Principal Scientist and Associate professor (AcSIR) at Pharmaceutics & Pharmacokinetics Division, CSIR-Central Drug Research Institute Lucknow where for about 15 years he has been studying pharmacokinetics and biopharmaceutics of potential candidate molecules of CSIR-CDRI drug R&D pipeline (in addition to marketed drugs/metabolites/natural products) and deciphering the molecular mechanism(s) of ADME/disposition thereof. He is also registered patent agent with Indian patent office New Delhi. He has been given the additional charge as course coordinator (pharmaceutics) at the National Institute of Pharmaceutical Education & Research (Raebareli, India) which is a postgraduate institute of national importance of Govt. of India. He had also worked as visiting scientist at UNC Eshelman School of Pharmacy, University of North Carolina at Chapel Hill, NC, USA in 2013-14 and Humboldt Research Fellow at University of Cologne Hospital's Centre for Pharmacology, Cologne, Germany in 2018-19. He has also won many awards and accolades like Young Scientist Award 2013-14 from State Government of Uttar Pradesh, India, Technology Award for Life Sciences-2019 from Council of Scientific and Industrial Research, Govt. of India, the Shakuntala Amir Chand Prize 2019 for Young Scientist by the Indian Council of Medical Research (ICMR), Govt. of India, Young Pharmaceutical Analyst Award 2012 from Indian Drug Manufacturer's Association; DBT- Cutting-edge Research Enhancement & Scientific Training (DBT-CREST) Award 2011-12 from Dept. of Biotech. Govt. of India, Junior Investigator Award 2017 from Safety Pharmacological Society USA and ISMAS Young Mass Spectroscopist Award 2013 from Indian Society for Mass Spectrometry etc. He has more than 100 research papers in highly reputed peer reviewed international journals and also serving as Section editor, Editorial Board Member, and reviewer of many highly reputed peer-reviewed international journals. He has been elected member to Global Young Academy under the aegis of German National Academy of Sciences Leopoldina Halle Germany, Indian National Young Academy of Sciences and admitted as Fellow of Royal Society of Biology (UK), Royal Society of Chemistry (UK) and Higher Education Academy (UK). He is one of the co-leads of Science Diplomacy in South Asia working group of Global Young Academy (2020-2021).

Corresponding Editor's Email: wahajuddin@gmail.com.

Dr. Ravindra Varma Alluri

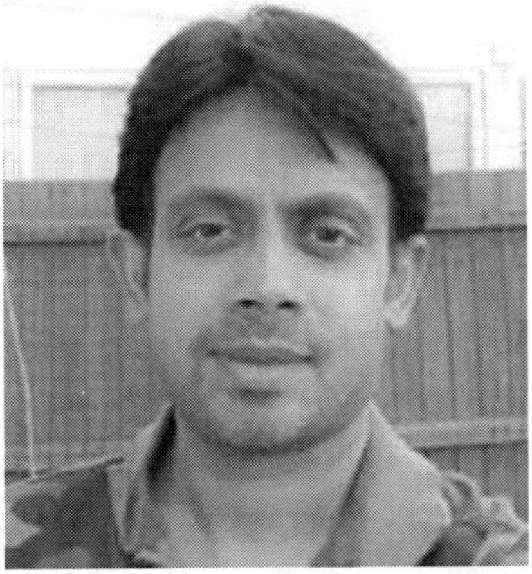

Dr Ravindra is an Associate Principal Scientist (Systems Medicine) at AstraZeneca, United Kingdom. He did his Postdoctoral research in drug transporters at University of North Carolina at Chapel Hill, NC, USA. He has around 18 years of experience in the field of drug metabolism and pharmacokinetics and in silico modelling (statistical, mechanistic and PBPK). During his tenure, he worked with several Pharmaceutical companies, where he made significant contributions to the advancement of candidate drugs into clinical development by developing several key DMPK assays, modelling approaches and strategies. He led DMPK teams, worked extensively in the field of drug transporters, transporter-enzyme interplay and drug-drug interactions. He has developed/applied mechanistic and Physiological Based Pharmacokinetic (PBPK) modelling approaches to investigate the role of efflux transporters and enzymes in altering oral drug absorption and disposition. As a member of IQ Consortium, he has contributed to advancing the application of PBPK models for predicting the impact of food on oral drug absorption. He has mentored students, post-docs and colleagues throughout his industrial career and his tenure as a post-doctoral research associate. He presented his research at several scientific meetings such as AAPS, DMDG and GRC. He has 11 publications, including 2 book chapters.

Dr. Rahul Dev Jayant

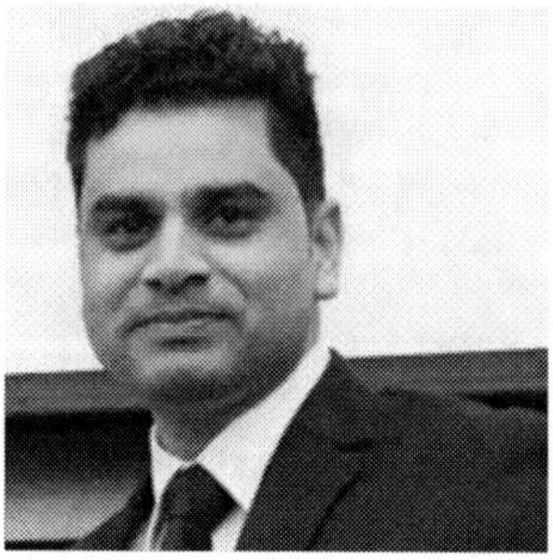

Dr. Jayant, Assistant Professor (Tenure-Track) at the School of Pharmacy, Department of Pharmaceutical Science (TTUHSC, Amarillo). Dr. Jayant obtained his Ph.D. in Biomedical Engineering from the Indian Institute of Technology-Bombay (IITB, Mumbai) and Master of Technology (M. Tech.) in Pharmaceutical Technology Biotechnology from National Institute of Pharmaceutical Technology and Research (NIPER, Mohali), India. He has over ten years of experience working at the interface of biomedical engineering, material science, microfluidics, pharmaceutical science, and nanoformulation development for the clinical and biomedical applications. In his current research, he is working on the development of the CRISPR based gene therapy and nanotechnology-based drug delivery approaches for personalized nanomedicine applicable to neuroAIDS and drug abuse treatment. His lab is also working on the development of bioengineering platform technologies using a 3D-printed-cerebral organoid-on-a- chip platform system to study the effect of drug abuse, alcohol exposure, or HIV-1 infection on early-stage brain development and drug neurotoxicity testing. His lab is funded by NIH, a private foundation, and internal pilot grants. He has published (50) high-quality research papers in peer-reviewed scientific journals, holds 1 US patent, co-edited one book on Personalized Nanotherapeutics (Springer), and 15 book chapters. He has presented his work in many national and international scientific meetings related to HIV Nanomedicine, Drug abuse, Neuroimmune Pharmacology, Novel Drug Delivery systems, etc. Many prestigious awards have recognized Dr. Jayant's innovative research, e.g., Young Investigator Award by Society for Brain Mapping & Therapeutics (SBMT), Junior Investigator Research Award by Society for Personalized NanoMedicine (SPNM), Arthur-Falek Outstanding Presentation Award by Society for NeuroImmune Pharmacology (SNIP) and AAPS-Manufacturing Science and Engineering award and other conference travel awards. He is also serving as Associate editor, Consulting Editor, Editorial Board Members, and reviewers of many reputed high-impact scientific journals. Dr. Jayant is also an active member of several international scientific societies/ organizations (SNIP, SPNM, SBMT, and AAPS).

INDEX

C

D

J

K

L

M

N

O

P

Q

R

S

T

U

V

W

X

Y

Z